TRAIN LIKE A PRO

Matthew S. Ibrahim

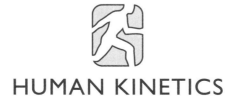

Library of Congress Cataloging-in-Publication Data

Library of Congress Cataloging-in-Publication information is available. LCCN 2025012925 (print).

ISBN: 978-1-7182-2251-9 (print)

Copyright © 2026 by Matthew S. Ibrahim

Human Kinetics supports copyright. Copyright fuels scientific and artistic endeavor, encourages authors to create new works, and promotes free speech. Thank you for buying an authorized edition of this work and for complying with copyright laws by not reproducing, scanning, or distributing any part of it in any form without written permission from the publisher. You are supporting authors and allowing Human Kinetics to continue to publish works that increase the knowledge, enhance the performance, and improve the lives of people all over the world.

To report suspected copyright infringement of content published by Human Kinetics, contact us at **permissions@hkusa.com**. To request permission to legally reuse content published by Human Kinetics, please refer to the information at **https://US.HumanKinetics.com/pages/permissions-translations-faqs**.

This publication is written and published to provide accurate and authoritative information relevant to the subject matter presented. It is published and sold with the understanding that the author and publisher are not engaged in rendering legal, medical, or other professional services by reason of their authorship or publication of this work. If medical or other expert assistance is required, the services of a competent professional person should be sought.

The web addresses cited in this text were current as of February 2025, unless otherwise noted.

Senior Acquisitions Editor: Diana Vincer
Developmental Editor: Cynthia McEntire
Managing Editor: Kevin Matz
Copyeditor: Emily Bartlett Hines
Proofreader: Lindsay Majer
Permissions Manager: Laurel Mitchell
Senior Graphic Designer: Julie L. Denzer
Graphic Designer: Denise Lowry
Cover Designer: Keri Evans
Cover Design Specialist: Susan Rothermel Allen
Photograph (cover): Maddie Meyer/E+/Getty Images
Photographs (interior): © Human Kinetics, unless otherwise noted
Photo Production Manager: Jason Allen
Senior Art Manager: Kelly Hendren
Illustrations: © Human Kinetics, unless otherwise noted
Printer: Sheridan Books

Printed in the United States of America   10 9 8 7 6 5 4 3 2 1

The paper in this book is certified under a sustainable forestry program.

Human Kinetics
1607 N. Market Street
Champaign, IL 61820
USA

United States and International
Website: **US.HumanKinetics.com**
Email: info@hkusa.com
Phone: 1-800-747-4457

Canada
Website: **Canada.HumanKinetics.com**
Email: info@hkcanada.com

Human Kinetics' authorized representative for product safety in the EU is Mare Nostrum Group B.V., Mauritskade 21D, 1091 GC Amsterdam, The Netherlands.
Email: gpsr@mare-nostrum.co.uk

E9179

I would like to dedicate this book to my wife, Alyssa, and my daughter, Giuliana. Without them, this wouldn't be possible.

CONTENTS

Preface vii • Acknowledgments ix

1 The Truth About Training Like an Athlete   1

Training your ability to control your body is a key part of athleticism in competitive sports and lifelong fitness in life off the field. Becoming more athletic in your training will lead to more strength, power, speed, and agility.

2 Developing Athletic Strength and Power   9

Strength training aims to improve the durability and resilience of muscles and body structures such as bones, tendons, and ligaments. A balanced training approach that incorporates power and speed leads to optimal performance in sports and life.

3 Developing Change of Direction and Agility Skills   15

Change of direction and agility skills are key for competitive athletes and non-competitive trainers. In this chapter, you will discover training strategies, motor learning strategies, and drills to improve body control, balance, and coordination.

4 The Science of Conditioning   33

Conditioning enhances stamina and cardiovascular endurance and is a key component of any well-rounded training program. Learn about the three energy systems and how they work together to provide the boost you need to improve aerobic and anaerobic conditioning.

5 Warm-Up Exercises   39

Warming up is more than stretching. A proper warm-up prepares the body for the workout to come, awakening mobility, flexibility, stability, and activation. You will find more than 60 exercises to help you build a safe, effective warm-up.

6 Strength Exercises   109

Improve strength with more than 85 exercises. You will find variations that use free weights such as kettlebells and barbells, body weight, exercise bands, cable machines, physioballs, and more.

7 Plyometrics and Power Exercises   197

Discover your inner athlete through 19 exercises that use jumps, hops, bounds, and skips to challenge your ability to move quickly and powerfully. Variations use exercise bands, medicine balls, or just your own body.

8 Change of Direction, Agility, and Speed Exercises   219

Being able to accelerate and decelerate safely and efficiently is a highlight of athleticism. The nine drills in this chapter will develop first-step speed, dynamic change of direction, explosiveness, and tempo.

9 Conditioning Exercises and Protocols   229

The programs described in chapters 10 through 13 include a conditioning day in each phase. This chapter reviews the conditioning exercises and protocols required for these programs.

10 The Train Like a Pro Training Program   235

This 12-week program includes three consecutive phases of four-week training blocks that build off each other. The goal of this program is to tap into your inner athlete and develop a stronger, faster, more powerful version of yourself. Using the rate of perceived exertion scale and the concept of reps in reserve, you will customize the program to fit your body and needs.

11 The GPP/Hypertrophy Training Program   253

The goal of this 12-week program is to develop general preparedness and hypertrophy, or muscle size.

12 The Strength Training Program   269

To increase your overall strength, follow this 12-week training program focused on strength development.

13 The Power Training Program   285

The final program is focused on power development through a 12-week program. Discover the more powerful, explosive version of yourself.

Exercise Finder 301 • About the Author 307
Earn Continuing Education Credits/Units 308

PREFACE

Remember when you were a kid and playing sports was the single most important thing to you? Better yet, do you member that feeling of scoring the game-winning goal, hitting the buzzer-beating shot, or forcing overtime with a touchdown catch with only seconds remaining on the clock?

All these moments share one thing in common: athleticism. Training to keep your overall athleticism should never come to an end. In fact, it might be the most important thing you can focus on when it comes to your overall health and performance in life.

As I move through my third decade around the sun, I can't help but think back to playing sports as a kid and wanting to keep that feeling of athleticism; I don't want to lose it now. Whether I was playing organized soccer or basketball in various leagues, playing street hockey or backyard football with my brothers and neighbors, or even participating in track and field on the high school team, I have many fond memories of playing sports and being able to show off my athleticism. I bet you have these memories as well, which is exactly why I wrote this book.

Most people think that training for athletic performance is exclusively for athletes participating in elite, collegiate, or professional sports. This couldn't be further from the truth. All humans are athletes since we all have the ability to control our body in space. Ultimately, that's what athleticism comes down to. If you can control your body in space, you can develop your athleticism. When you develop quality strength, power, speed, and agility—all of which represent the primary pillars of athletic performance—you're unlocking your inner athlete and reaching the pinnacle of your overall health.

This book is all about helping you find your inner athlete, tap into your full athletic potential, and most importantly, become the best version of yourself. Most training programs out there in the marketplace focus too heavily on strength, power, and speed. These are definitely qualities and skills that you want to possess. However, it's also important to think long-term and focus on the additional qualities and skills that will help you take a more well-rounded approach. This book helps you turn over every stone when it comes to championing your health and performance. Not only will this book help you build strength, improve power, and develop speed, but it will also help you improve joint mobility, muscle flexibility, stamina, endurance, conditioning, multidirectional movement skills, and recovery. This is what makes my approach unique. I take a holistic approach to your health and performance so that you can keep doing the things you love and train in a challenging, yet sustainable way.

In this book, we'll take a deep dive into a variety of areas that will help you improve your overall athleticism while focusing on health and performance. Each chapter will have a specific focus area to help you better understand basic training principles, all while helping you develop the skills you need for long-term success in your training. The beginning chapters break down the truth about training like an athlete for both strength and power. After that, we'll move onto developing skills in change of direction, reactive agility, and conditioning. Then we'll cover a variety of movements and exercises in the areas of the warm-up, plyometrics, power development, change of direction, agility, speed, and conditioning. Finally, we'll come to the best part: the training program chapters. The first training program chapter is a culmination of every topic in the book, while the remaining three focus on building muscle, strength, and power, respectively.

Now, can you think back again to when you were just a kid shooting hoops with your friends, about to race the fastest kid in the neighborhood, or playing in the high-school football championship game? I bet that your goal was to become the champion of your sport. Now your goal should be to become the champion of your life. Pick up this book and begin applying these athletic performance concepts to start winning today.

ACKNOWLEDGMENTS

Sitting down to write this is emotional for me. I never thought that I would truly be here with this type of opportunity while being able to share my message with people around the world. When you consider my past, my failures in life, and the many hurdles I've overcome, it makes me appreciate everything even more. Whether it was failing during my undergraduate studies in a six-year span with a cumulative GPA of 2.961, being put on academic probation during that time, or taking over three years of graduate school applications to finally get accepted, being able to write all of this makes it all worth it to me. The most important part about all of this, though, is the people around me on my path. In other words, without my beloved family, close friends, and colleagues, I simply would not be here right now doing this. I would like to take this time to acknowledge these special people in my life.

To my wife, Alyssa. You will never truly understand the magnitude or depth of my love for you. I know that I've said this time and time again, but it's important for you to know what you mean to me. You've stood by me through thick and thin since July 5, 2012. No matter what came my way, you were there to support me, show me unconditional love, and demonstrate an unequivocal level of compassion. You are kind, thoughtful, caring, and above all else, you push me to be more and do more daily. The thought of you, alone, continues to make me want to be a better person, a better companion, a better family member, and a better friend. Thank you for always believing in me and making me dig deeper. For that, I am eternally grateful. I love you, always and forever.

To my daughter, Giuliana, born on September 17, 2024. You have lit up our life ever since coming into this world, and most importantly, you've made your daddy so proud of your accomplishments and milestones so far. Your beautiful smile, your laugh, your energy and your soft touch have all taught me a valuable lesson in life: slow down and live in the moment. I love you more than you will ever know, and I look forward to raising you alongside the best mommy in the world.

To my mom, Maria, and dad, Sam. I know that the first two decades of my life beginning on January 19, 1989, weren't smooth sailing by any means. I know that, more than anyone, you've seen me fail in life and in academics, on several occasions. I also know that I made it challenging, at times, for you to see the bigger picture of why I was doing what I was doing. I thoroughly appreciate the mental fortitude you taught me. Moreover, I appreciate how you gave me strength, both physical and mental, to be able to persevere through failures and chase my goals. I think of how you both immigrated here to the United States during your early years in life, and together, worked toward building a family. To that end, I thank you for sacrificing so much for me and my brothers, Michael and John, from the very beginning. You always put us first, no matter what. Your level of sacrifice, dedication, and commitment to our overall well-being will never be forgotten. Thank you both for pushing me, both directly and indirectly. Your belief in me has always been a constant reminder of being more and doing more. I love you both to the moon and back.

To my brothers, Michael and John. You may not know this, but you both push me to be better. Your level of support over the years has been instrumental in opening doors and avenues for me that I never thought possible. I have continued to lean on you both for guidance, mentorship, and support, and you have never let me down. I want you both to know how much I love you. There is nothing I wouldn't do for you, either.

To my family on my wife's side: my mother-in-law, Judi; father-in-law, Frank; sister-in-law, Nicole; brother-in-law, Manny; and niece, Isla. Judi and Frank, I love you both immensely. You have always supported me on my path, given me encouragement, and believed in me. I have always felt better knowing that I have you both by my side. Thank you for making me a better person. Nicole and Manny, I appreciate you both for always rooting me on in my career. No matter what I was doing, you've always made it a point to cheer me on, support my work, and believe in me. I love you both very much. Isla, thank you for making me an uncle. I love you very much.

To my sisters-in-law, Holly (Michael's wife) and Daria (John's wife). Over the years, I have had several conversations with you both on an individual level about my work, my career path, and my dreams. Time and time again, I've been met with unconditional support, love, and encouragement. You may not know this, but I think back to these moments all the time. Thank you both for believing in me. I love you both so much. To my goddaughter, Ellie, and niece, Penelope. Thank you for making me a godfather and an uncle. Your presence brings me so much joy, and I love being able to mentor you in life. Ellie, thank you for always wanting to "do exercise" with Uncle Matthew. You may not know this yet, but I truly cherish these moments together. I love you both very much.

To my mentor, Victor Kizer. You took a chance on me several years ago, and for that, I am eternally grateful. I have always been amazed at your ability to be a people-person, to allow others into your life, and to be an incredible friend. Beyond that, I have always been in awe of your ability to be an amazing human being. You have always been a source of encouragement for me, one that continues to provide support, guidance, and mentorship. Thank you for always believing in me, and for giving me a platform to share my message. I love you, man.

To my dear friends and colleagues, Brad Leshinske, Darrin Smith, Jack Dustin, and Jeff Stern. Each of you have had a profound impact on my career, the way that I think, the way that I approach problem-solving, and most importantly, the way that I treat others. I am beyond lucky to call you all respected colleagues. More importantly though, I am forever indebted to be able to call you all dear friends. Thank you for always believing in me and acting as my support system. Your presence in my life has been incredibly valuable.

To the man who opened the door for me in strength and conditioning, Mike Boyle. Mike, without my internship at MBSC back in the fall of 2011, I don't know if I would have received half of the opportunities that came after that. You have always had a positive impact on my career as a strength and conditioning coach, but more importantly, as a person. You changed the way that I view relationship-building within the strength and conditioning profession, and how to pay it forward to the next generation of coaches. Thank you for all that you do and for giving me the opportunity early on in my career. I will never forget how giving and kind you are. Thank you, my friend.

To my dear friends, colleagues, and students at Endicott College. Thank you to Dr. Brian Wylie and Jack Dustin for allowing us to use the Athletic Performance Center weight room. Thank you to the amazing demo athletes featured all throughout this book: Annie Siemasko, Elijah Harris, Elizabeth Lentino, Grace Kolis, Katrina Haddad, Logan Batchelor, Michael Canney, Rachel DiFronzo, Tallon Craver, and Zachariah Twardosky. Without you all, this book would simply not be possible.

Lastly, I'd like to thank Korey Van Wyk. You reached out to me back in July of 2022 with the crazy idea of having me author this book. Fast-forward to right now, and I continue to feel grateful for the opportunity. Thank you for opening the door, giving me this opportunity, and believing in me. I appreciate you very much, my friend.

CHAPTER 1

The Truth About Training Like an Athlete

Close your eyes for a moment and think back to when you were a kid. You're watching your favorite team play on TV. It just so happens that you're also watching your favorite player. For me, this was Michael Jordan on the Chicago Bulls in the NBA in the 1990s. Think of how your favorite player moved in their sport, how they played the game, how effortless they made it seem to you—and, most notably, how they just seemed to exude athleticism. This is how I felt watching Jordan play basketball. It was difficult to put the words together to describe what I was seeing. Athleticism is an elite display of balance between multiple physical qualities through graceful and efficient movement. When everything clicks for an athlete, it's awesome to watch.

When we take a closer look at these amazing feats of athleticism from athletes across the spectrum of sports, we begin to realize that these physical qualities—or pieces of the athletic puzzle—can be broken down and better understood. From a physiological standpoint, qualities that immediately come to mind when thinking about elite athleticism are related to strength, power, change of direction, and agility. All these qualities, when put on display within the context of sports and athletics at elite levels, are amazing to watch. However, they are also amazing to experience as a doer. We are all athletic to some extent, and we all have the ability to show off our athleticism within the context of sports, athletics, training, and performance.

The best part about training like an athlete is that it's for everyone. It's not just for the best athletes in the world; it's for you, too! More importantly, it's a mindset, it's a shift in thinking, and it's about adopting a holistic approach to champion your overall health and performance. By using the same strategies and tactics in your training as athletes do, you can train to become more athletic. However, training like an athlete starts by understanding what all of it means to adopt this type of holistic approach in your mind so that you can become a champion of your health and your performance. This is how you'll begin to develop a strategic plan. That's the next step in this process.

WHY TRAIN LIKE AN ATHLETE?

Athleticism is hard to define, yet we know it when we see it. In its simplest form, athleticism can be defined as your ability to control your body. We often associate athleticism with physical qualities such as strength, power, speed, and agility, traits displayed by elite athletes. Although each of these physical qualities can be expressed in different ways, they all overlap at the intersection of body control. An individual who can control their body in space at an elite level through efficient movement that looks crisp to the naked eye is what we often think of as athleticism. Have you ever seen Michael Jordan explode off the basketball court with otherworldly power and glide through the air for an attack on the rim? Maybe you've watched Serena Williams smash through the ball with an immense level of power in a serve on the tennis court? What about seeing Lionel Messi dribble with speed, agility, and precision as he reacts to defenders and evades their slide tackles on the way to the net? Did you ever catch Mia Hamm as she dominated her competition on the pitch through speed and strategic balance on her path toward a goal? All these athletes will forever live on in our minds as displaying athleticism to the highest degree. The one thing they all have in common? Body control.

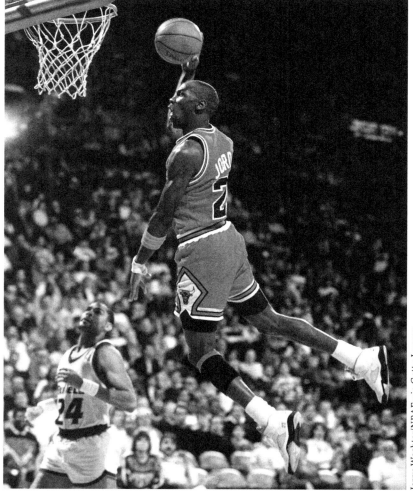

| Training strength, power, speed, and agility makes it look easy for Jordan.

Body control is not exclusive to the athletes who play competitive sports at the high school or collegiate level or competitive athletes in semi-professional and professional sports. The fascinating thing about body control is that every single human has the ability to master it, own it, and dominate it. Strength, power, speed, and agility—all key physical qualities of athleticism—are skills that take time to develop, but that help you improve your ability to control your body. By working on developing and improving your current levels of strength, power, speed, and agility, you are ultimately becoming more athletic. This means that we are all athletes.

You're likely reading this and finding it hard to believe that you can jump like Michael Jordan, serve like Serena Williams, be agile like Lionel Messi, or sprint like Mia Hamm. However, the goal is not to be like them. Rather, your goal is to be the best version of you. More specifically, you should be laser-focused on improving your individual ability to jump, sprint, rotate with power, and be agile and reactive. Unlocking your inner athlete requires first believing in your ability to get there.

A common misconception when it comes to training like an athlete is that your level of competition determines your training style. We might find ourselves thinking, "Am I an athlete who plays a competitive sport?" If the answer is "yes," we're more likely to see the need to train like an athlete for whichever sport we are playing at a competitive level. Someone on the other side of the coin might think, "Well, I don't play a sport at all at any level, so I don't need to train like that." This is where I believe we go wrong. Thinking that we "shouldn't" or "don't need to" train like an athlete if we don't play a sport or compete at any level might deter us from building and improving our ability to control our body. Although training with the intent of becoming more generally fit and healthy is an admirable goal, I believe that we can check off both these boxes while also becoming more athletic in our training. This shift in our thought process, in the way that we view training, and most importantly, in the way that we believe in our abilities is a major catalyst in achieving athleticism. Self-efficacy—your belief in your ability or capacity to complete a task or execute a behavior—is a monumentally important skill that you can harness with your mind and your body to improve in each of the following physical qualities, one by one: strength, power, speed, and agility. Improving your self-efficacy, a primary pillar in behavior change, is the cheat code to success in this arena.

Let's face it: We all have a competitive side. Think of how we act at our job, in our studies in school, or even growing up alongside our siblings. I'm positive that there have been countless times in your life where you competed at something outside of sports and athletics, which leads me to believe you can tap into this side of yourself to kick-start the process of improving your athleticism. Couple this with improving your self-efficacy, and you have a potent recipe for becoming stronger, more powerful, faster, and more agile. Instead of shying away from your competitive side, you should lean in, embrace it, and prioritize it. When you do that, you unlock all the possibilities in your athletic performance. You unlock doors that may have been closed for years. You gain access to rooms that have gone unoccupied. Most importantly, you get in the game. The game may not be a sport—you still have the game of life to compete in. Wherever your game takes place, you can start at any point and start improving in all these areas of athleticism.

Training like an athlete is a mindset. It goes far beyond the sets and reps you'll do in the gym, field, or court. It comes down to your willingness to let go of your previous beliefs about training, and instead, tap into your athletic potential. When you do that, you'll reach your inner athlete. You'll reach a side of you that understands the importance of self-efficacy and a competitive edge that helps you achieve greatness in your own athletic performance. Don't be mistaken, though; this isn't about gimmicks, fancy exercises, or flashy drills that fill up your social media feed. It's about putting in the work, remaining consistent in your training, and performing tried-and-true athletic movements that have stood the test of time.

PHYSICAL QUALITIES OF ATHLETICISM

When we talk about athleticism, we think of strength, power, speed, and agility. But what do each of these qualities really mean? Why are they important and how are they related to athleticism? The answer to those questions ultimately comes down to how you view yourself and whether or not you truly believe that you are an athlete. Every single human is an athlete—keeping that at the forefront of our minds helps us to paint a clearer picture of why we train.

Strength

Imagine building enough strength to feel confident in your ability to produce or resist force, without hesitation, at any time. Carrying groceries from the car to your house, lifting heavy boxes when moving to a new home, or moving furniture in your office are abilities related to your overall athleticism. When it comes to strength, the real goal is being strong enough. We aren't necessarily chasing maximum strength here—instead, the aim should be enough strength for whatever you're tasked with on the court, in the field, or in your daily life. Beyond building muscular strength, it is also crucial in athletic performance to have strong bones, ligaments, and tendons, all of which are important support structures in your body. Building strength to produce and absorb force is one of the main components of athleticism. Producing force relates to how powerful you can become, and absorbing force relates to how well you can harness and control power. This leads us to the next component: power.

Power

Power is a physical quality that allows us to exert and absorb force quickly. You can think of power as simply using your strength rapidly. The cool thing about strength and power is that these physical qualities have a ton of overlap in training and in life. Power is a hallmark trait of athleticism, and we should never lose sight of it in training. Explosiveness lives in dunking a basketball, kicking a soccer ball, spiking a volleyball, taking a slapshot, and many other feats of athleticism that we see demonstrated across a broad spectrum of sports. In daily life, maintaining and even improving your power throughout the lifespan makes physical daily tasks much easier to perform. If strength is the hammer, then power is the nail gun. They both get the job done, but power is faster. This is a very simplistic way to view these physical qualities, but can help you understand the rationale behind building them. Power is a quality that, once harnessed, can allow you to do some pretty cool stuff both in and out of the weight room.

Speed

Have you ever heard the phrase "Speed kills"? Think of some of the fastest people in the world: Usain Bolt, Ali Krieger, Tyreke Hill, Shell-Ann Fraser-Pryce. When you watch them sprint, regardless of which sport they play, it might appear as though they're gliding above the ground. Fast people make speed look really easy.

The "speed kills" phrase is right on target. A difference in speed that seems tiny on paper can make a world of difference on the court, in the field, and even in the game of life. In other words, if you are even just minimally faster than your competition (or than yourself from the past), this will help to boost your overall athleticism.

Strength and power, both intimately related to the application of force, are also closely related to speed. Each physical quality builds off the previous one—if you train to develop power, you're developing speed too. This means improving your overall athleticism might be easier than you originally thought.

Agility

The last component in athleticism is related to your ability to be reactive. Think of Barry Sanders when he would fake one way to the defender and then run in the opposite direction. Think of Caitlin Clark when she jab-steps and then launches a three-point shot into the net. Reacting to a defender trying to tackle you at game speed is what we call agility. Being agile—able to change directions with precision and efficiency—is a way to show off all the previously mentioned qualities (strength, power, and speed) all at once. When you break down each sport, you'll begin to see how often each athlete has to react to something. That could be a ball, a defender, a reflection, a change in possession, or one of many other things. It's clear why the quality of agility is important to becoming more athletic. But agility isn't exclusive to competitive athletes at the high school, collegiate, semi-professional, or professional levels. Agility, along with strength, power, and speed, is truly for everyone. In daily life, moments that require you to react quickly happen all the time, which is one of the reasons it's beneficial to improve in these areas. Quicker reactions equal more overall athleticism.

The real question isn't whether building strength, power, speed, and agility are right for you. Instead, ask yourself whether you're ready to build them the way an athlete does.

BUILDING ATHLETICISM

Athleticism is a combination of strength, power, speed, and agility. The delicate balance between these physical traits is what boosts your overall athleticism, and more importantly, helps you remain athletic. A primary foundation of athleticism is strength—your ability to exert force. You can develop strength through a variety of modalities in a gym or weight room.

From a scientific standpoint, building strength is all about progressive overload, a term that means exactly what it sounds like: an increase in load over time in a progressive manner. You're essentially increasing the mass you lift or move gradually over a period of time, making you stronger. This is one of simplest concepts to grasp in the science of building strength. It's easy to apply and nearly always works. As an example, think of the deadlift. Imagine that your goal is to build a stronger overall trap bar deadlift, with a current personal record of 225 pounds for five reps and a goal of achieving five reps at 315 pounds. The difference is 90 pounds. Let's say you're not necessarily in a rush, but you'd like to achieve this goal in a reasonable time frame. Using simple math, you can break down this goal on a weekly basis by attempting to increase the weight lifted by 7.5 pounds each week for a period of 12 weeks (roughly three months). This is a simple example of progressive overload in the context of increasing strength in your trap bar deadlift. Is this the only way to apply this concept? Of course not. However, it shows how you can improve your overall strength through small increases.

From a physiological standpoint, I always find it easiest to explain power as *fast strength*. We know that strength is your ability to exert or produce force. Power, on the other hand, is your ability to exert or produce force in a fast and explosive manner. This means that there is a time component associated with power. Typically, someone who is strong is also powerful, but there are certainly outliers.

When training to improve strength, you should primarily focus on technique, form, and a controlled tempo. When training to improve power, you should perform a given movement fast and explosively. That's the differentiator. A classic example of improving power can be seen in the kettlebell swing, where the ultimate goal is to perform the movement explosively through the hip hinge pattern. This allows you to improve lower body power in your hips and the surrounding muscles (i.e., hamstrings and glutes).

Training to develop speed is much easier than you think. To train to be fast, you must not only train at fast speeds, but do so both moving in a straight line and changing directions. This is the primary difference between someone who is fast and someone who is fast with athleticism. It's important to train in the way that you want to perform. If you are a track and field sprinter, you typically run in a straight line, but all other sports take place in all directions (i.e., they are multidirectional). When you want to improve speed, sprint in a straight line, sprint on a curved lined, and lastly, sprint while changing directions. Learning how to change directions effectively and react quickly is key, which brings us to our next topic.

Change-of-direction ability and agility are often confused when athletes are considering how to train for each quality from a physiological standpoint. When you watch your favorite athletes play in their sports, it's clear that they can change directions efficiently while also reacting quickly and being agile in their body movements. There is a good amount of overlap between the qualities of direction change ability and agility. But there's one key factor that helps to better understand the differentiating factor between the two. Think back to when you were a kid playing youth or high school sports. Do you ever remember your coach providing very specific coaching cues, instructions, and guidance on how to complete a practice drill? For instance, did your coach ever set up some cones on the field and then instruct you to sprint from cone to cone, and then have you perform exactly what they had instructed you to do? This is an example of change-of-direction ability. It requires no reaction to any sort of external stimulus, but it sharpens your ability to change directions quickly and efficiently based on specific coaching instructions. Conversely, imagine a similar scenario with cones and maybe a defender where the primary objective is to react to some sort of external stimulus. An external stimulus could be anything from a coach yelling out a color or number to you having to react to the direction a defender moves. That's true agility—your ability to change directions quickly, led by an external stimulus. That is the primary difference.

In training, it makes the most sense to first improve your ability to change directions. There are many ways to train for this, so long as you follow what was outlined previously: Specific instructions must be provided, and the drill must be without any sort of reaction component. The goal for you as the athlete would be to master change-of-direction drills, steadily improving your ability over time until you perform them with ease. Once you've mastered the ability to change directions with drills that do not require any sort of reaction, you can take a deep dive into reaction-based agility drills. Knowing that agility drills will be more challenging, be sure to ease your way into them over time by steadily increasing the overall intensity or challenge. When you have an adequate level of strength and power, performing both change-of-direction drills and agility drills becomes much easier. This is why it's important to incorporate all the aforementioned elements of overall athleticism into your training.

MIMIC HIGH-LEVEL ATHLETES FOR HIGH-LEVEL RESULTS

High-level athletes treat the preparation for their sport as a job because it is their job. Now, this certainly won't be the case for everyone. Training your body to become more athletic doesn't have to be treated this way. However, what should resonate with everyone is the level of focus and attention to detail that high-level athletes bring to training for their sport. This is evident to viewers on game day when we see how dialed in an athlete is, how sharp they look, or even the intent look on their face. The secret is that this level of focus and attention to detail doesn't just show up on game day. Rather, it starts with preparation—anything the athlete does to prep for game day. A large portion of this comes down to their training, which is primarily based on the physical qualities we've already discussed: strength, power, speed, change of direction, and agility.

What we can all take from how high-level athletes train is their sharpened level of focus and heightened attention to detail. These little things, when combined, truly have an impact on your level of athleticism. Anyone would benefit from dialing in their focus, paying close attention to even the smallest details, and approaching their training like a high-level athlete. If your goal is to improve your overall athleticism, this approach will put you on the fast track to success in your training and improvement in key areas.

TRAIN ALL ASPECTS OF ATHLETICISM

I love building strength just as much as the next person. Strength has a carryover effect in many other physical qualities, such as power, sprinting, mobility, and flexibility. Truthfully, if you have time to do only one thing in your training, focusing all your efforts on strength isn't the worst idea. However, this is also where most people go wrong. They simply focus on how strong they can become. As with many things in life, there is a limit to how strong you can get based on genetics, anatomy, physiology, chronological age, and even training age. Most people will find a ton of success early in the process of building strength, especially if they are relatively new to training. However, there is often a plateau or leveling off when the athlete reaches their unique maximal or near-maximal levels of strength. After that, most people continue trying to build more strength, only to realize that it becomes more challenging the stronger you are. Unless your goal is to be the strongest human on the planet or the strongest lifter in a powerlifting competition, I would suggest avoiding this path.

Instead, remember that while it's a great idea to build strength throughout the body, the strength you build must also transfer into the other important areas of athleticism: power, speed, change of direction, and agility. If your strength doesn't transfer well into these areas, dial down the strength and dial up in the other areas.

If your goal is to become more athletic, it's important to focus your efforts across the board in each of the key physical qualities in athleticism.

Many athletes overlook this. They forget to add exercises to their training programs that focus on jumping, landing, power training, sprinting, change of direction, and agility. Some of the hallmark exercises to improve in these areas are much simpler than you would think. For example, a variety of jumping, hopping, and bounding exercises emphasize producing force by pushing off the ground and absorbing force via landing. When it comes to power development, there are a variety of simple exercises to help boost your lower and upper body power through the use of weights, bands, and medicine balls. Lastly, for speed, change of direction, and agility, you'll have dedicated sections and days of your training program to refine your skills in these areas to improve your athleticism!

CHAPTER 2

Developing Athletic Strength and Power

When it comes to strength, most people think only of bigger muscles. When it comes to power, people tend to think of how explosively they can exert their strength or force. While all of this is good and well, developing strength and power involves much more than just the size of your muscles or your level of explosiveness.

It's important to consider how the development of strength and power in the weight room can provide more durability and resilience to the other major support structures in the body, such as your bones, ligaments, and tendons. We can see the size of muscles as they grow over time in response to strength and power training. However, it isn't as easy to visualize the other major support structures—such as your bones, ligaments, and tendons—from a growth and development standpoint since they are deeper in the human body and don't have the physical growth capacity of muscles. When it comes to building strength and power, it is critical to think of these major support structures as pieces of the puzzle.

TRAINING FOR STRENGTH

There are many ways to increase your overall muscle size, also known as muscle mass. But having bigger muscles isn't necessarily the goal when it comes to training like an athlete. While it's important to develop muscle mass via strength training and power training, athletes must consider how much muscle mass is enough based on the sport or position they play. We also have to consider the purpose of building muscle mass and how we plan to use it. Bigger isn't always better. When it comes to improving overall athleticism, I'd suggest building muscle mass to the extent that you have the strength and power to display the needed skills in any sort of athletic or recreational endeavor. With that in mind, we can focus on how to effectively develop strength, muscle, and power in training. For example, if your goal is to develop maximal strength, you'll likely want to hover around 90%-100% of your maximum effort performing one to five repetitions, while general strength can be obtained at 80%-90% of your maximum effort at five to eight repetitions. If your goal is to build muscle and maximize hypertrophy, it will be more effective to operate at 65%-80% of your maximum effort at 8-15 repetitions. Lastly, for power, aim for roughly 85%-95% of your maximum effort at around three to five repetitions.

Your skeletal structure plays a major role in allowing you to both absorb and produce force. Bone mineral density is an important factor when training for strength and power because stronger bones means that you have a greater ability to generate and transmit force. Consider bones as the major connectors of each of the joints in your body. Ligaments—another major support structure in the body—help to connect bone to bone and are equally important. Ligaments are what we call avascular, meaning that they lack blood supply, so they are slower than muscle to respond to training. However, we can still strengthen them and increase their ability to withstand and produce force.

Tendons are the last piece of the puzzle when it comes to building "body armor" to increase your overall durability and resilience. Tendons connect muscles to bones, so you can also directly strengthen them through training that focuses on strength and power development. Tendons respond especially well to exercises that emphasize the eccentric (lowering aspect) component of a movement and also the isometric (static aspect) component. An additional consideration when it comes to strengthening tendons is the amount of time spent under tension in an exercise. Think of time under tension as the amount of time a muscle is being challenged by resistance, whether from your own body weight or an external load such as a dumbbell. Either way, the more time your muscles spend under tension and being challenged by resistance, the more they grow and adapt. It is important to use strength and power training as a way to improve your durability and resilience in the bones, ligaments, tendons, and muscles for a training approach that turns over every stone. This will help you to increase muscle mass, improve bone mineral density, and improve your ability to generate force. You'll be stronger, more durable, and even more resilient to everything life throws at you, from grocery carrying (seriously!) to flag football and even some weekend recreational tennis. Training for athleticism will help you become a high performer for life!

How Strong Is Strong Enough for Athletic Performance?

How strong is strong enough? The question of strength often comes up when discussing training for the purpose of improving athletic performance. If your goal is to become the strongest human being on the planet, building strength and muscle should obviously be your priority. However, this isn't the goal when it comes to improving your overall athleticism. Being strong enough in sports and life is the goal. In other words, if your goal is to dunk a basketball, build the necessary amount of strength to achieve that task. If your goal is to push a wheelbarrow up a steep hill, develop enough strength to do that. If your goal is to carry heavy grocery bags in both hands for a half-mile walk, then build enough strength to do that. Remember: Keep the goal the goal. Being strong enough for the specific task or goal should be your primary objective. Strength isn't just displayed in a one-rep maximum in the gym. Rather, varying levels of strength are everywhere in sports and in life! Sure, there are certain positions in certain sports that require a maximum level of strength. There also may be occupations in life that require a similar output. But strength alone isn't enough. It's important to be strong and powerful. If your goal is to move, perform, and feel like an athlete, you need a balanced combination of strength, power, speed, and agility for overall athleticism.

TRAINING FOR POWER

Power development is often associated only with athletes who participate in competitive sports. While developing power is certainly important for these athletes, it is also important for everyone in life. When we talk about power training, we must consider the importance of plyometrics and sprinting. Plyometrics is another word to describe training that involves jumping and the use of power. Specific examples of plyometrics are jumps, hops, and bounds. Plyometrics is best performed in short bouts of high-intensity efforts for maximum gains. Performing continuous box jumps for one minute is not considered power training or plyometrics, simply based on the fact that fatigue will begin to set in after 10-20 seconds. It's also important to keep power training and plyometrics near the beginning of your training session, directly after the warm-up and before the strength training exercises. Sprinting, on the other hand, is a much more common term that refers to running at maximum speed. Again, performing sprinting exercises is best suited near the beginning of the training program, when you're feeling fresh and energized, since it requires you to operate a high intensities.

Incorporating plyometrics and jumping exercises into our training program improves our ability to produce force quickly and efficiently. This aspect of fitness—how rapidly we can produce force—is referred to as the rate of force development. Think of your favorite athlete in your favorite sport. Now think of that athlete performing any sort of movement or activity that requires power or an explosive action. Consider a basketball player jumping up to dunk the ball at the rim. To complete this move, it's important for that player to perform at a high rate of force development with respect to their jumping ability. Rate of force development in sports is critical because time is of the essence; you have a very small window of time to produce a lot of force. Maybe the player is coming down from a rebound and needs to jump again right away so the ball isn't stripped. This is a simple way to understand this concept.

Do I Need Power?

You may be thinking, "Power isn't for me since dunking a basketball isn't my job." Here's why power *is* for you.

When someone assumes power development is for the purpose of playing sports only, they're thinking about power in the wrong way. There are situations in life outside of sports that require you to exert your power in a fast and efficient manner. For example, have you ever had to sprint to catch the bus for work? Have you ever crossed a pond or stream and had to jump from one rock to the next? Have you ever had to dodge to the side to get out of the way of an oncoming car or bicycle? I understand that these are extreme examples. However, there are plenty of other situations that require you to exert power outside of sports.

The flip side of the coin is your ability to harness your power and absorb force. We can see this in the examples of slowing down, landing, and decelerating—all important when it comes to improving your power and overall athleticism outside of sports.

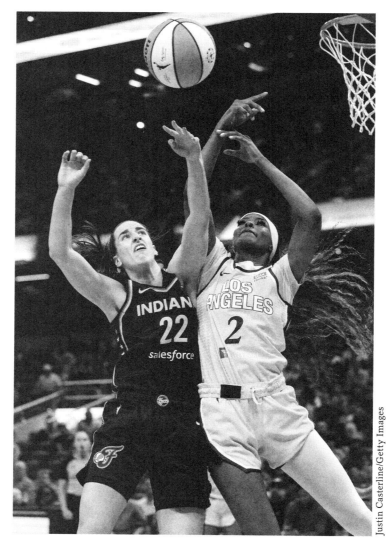

Plyometric training improves your ability to produce explosive power, which is important when you need to battle for a rebound.

It's also important to increase the exact opposite skill: your rate of force acceptance. Consider how rapidly that basketball player must land on the ground after the dunk. That ability to come to a stop after rapid motion with complete body control is your rate of force acceptance. Increasing your ability to produce force (rate of force development) and absorb force (rate of force acceptance) are key to developing athleticism.

We can develop power through many different movements, exercises, and modalities. Power training often takes place through a variety of jumping exercises or movements that incorporate familiar training equipment such as barbells, dumbbells, kettlebells, and medicine balls. When training for power, it's important to address the lower body, core, and upper body. Making sure that you're building power through exercises that help you exert force fast throughout your entire body will also increase your overall athleticism.

> ## Will Strength Training Make You Slower?
>
> You won't lose speed or power through strength training unless your program includes only exercises that build strength. If your overall training program includes a variety of strength training exercises, power training exercises, speed training exercises, and agility training exercises, you have a balanced program that will help you improve in all areas.

TRAINING FOR SPEED

Sprinting is a crucial component of athletic development that often gets forgotten within the process of training. I live in New England, which means that we have only a few nice months throughout the year with weather that allows us to sprint outdoors. However, during the colder months, we still have access to indoor facilities that allow us to continue improving our ability to sprint. No matter your situation, you can always figure out a way to sprint. The cool thing about sprinting is that it's not about trying to become the fastest man or woman on the planet. Instead, think about your intent of becoming faster. When you sprint frequently at or near top speed, you're becoming faster and more powerful—beneficial qualities for your long-term health and performance. Improving your ability to produce and absorb power and force, including through sprinting, are key components of your overall athleticism.

CHAPTER 3

Developing Change of Direction and Agility Skills

Remember when you were a kid on the playground at school playing tag? Your heart is pounding, you have beads of sweat running down the sides of your face, you're trying to catch your breath, and you're thinking about your next move. You didn't know it, but you were working hard to develop both change of direction ability and agility.

It's important to understand the value of change of direction ability and agility within the context of sports. Sports exist on a continuum of movements and actions that happen at the speed of light. Split-second decisions are constantly being made, and athletes carry out those decisions in fast-forward. This continuum of movement relates to the process of acceleration, deceleration, and reacceleration. To paint a clear picture, let's review a sample scenario. If you were a fan of the NFL back in the 1990s, you remember how elusive and shifty Barry Sanders was. Imagine that the quarterback hands off the ball to Sanders. Now, Sanders' ideal move is to find a gap or hole in the defense and exploit it by running through it toward the end zone. In essence, he needs to run either straight forward or forward at an angle with speed and acceleration. Next, he is met by an incoming defender coming from his right side. He needs to think on his feet, literally, and make a split-second decision to evade the defender and avoid being tackled. What does Sanders do? He stops dead in his tracks by planting his left foot in the field and jukes right, barely missing the incoming defender's tackle. That represents the deceleration end of the continuum. Lastly, and most importantly, Sanders needs to turn the burners back on as fast as possible, speeding up again as he runs like hell toward the end zone. This is one of many examples in sports of the need to accelerate, decelerate, and reaccelerate. If you have a free moment, visit YouTube and watch some of Barry's highlight clips from the 1990s. Agility personified. But it's not limited to football legends—stuff like this happens all the time across all sports.

Agility, fast reaction, and the ability to change directions rapidly are also important for non-competitive folks in daily life. Whether you're playing pick-up basketball with your friends or recreational tennis on the weekends at the tennis club, or even chasing your kids around, these athletic qualities are important for everyone. These skills decline over time at a faster rate when we don't train them, which is yet another reason to keep them in the mix!

CHANGE OF DIRECTION VERSUS AGILITY

These two terms overlap and frequently get confused in the context of sports. The problem is that they look eerily alike, which makes it challenging to understand the true difference. Interested in knowing the difference in a simple way? It all comes down to a rehearsed pattern versus a reaction to an external stimulus. When something is rehearsed, it means that you as the athlete understand exactly what you need to do, where you need to go and how to get there. For example, consider a scenario where you set yourself up in a sprinter's stance at the 50-yard line on a football field. The coach instructs you to sprint 10 yards forward, stop on a dime once you've reached the 40-yard line, turn around, and then immediately sprint back to the starting point (50-yard line). Before performing this activity, you discussed every single element and step, and most importantly, you did not need to react to anything at all. You simply had to complete the drill as instructed and rehearsed. That is a prime example of a change of direction drill where the emphasis is on following instructions based on a rehearsed pattern that excludes any sort of reaction.

Now, let's use the same scenario, but with an additional wrinkle. Again, you set up in a sprinter's stance at the 50-yard line on a football field. This time, though, when you are instructed to sprint 10 yards forward to the 40-yard line, there is

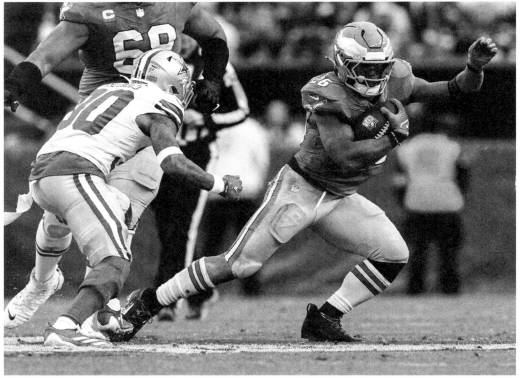

| Training change of direction ability is crucial in sports like football.

another athlete standing directly in front of you. It's your job to react to this other athlete. Your reaction will be based on a variety of cues the athlete at the 40-yard line can choose from. This athlete can use hand signals (i.e., left or right), verbal cues (i.e., shouting out either "left" or "right"), and even physical cues (i.e., short and quick step toward either the left or the right). In addition, verbally shouting out colors or numbers can be a cue. There's a ton of variety, and you can truly be as creative as possible. However, the most important component, the one that truly makes this agility, is the presence of an external stimulus (i.e., cue) that forces you to use your decision-making skills to decide and react. In sports, this happens all the time through a variety of plays and examples, such as a ball deflection in football, a defender moving off the base in baseball, players chasing down a puck in hockey, and even a goalie saving a penalty kick in soccer.

Is it Agility or Change of Direction?

Watch an NFL combine. You'll notice a drill called the Pro Agility Test, sometimes called the 5-10-5 Shuttle or 20-Yard Shuttle. During this drill, the athlete is asked to change directions rapidly in the fastest time possible. We spectators can see how quickly, rapidly, and efficiently an athlete can change directions in a very short period of time, that is clear. However, this specific test is commonly used in the NFL, in other pro sports, and even in some colleges and high schools to test an athlete's agility. That's a misconception and not entirely true. When it truly comes down to it, the Pro Agility Test does not incorporate any sort of external stimulus that challenges the athlete to think quickly on their feet and react rapidly through a lightning-quick decision. This is why, in my opinion, the Pro Agility Test highlights more of the change of direction abilities of any athlete and not necessary any sort of reactive ability.

An alternative would be to instead challenge an athlete with a mirror drill. A mirror drill forces one athlete to mirror exactly what another athlete is doing, whether it be sprinting, shuffling, backpedaling, or anything else they can think of. Performing a mirror drill in tight spaces while keeping each athlete within arms' reach of one another would most certainly allow the skill of agility to truly be on display.

TRAINING CHANGE OF DIRECTION AND AGILITY

When playing competitive sports in middle school, high school, and even in college for some, it's rare to think about how these movements in sports keep you athletic, quick, and reactive. This is probably because players are simply having fun and playing the sports they love. In addition, they are likely thinking more about the next play, the next shot, or the next move rather than the importance of consistent exposure to changing directions and reacting for the purpose of improving athleticism. This is why it becomes super important for you to continue doing these things in your training, regardless of whether you're playing sports competitively or not. Some might play pick-up, club, or recreational sports after college. Others may just focus their efforts on training and staying fit simply because that is their goal.

Most people who take their fitness seriously have the lifting thing down pretty well. They might lift weights regularly each week on three or four days to build strength and muscle. However, this is where most people stop. They figure that they're still in the gym lifting weights and building strength, and that all that athletic stuff they did back in high school is simply going to carry with them.

Unfortunately, this isn't how it works at all. If your goal is to stay or become as athletic as possible, then keeping current with your change of direction ability and agility is an absolute must. In essence, continue doing things each week in your overall training routine that challenge your ability to change directions efficiently and react quickly. The best part is that there are literally hundreds of exercises, drills, and activities that can help you do this. When you do all of these things consistently, it keeps your body fine-tuned for any type of physical activity and athletic endeavor, regardless of whether that's playing pick-up basketball with your friends down by the park, jumping in on your kid's game of tag in the backyard, or even joining your local tennis club for some sets.

When implementing change of direction and agility drills, it's important to understand how to incorporate them in such a way that allows you to learn, develop, and grow. For example, although agility drills and exercises are more fun and challenging, from a pure learning standpoint, it makes much more sense to begin with change of direction drills and exercises. As stated earlier, change of direction drills and exercises are rehearsed through instruction and guidance. This means that there is no guessing or reacting. It's much easier to complete these types of drills with precision and efficiency since the components of thinking and reacting have been removed. Consider change of direction drills and exercises as the training wheels to a bike. Work them in as much as possible until you've mastered the patterns and movements with a supreme level of efficiency and precision. Then, once that happens, remove the training wheels and jump into exercises and drills that require you to react to some sort of external stimulus, which represents agility. The cool thing about agility is that it most reflects in-game situations in sports since reactions are routine in those environments. In some scenarios, you may not have another athlete or partner to work with when it comes to agility, which is certainly understandable. However, this shouldn't stop you from working in agility drills, since it all really comes down to your creativity.

As discussed previously, change of direction ability and agility are separated by the emphasis on either rehearsing or reacting. When performing a change of direction drill, you know exactly what the task is and how to perform it. This is why it's crucial for you to understand proper form and technique before performing change of direction drills. However, once you have developed a level of proficiency in change of direction drills, it's time to increase the overall challenge by adding some sort of external stimulus to force a reaction. Ultimately, this type of drill falls under the category of agility, which is more challenging than change of direction ability. Will you change direction rapidly during agility drills? Absolutely! However, the reactive component forces you to use perceptual skills to react rapidly and accurately. In essence, it's decision-making ability on display in the flash of an eye. That is true agility.

Change of direction drills and agility drills can certainly be implemented within a traditional weight room or gym, especially if you have areas of open space that allow freedom of movement. If you have access to large areas of indoor turf and space, I strongly encourage you to take full advantage of this and get your drills done within these environments. Programming of change of direction and agility may need to be based on general indoor gym access, space, and time. If accessible and when the weather allows for it, I always find it more valuable to get outside. Although performing change of direction drills and agility drills outdoors is my personal preference, both indoors and outdoors are viable options. In the diagrams that follow, you'll be able to visualize what we've been discussing, and most importantly, see ways in which you can begin building more athleticism in the areas of change of direction and agility.

When it comes down to physical changes you'll make when training both change of direction and agility, the number one thing that you'll notice is that you'll be much quicker to react. Along with quick reaction times, your body will feel more fluid when changing directions and you'll be able to move with more ease as well. Think of something as simple as turning the lawnmower around when mowing the lawn, which would be a low-intensity example of physical changes you'd make where this action would be much easier to complete. As an example of this on the other end of the spectrum at high intensity, you'll notice your improved quickness and reaction time during something like pick-up basketball or even recreational tennis at your local tennis club.

Change of Direction and Agility Drills on a Dime

You don't have access to any sort of fancy equipment? No problem. You can still perform change of direction and agility drills, and most importantly, improve in each category. Anecdotally, I've seen people use balloons and even tennis balls to get the job done. Blow a balloon up, smack it as hard as possible and continue to do so without ever letting it touch the floor. This will likely look like a cat and mouse game of chase. However, if that's too easy, blow up two or even three balloons and keep going. Trust me, it will begin to become much more challenging than you may have initially anticipated.

As for the tennis ball scenario, find a wall, step back about 10 to 15 feet and throw it as hard and as fast as possible off the wall. Your next move is to gather the tennis ball without ever letting it bounce more than once. Too easy? Move in closer. Too challenging? Back up a bit.

The balloon and tennis ball scenarios are merely examples of agility activities you can incorporate. But, again, be creative and use whatever makes the most sense to you. We will visit more specific examples later in this book.

LEARNING CHANGE OF DIRECTION AND AGILITY DRILLS

When it comes to drills and learning, we must appreciate the importance of starting simple and then advancing to complex. This is why it's crucial to master change of directions drills first and then work your way to agility drills. Table 3.1 presents a novice series of drills that can be performed to master your skills and abilities in change of direction and in agility.

Table 3.1 Novice Series: Change of Direction and Agility

	Level 1	Level 2	Level 3	Level 4
Change of direction (rehearsed)	5-yard sprint and rehearsed stop	5-yard sprint, rehearsed stop and go	5-yard sprint and rehearsed Y-turn	5-yard sprint and rehearsed T-turn
Agility (reactionary)	Sprint and reactionary stop	Sprint and reactionary Y-turn	Sprint and reactionary T-turn	N/A

Breaking down levels of difficulty as it pertains to change of direction skills and agility skills, it all comes down to the simplicity versus complexity of a drill. When a drill is simple, requires only a few steps, and minimizes the need for the individual to think and react, this would be deemed novice. Over time, we can layer on more challenges and components of a drill to enhance the overall complexity, in addition to adding a reactive aspect, which would be deemed advanced. The best part about this entire process from novice to advanced is that each drill is scalable from change of direction (simple) to agility (complex), which makes training that much easier!

The advanced series outlined in table 3.2 consists of exercises that build off what you completed in the previous phase in the novice series. Again, it is intended to perform these exercises in the order of sequence from novice to advanced so that you're increasing your ability to rapidly change directions and react with agile body movements over time. The best way to approach these drills is start out with the novice series, and if it ever feels too easy and you're able to complete them with ease, simply move on to the advanced series. However, if when performing the novice series, your movement is not crisp and quick, then stay there until you've improved.

Table 3.2 Advanced Series: Change of Direction and Agility

	Level 1	Level 2	Level 3	Level 4
Change of direction (rehearsed)	5-yard sprint to rehearsed curved run	5-yard backpedal to rehearsed turn and sprint	5-yard lateral shuffle to rehearsed turn and sprint	N/A
Agility (reactionary)	5-yard partner chase and hip tap reactionary T-turn (sprinter reacts to chaser)	5-yard partner chase and verbal reactionary T-turn (sprinter reacts to chaser)	5-yard partner chase and non-verbal reactionary T-turn (chaser reacts to sprinter)	5-yard partner chase and verbal reactionary T-turn (chaser reacts to sprinter)

5-YARD SPRINT AND REHEARSED STOP

For this exercise, all you'll need is two cones separated 5 yards apart where cone A is at the baseline and cone B is 5 yards out in front (figure 3.1). Set yourself up in a two-point sprint stance at cone A the same way a track and field sprinter would in the blocks, but instead with both hands just out in front of your hips. You'll want to hinge your hips back, and sink down and forward just slightly as well. Now, once you're ready, sprint as fast as possible forward for 5 yards from cone A to cone B, and then stop at cone B with as much body control as possible. Your goal is to sprint fast and stop fast.

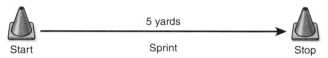

Figure 3.1 5-yard sprint and rehearsed stop.

5-YARD SPRINT, REHEARSED STOP AND GO

For this exercise, all you'll need is two cones separated 5 yards apart where cone A is at the baseline and cone B is 5 yards out in front (figure 3.2). (You may also want to set up a third cone a further 5 yards from cone B.) Set yourself up in a two-point sprint stance at cone A the same way a track and field sprinter would in the blocks, but instead with both hands just out in front of your hips. You'll want to hinge your hips back, and sink down and forward just slightly as well. Now, once you're ready, sprint as fast as possible forward for 5 yards from cone A to cone B, stop on a dime as controlled as possible at cone B, and then sprint for 5 more yards forward. Your goal is to sprint fast, stop fast, and then sprint fast again.

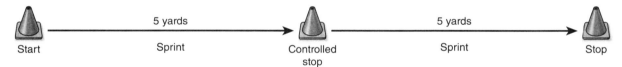

Figure 3.2 5-yard sprint, rehearsed stop and go.

5-YARD SPRINT AND REHEARSED Y-TURN

For this exercise, all you'll need is four cones. Cone A is on a baseline, cone B is 5 yards straight ahead, and cones C and D are set at 45-degree angles from cone B, one to the right side and one to the left (figure 3.3). The setup should look like the letter Y. Set yourself up in a two-point sprint stance at cone A the same way a track and field sprinter would in the blocks, but instead with both hands just out in front of your hips. You'll want to hinge your hips back, and sink down and forward just slightly as well. Now, once you're ready, sprint as fast as possible forward for 5 yards from cone A to cone B. Once you get to cone B, your job is to redirect your body and angle off at 45 degrees to the right side in order to continue sprinting to cone C. This quick maneuvering of your body through the redirection is a hallmark skill of change of direction ability. In the Y format, this makes it relatively easy to work on. Complete all reps on the right side, and then complete all reps on the left side.

NOVICE SERIES: Change of Direction and Agility

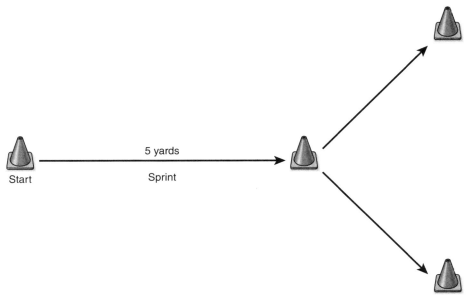

Figure 3.3 5-yard sprint and rehearsed Y-turn.

5-YARD SPRINT AND REHEARSED T-TURN

For this exercise, all you'll need is four cones. Core A is on a baseline, cone B is 5 yards straight ahead, and cones C and D are set out at 90-degree angles from cone B, one to the right side and one to the left side (figure 3.4). This setup should look like the letter T. Set yourself up in a two-point sprint stance at cone A the same way a track and field sprinter would in the blocks, but instead with both hands just out in front of your hips. You'll want to hinge your hips back, and sink down and forward just slightly as well. Now, once you're ready, sprint as fast as possible forward for 5 yards from cone A to cone B. Once you get to cone B, your job is to redirect your body and angle off at 90 degrees to the right side in order continue sprinting to cone C. This quick maneuvering of your body through the redirection is a hallmark skill of change of direction ability. In addition, this T format is the much more challenging version than the Y format, since the turning angle is much greater. Complete all reps on the right side, and then complete all reps on the left side.

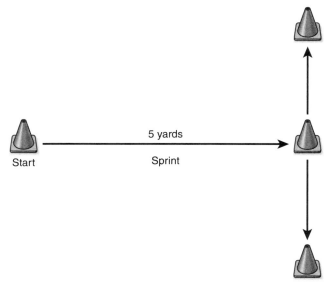

Figure 3.4 5-yard sprint and rehearsed T-turn.

SPRINT AND REACTIONARY STOP

For this exercise, you'll need a training partner to react to, which is the primary objective of the drill. You'll need two cones, separated 5 yards apart; cone A is at the baseline, and cone B is 5 yards out in front (figure 3.5). Set yourself up in a two-point sprint stance at cone A the same way a track and field sprinter would in the blocks, but instead with both hands just out in front of your hips. You'll want to hinge your hips back, and sink down and forward just slightly as well. Now, once you're ready, sprint as fast as possible forward for 5 yards from cone A to cone B. Your training partner will use any of the following coaching instructions to tell you which side to angle your body to when stopping at cone B: verbal left, verbal right, hand signal left, or hand signal right. Your job is to react to the coaching instruction as quickly and with as much body control as possible with a hard stop at cone B and angle your body in the direction required. Complete the prescribed number of reps within the training program.

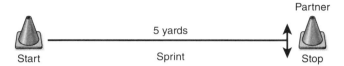

Figure 3.5 Sprint and reactionary stop.

SPRINT AND REACTIONARY Y-TURN

For this exercise, you'll need a training partner to react to, which is the primary objective of the drill. You'll need four cones, separated 5 yards apart each. Cone A is on a baseline, cone B is 5 yards straight ahead, cone C is set out at a 45-degree angle on the right side, and cone D is set out at a 45-degree angle on the left side, all of which should look like the letter Y (figure 3.6). Set yourself up in a two-point sprint stance at cone A the same way a track and field sprinter would in the blocks, but instead with both hands just out in front of your hips. You'll want to hinge your hips back, and sink down and forward just slightly as well. Now, once you're ready, sprint as fast as possible forward for 5 yards from cone A to cone B. Your training partner will use any of the following coaching instructions to tell you which side (cone C on the right side or cone D on the left side) to react and sprint toward: verbal left, verbal right, hand signal left, or hand signal right. Your job is to react to the coaching instruction as quickly as possible with a rapid redirection with your body and angle off at 45 degrees to the required side (cone C on the right side or cone D on the left side). Complete the prescribed number of reps within the training program.

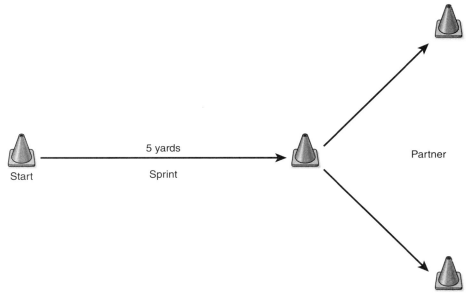

Figure 3.6 Sprint and reactionary Y-turn.

SPRINT AND REACTIONARY T-TURN

For this exercise, you'll need a training partner to react to, which is the primary objective of the drill. You'll need four cones, separated 5 yards apart each. Cone A is on a baseline, cone B is 5 yards straight ahead, cone C is set out at a 90-degree angle on the right side, and cone D is set out at a 90-degree angle on the left side, all of which should look like the letter T (figure 3.7). Set yourself up in a two-point sprint stance at cone A the same way a track and field sprinter would in the blocks, but instead with both hands just out in front of your hips. You'll want to hinge your hips back, and sink down and forward just slightly as well. Now, once you're ready, sprint as fast as possible forward for 5 yards from cone A to cone B. Your training partner will use any of the following coaching instructions to tell you which side (cone C on the right side or cone D on the left side) to react and sprint toward: verbal left, verbal right, hand signal left, or hand signal right. Your job is to react to the coaching instruction as quickly as possible with a rapid redirection with your body and angle off at 90 degrees to the required side (cone C on the right side or cone D on the left side). Complete the prescribed number of reps within the training program.

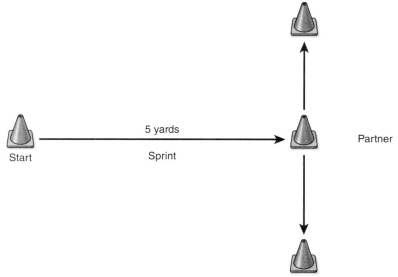

Figure 3.7 Sprint and reactionary T-turn.

5-YARD SPRINT TO REHEARSED CURVED RUN

For this exercise, all you'll need is two cones, separated 5 yards apart; cone A is at the baseline, and cone B is 5 yards out in front. Set yourself up in a two-point sprint stance at cone A the same way a track and field sprinter would in the blocks, but instead with both hands just out in front of your hips. You'll want to hinge your hips back, and sink down and forward just slightly as well. Now, once you're ready, sprint as fast as possible forward for 5 yards from cone A to cone B. Once you arrive at cone B, begin to angle your body off toward one side and continue sprinting along a curved line toward the right side similar to that of the McDonald's golden arches for 5 to 10 more yards (figure 3.8). (You may want to set up a third cone at the 5- or 10-yard mark.) Your goal is to sprint fast and maintain body control throughout the entire movement from the initial sprint through the transition in directions while still sprinting. Complete all reps on one side, switch sides, and repeat.

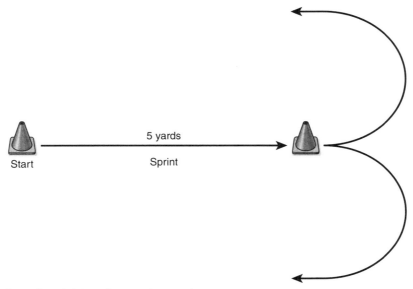

Figure 3.8 5-yard sprint to rehearsed curved run.

5-YARD BACKPEDAL TO REHEARSED TURN AND SPRINT

For this exercise, all you'll need is two cones, separated 5 yards apart; cone A is at the baseline, and cone B is 5 yards out in front. Set yourself up in an athletic position while hinging your hips back, bending both knees, and sinking down and forward just slightly as well. Keep both hands active and make sure to be facing backward so that the cones are behind you. Now, once you're ready, stay low and backpedal as fast as possible for 5 yards from cone A to cone B. Once you arrive at cone B, your job is to quickly rotate and open up your hips while turning toward the left side, and then, sprint for the remaining 5 to 10 yards (figure 3.9). (You may want to set up an additional cone to indicate the 5- or 10-yard distance.) Your goal is to move fast and maintain body control throughout the entire movement from the initial backpedal through the transition in directions and the final sprint. Complete all reps on one side, switch sides, and repeat.

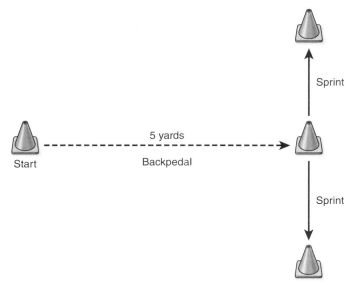

Figure 3.9 5-yard backpedal to rehearsed turn and sprint.

5-YARD LATERAL SHUFFLE TO REHEARSED TURN AND SPRINT

For this exercise, all you'll need is two cones, separated 5 yards apart; cone A is at the baseline, and cone B is 5 yards out in front. Set yourself up in an athletic position while hinging your hips back, bending both knees, and sinking down and forward just slightly as well. Keep both hands active and make sure to be positioned where both cones are on your left-hand side. Now, once you're ready, stay low and lateral shuffle as fast as possible for 5 yards from cone A to cone B. Once you arrive at cone B, your job is to quickly rotate and open up your hips while turning toward the left side, and then, sprint for the remaining 5 to 10 yards (figure 3.10). (You may want to set up an additional cone at the 5- or 10-yard distance.) Your goal is to move fast and maintain body control throughout the entire movement from the initial lateral shuffle through the transition in directions and the final sprint. Complete all reps on one side, switch sides, and repeat.

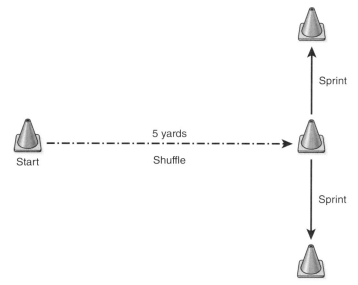

Figure 3.10 5-yard lateral shuffle to rehearsed turn and sprint.

5-YARD PARTNER CHASE AND HIP TAP REACTIONARY T-TURN (SPRINTER REACTS TO CHASER)

For this exercise, you'll need a training partner to react to, which is the primary objective of the drill. In this situation, you are the sprinter who will react to your partner and your partner is the chaser. You'll need two cones, separated 5 yards apart; cone A is at the baseline, and cone B is 5 yards out in front. Set yourself up in a two-point sprint stance at cone A the same way a track and field sprinter would in the blocks, but instead with both hands just out in front of your hips. You'll want to hinge your hips back, and sink down and forward just slightly as well. Your partner will set up in the same position, but directly behind you within arm's reach. Now, once you're ready, sprint as fast as possible forward for 5 yards from cone A to cone B. Once you arrive at cone B, your partner's job is to tap your hip on the right side or left side (this is a non-verbal cue), which you will need to react to by sprinting toward the right side or left side. For example, if your partner taps your hip on the right side, you'll need to sprint to the right side. In terms of the direction to sprint in, this is where the T-turn (figure 3.11) comes into play where you'll need to angle your body off at a 90-degree angle and sprint in that direction, which requires a sharp turn and body control in a tight space. Your goal is to move fast and react quickly here to demonstrate your ability to rapidly change directions and remain agile. Complete the prescribed number of reps within the training program.

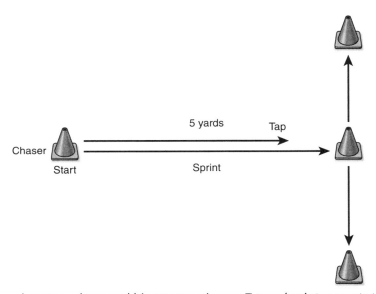

Figure 3.11 5-yard partner chase and hip tap reactionary T-turn (sprinter reacts to chaser).

5-YARD PARTNER CHASE AND VERBAL REACTIONARY T-TURN (SPRINTER REACTS TO CHASER)

For this exercise, you'll need a training partner to react to, which is the primary objective of the drill. In this situation, you are the sprinter who will react to your partner and your partner is the chaser. You'll need two cones, separated 5 yards apart; cone A is at the baseline, and cone B is 5 yards out in front. Set yourself up in a two-point sprint stance at cone A the same way a track and field sprinter would in the blocks, but instead with both hands just out in front of your hips. You'll want to hinge your hips back, and sink down and forward just slightly as well. Your partner will set up in the same position, but directly behind you within arm's reach. Now, once you're ready, sprint as fast as possible forward for 5 yards from cone A to cone B. Once you arrive at cone B, your partner's job is to verbally yell out loud "right" or "left" (verbal cue), which you will need to react to by sprinting toward the right side or left side. For example, if your partner yells out loud "right", you'll need to sprint to the right side (figure 3.12). In terms of the direction to sprint in, this is where the T-turn comes into play: You'll need to angle your body off at a 90-degree angle and sprint in that direction, which requires a sharp turn and body control in a tight space. Your goal is to move fast and react quickly here to demonstrate your ability to rapidly change directions and remain agile. Complete the prescribed number of reps within the training program.

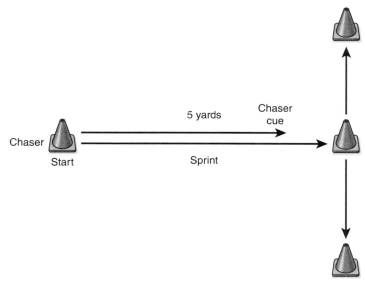

Figure 3.12 5-yard partner chase and verbal reactionary T-turn (sprinter reacts to chaser).

5-YARD PARTNER CHASE AND NON-VERBAL REACTIONARY T-TURN (CHASER REACTS TO SPRINTER)

For this exercise, you'll need a training partner to react to, which is the primary objective of the drill. In this situation, you are the sprinter, and your partner is the chaser. You'll need two cones, separated 5 yards apart; cone A is at the baseline, and cone B is 5 yards out in front. Set yourself up in a two-point sprint stance at cone A the same way a track and field sprinter would in the blocks, but instead with both hands just out in front of your hips. You'll want to hinge your hips back, and sink down and forward just slightly as well. Your partner will set up in the same position, but directly behind you within arm's reach. Now, once you're ready, sprint as fast as possible forward for 5 yards from cone A to cone B. Once you arrive at cone B, your job is to make a quick decision by sprinting toward the right side or left side, and your partner's job is to quickly react to your decision by chasing you in the direction you chose to sprint in (this is a non-verbal cue). For example, if you chose to sprint to the right side, your partner would need to chase you by sprinting to the right side. In terms of the direction to sprint in, this is where the T-turn (figure 3.13) comes into play: You'll need to angle your body off at a 90-degree angle and sprint in that direction, which requires a sharp turn and body control in a tight space. Your goal is to move fast and react quickly here to demonstrate your ability to rapidly change directions and remain agile. Complete the prescribed number of reps within the training program.

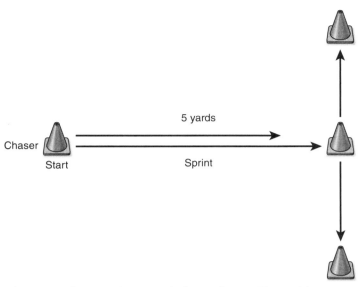

Figure 3.13 5-yard partner chase and non-verbal reactionary T-turn (chaser reacts to sprinter).

5-YARD PARTNER CHASE AND VERBAL REACTIONARY T-TURN (CHASER REACTS TO SPRINTER)

For this exercise, you'll need a training partner to react to, which is the primary objective of the drill. In this situation, you are the sprinter, and your partner is the chaser. You'll need two cones, separated 5 yards apart; cone A is at the baseline, and cone B is 5 yards out in front. Set yourself up in a two-point sprint stance at cone A the same way a track and field sprinter would in the blocks, but instead with both hands just out in front of your hips. You'll want to hinge your hips back, and sink down and forward just slightly as well. Your partner will set up in the same position, but directly behind you within arm's reach. Now, once you're ready, sprint as fast as possible forward for 5 yards from cone A to cone B. Once you arrive at cone B, your job is to verbally yell out loud "right" or "left" (verbal cue), which your partner will need to react to by sprinting toward the right side or left side. For example, if you yell out loud "right", your partner will need to sprint to the right side. In terms of the direction to sprint in, this is where the T-turn (figure 3.14) comes into play: You'll need to angle your body off at a 90-degree angle and sprint in that direction, which requires a sharp turn and body control in a tight space. Your goal is to move fast and react quickly here to demonstrate your ability to rapidly change directions and remain agile. Complete the prescribed number of reps within the training program.

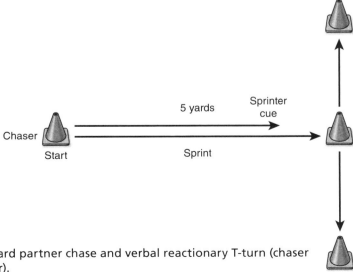

Figure 3.14 5-yard partner chase and verbal reactionary T-turn (chaser reacts to sprinter).

PROGRESSIVELY BUILDING BODY CONTROL FOR ATHLETICISM

When we talk about what it takes to be an athlete, it all comes down to body control for me. Can you control your body in space to remain stable and balanced? Can you coordinate quick and efficient movements without wasting much time at all to think and decide? Lastly, can you change directions rapidly and react quickly to any sort of stimulus or challenge around you? These are questions that constantly run through my mind as it pertains to remaining athletic and expressing qualities that make you feel like an athlete.

From the standpoint of balance and stability, we often associate these terms with strength and force. The presence of strength and force are certainly part of the overall athletic puzzle when it comes to balancing and stabilizing. However, this is more related to being able to, for example, balance on one leg and stabilize in that stance or position. Although this is certainly part of the equation, I believe it's important to think beyond this type of scenario, and instead, toward viewing how an athlete stays balanced and stable in sports. For example, have you ever watched a volleyball game? Take a closer look at each of the players on defense as the opposing offensive player prepares for a serve. Notice how these athletes on defense keep a rhythm with their body as they gently sway side to side or front to back. This constant state of rhythm literally keeps them on their toes, ready to react at any instant and in a state of both balance and stability. Sometimes, in the sport of basketball, you'll even notice this rhythm through slight and subtle up and down bounces where the athlete's feet don't necessarily leave the floor, but it's evident that rhythm, balance and stability are being used to prepare for the next move or the next play. This component of sports and athletics has always fascinated me. It truly identifies an athlete's ability to react, stop on a dime, change directions and even change gears in an instant. This unique lens allows us to see the athlete in their element, ready for the next play, the next move, or the next call. The best part? You can be that athlete, too. You have everything it takes to train to be just as athletic, reactive, and quick with your direction changes.

Consistency, Not Intensity

The key to change of direction and reactive agility drills isn't about how intense you are; it's more about consistency. Like any skill, building change of direction ability and agility takes time, hard work, and tons of reps to truly master. Consider these both as skills in athleticism that you're chasing down in hopes of refining and improving in. Consistency is the name of the game here through weekly exposure to exercises and drills that allow you to first learn how to change directions rapidly under a rehearsed pattern and then eventually react quickly to an external stimulus. Don't worry about the intensity when you first begin implementing these drills and exercises. First, focus on controlling your body in space, staying balanced and organized with your body, and most importantly improving in your quickness over time. The intensity will come later down the line once you're up to speed and have accrued tons of reps! Again, consistency is the name of the game.

The next aspect to consider is within the realm of coordination. Put more literally, how quickly and efficiently can you execute or string together specific movements to complete a task? When we watch athletes play sports in person or on TV, we don't necessarily think about these aspects. We just simply watch them play their sport and spend time in constant awe of what they can do with their bodies. Coordination takes time to really master and plenty of reps to truly become precise. Consider how many times it took Steph Curry to shoot the basketball to truly master his shooting technique. He literally grew up in the game of basketball after spending his early childhood years watching his father play in the NBA. I've had to imagine that the basketball was placed in his hands at birth and that he started shooting at a very early age. What we see now is Steph routinely shoot a three-pointer and sometimes turn around and walk back down the court on defense since he's so supremely confident that it's going in without needing to look. That supreme confidence in his shooting ability, his ability to coordinate his entire body to take the perfect shot, doesn't just simply happen overnight. It takes time, dedication, and a ton of reps to truly master anything that requires coordination.

The stages of motor learning help us to better understand how we as athletes can efficiently coordinate our bodies and our minds to complete a task or movement. Through repetition, we're able to refine our technique and efficiency over time, thus helping us to improve our coordination. All of this ultimately ties into our ability to quickly change directions and react rapidly. There are three stages of motor learning that we must consider since this ultimately impacts our learning process when it comes down to tasks and movements. The first in these three stages is the cognitive stage, which covers what the athlete is to do. This is where the athlete begins to understand the skill, task, or movement, in addition to organizing all of the information and objectives that go into the completion of said skill, task, or movement. The next stage, the associative stage, is where the athlete learns how to complete the task. This is also considered the practice phase within the stages where the athlete begins chunking information together, to eliminate mistakes and improve focus. Lastly, the third stage in this process is known as the autonomous stage. This is where the athlete truly excels and enters a state of flow. Think back to Steph Curry being able to shoot the basketball, turn around and walk back down the court on defense without ever needing to visually see the ball go into the hoop. That's the ultimate flow state and ability to perform at a high level with respect to coordination and motor learning. In essence, the autonomous stage is habitual and routine. By following the three stages of learning, it allows us to better understand how you as the athlete can begin to improve in your abilities to first change directions rapidly through a rehearsed, instructed pattern without a reaction, and then advance into the more challenging agility drills that require you to react efficiently and quickly.

The Science of Conditioning

I'll never forget a commercial that was on TV back in 2008 when the Boston Celtics won the NBA Championship. At this time they had an absolutely stacked starting lineup (PG: Rajon Rondo, SG: Ray Allen, SF: Paul Pierce, PF: Kevin Garnett, C: Kendrick Perkins) and a ton of notable key players off the bench (Tony Allen, P.J. Brown, James Posey, Eddie House). The commercial that I can't seem to forget displayed Ray Allen running on a treadmill during what was seemingly a post-practice conditioning session. He wasn't sprinting. He wasn't walking. He was running at a relatively challenging yet moderate pace, shirtless and breathing fairly easily. That's the part that amazed me—he was breathing fairly easily! Here's a guy who was visibly at an elite level of body composition for his or any sport (i.e., ~6% to 8% body fat) and an impressive physical specimen. He had just finished a practice that was probably about two or three hours long and was now running on the treadmill. It was clear that he was already in shape but wanted to get an edge on his opponents on the court. Finding the time, energy, and effort for some extra conditioning on the treadmill seemed like an absolute must for him. Ray Allen was not only building his engine, improving his cardiovascular endurance and stamina; he was trying to last longer than his eventual opponent on the court. This commercial stays in my mind because it reminds me of how conditioning can help you as the athlete build the engine.

I think of level of conditioning as like a fire pit. Let me explain: Let's say that you start a fire by setting a match to a few wooden logs. The fire is lit and will likely remain lit for a period of time—maybe two to three hours. After those hours pass, the logs will likely be nearing their end and the flame will be producing much less heat than at the beginning. These flames are dying out in the same way that your energy dies out when you perform conditioning for long durations. In the fire scenario, your next move would be to add more logs and watch that flame reach a higher peak again. An athlete who possesses a high level of conditioning, generally speaking, can achieve higher peaks of flame and keep the flame lit for a longer period of time before needing to add more logs. This analogy is a way to better understand your level of conditioning. An athlete with a high level of conditioning has greater levels of stamina and cardiovascular endurance than one with a lower level, which means they can last longer. This also means that their heart is well conditioned, which will serve an athlete well during all types of training, physical activity, and recreational sport participation. On the opposite end of the spectrum, an athlete or individual who possesses a low level of conditioning won't be able to last long before needing to take a break and will have much lower levels of stamina and cardiorespiratory endurance. An athlete with high levels of stamina and cardiorespiratory endurance is far less likely to break down in technique in their training compared to an athlete with low levels and is thus at a decreased risk of injury.

AEROBIC AND ANAEROBIC CONDITIONING

When it comes to conditioning, we must first understand the three different energy systems at play. Energy systems can be thought of as the three different tanks your body draws from to complete a movement or exercise. Many people are aware of the three systems but think that your body switches between them by shutting off two tanks while one tank turns on. It's not that simple. Instead, all three of the energy system tanks are usually active to some extent, but based on the duration and intensity of the movement or exercise, one tank is supplying the bulk of the energy while the other two tanks take a back seat. The three energy systems are as follows: phosphagen system (anaerobic alactic system), glycolytic system (anaerobic lactic system), and oxidative system (aerobic system). You can think of the phosphagen system as your immediate source of energy (i.e., activities lasting less than 10 seconds), the glycolytic system as your short-to-moderate term source of energy (i.e., activities lasting predominantly between 10 seconds and 2 minutes), and lastly, the oxidative system as your long-term source of energy (i.e., activities lasting 2 minutes or more). Furthermore, the glycolytic system can be broken down into two subsystems: fast glycolysis (i.e., activities lasting between 10 and 30 seconds) and slow glycolysis (i.e., activities lasting between 30 seconds and 2 minutes).

Let's break this down even more. Some of the best examples of activities dominated by the phosphagen system are jumping up explosively to dunk a basketball, swinging the bat to hit a home run, taking a slapshot in hockey, sprinting a 40-yard dash, kicking a soccer ball toward the net, or even a powerful serve on the tennis court. Actions such as these are powerful and short-lived and require a period of rest or recovery directly afterward due to the high level of intensity used.

Activities dominated by the glycolytic system include a 500-meter kayak race, 400-meter sprint, and 400-meter swim. These activities require lower levels of power output compared to the phosphagen system, but they must be sustained for a longer period of time (i.e., between 10 seconds and 2 minutes versus less than 10 seconds).

Lastly, activities that draw on the oxidative system are those that take place over an extended period of time, over two minutes. The best example of activities where the oxidative system dominates are longer duration events such as marathon running, triathlon events, and even long distance cycling.

Aerobic conditioning could include activities such as an hour-long jog during which you operate at a low intensity for a long period of time. On the opposite end of the spectrum, anaerobic conditioning could involve 20-yard sprints repeated for six total sets with an adequate amount of time (i.e., 60-90 seconds) of rest in between each set. Both aerobic and anaerobic conditioning are crucial for competitive and non-competitive athletes to keep in their training programs for long-term health and performance. We've included all of this within all training programs in this book for you!

The Science of Conditioning 35

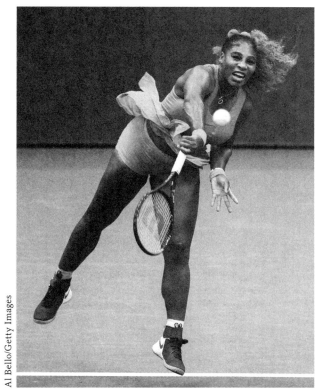
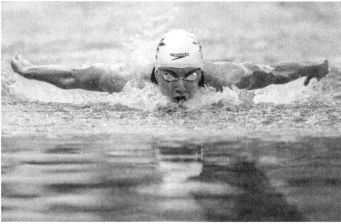
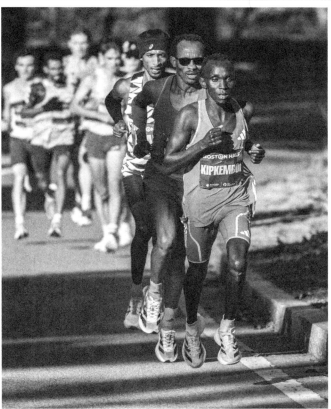

| The three energy systems: phosphagen, glycolytic, and oxidative.

Will Conditioning Lead to a Loss of Muscle Mass, Strength, and Power?

The idea that conditioning works against strength is a common misconception in the worlds of both general fitness and athletic performance. In fact, conditioning is simply part of sports. Watch a professional soccer match. The majority of the athletes can run for upwards of 90+ minutes during each game. Yes, they appear leaner than, for example, an average NFL running back. However, they still possess enough muscle mass to ward off defenders, they're still strong enough to kick a soccer ball upwards of 85 miles per hour, and they're still powerful enough to leap a few feet above the field to head the ball into the net. These levels of muscle, strength, and power are on display in many sports where athletes perform conditioning on a weekly basis in their practices and games.

For another example, let's take a look at ice hockey. Talk about muscle mass, strength, and power. These professional athletes routinely use their muscle mass, especially in their legs, to remain balanced and controlled on skates that are one eighth of an inch thick, their strength to check other players into and off the boards, and their power to take a slapshot upwards of 100 miles per hour. NHL players' conditioning is on full display each week, again, through a variety of practices, drills, scrimmages, and games. We could go on and on—the point is that it is very unlikely that you'll lose muscle mass, strength, or power with conditioning, as long as each separate quality is programmed properly with adequate levels of both rest and nutrition. A quality training program factors all these variables in, allowing you as the athlete to make gains across the board without losing anything.

AEROBIC OR ANAEROBIC: WHICH IS THE BEST CONDITIONING?

There's really no such thing as the best type of conditioning. It comes down to your specific training goals. If your goal is to become more athletic overall, then the first step is to build an aerobic base of conditioning, which helps to improve your overall cardiovascular health and stamina. This will allow you to recover more quickly between exercises within a single training session and between training sessions. By improving your aerobic conditioning, you're essentially improving how efficiently your heart works. The heart is a muscle, which is why it's important to break a sweat and challenge it through aerobic conditioning on a routine basis. Let's say, for example, you have goals of improving your overall athleticism. Whether your goal is to improve in strength, power, agility, or speed, having a more efficient cardiovascular system helps across the board. You'll not only improve your ability to recover quickly, but also reduce the risk of injury by being able to maintain technique and form for longer before feeling fatigued. This is an important component of aerobic conditioning that most people tend to forget. Can aerobic conditioning sometimes be boring? Absolutely! However, it is absolutely crucial to perform routinely to support the other athletic qualities you're after: strength, power, speed, and agility.

For best results, incorporate some form of aerobic conditioning one to two days per week for an average of 30-40 minutes each time. What you do within these sessions can vary. Whether you're a fan of traditional cardio machines (i.e., treadmill, elliptical, stair master, etc.), new-school cardio equipment (i.e., air bike, erg rower, ski erg, etc.), or getting outdoors (i.e., track, field, stadium stairs, etc.), there are plenty of options to choose from. The primary goal should be to maintain a challenging, yet manageable pace or level of intensity the entire time, somewhere in the ballpark of 130 to 150 beats per minute (bpm). Depending on how fit you are, this will likely place you at a rating of perceived exertion (RPE) of somewhere between 6 and 7 on a 10-point scale. On this RPE scale, 0 represents no intensity whatsoever (like being asleep) and 10 represents the maximum effort you could produce (like sprinting for your life while a lion is chasing you). Keep in mind that you can adjust both overall duration (volume) and RPE level (intensity) in a given session, keeping in mind that if intensity increases, volume must decrease. The opposite holds true as well: If intensity decreases, volume must increase. You can think of the RPE number (i.e., 5) as equivalent to a percentage of maximum effort multiplied by 10 (i.e., 50%). For example, if the program calls for RPE of 8, you should work at 80% of your maximum intensity.

Why is anaerobic conditioning different than aerobic conditioning? Anaerobic conditioning has to do with how long you can sustain repeated bouts of power at slightly higher intensity levels than you'd use in aerobic exercise. Aerobic conditioning calls for a longer duration of time at lower intensity levels compared to anaerobic conditioning. The latter requires greater levels of power output that are repeated over time with rest periods in between; each period of anaerobic output is much shorter than an aerobic conditioning session.

You can certainly do an aerobic conditioning session on the same day as a strength training session. However, this can eat up a lot of your time on that one day. This is why I always recommend performing your aerobic conditioning session on a day where it is the primary focus of your physical activity and a day off from strength training. The additional benefit of this scenario is that performing aerobic conditioning on its own training day supports the recovery process in your body. Now, life happens, so this type of schedule may not always be ideal. If you absolutely need to perform your strength training and aerobic conditioning sessions on the same day, my recommendation would be to either (a) perform strength first and conditioning second in one total session or (b) perform strength in the morning and then conditioning later in the day in a second session. When it comes to anaerobic conditioning, we have a bit more flexibility, especially since a typical session takes much less time to complete. More often than not, you can easily do your anaerobic conditioning session on the same day as your strength training session, at the end of the workout.

A typical equation for calculating your maximum heart rate is to take 220 bpm and then subtract your current age. For me, that looks like this: 220 bpm − 34 years old = 186 bpm. This equation tends to be fairly accurate and I often base my conditioning work on it. Knowing my estimated maximum heart rate (in this case, 186 bpm), I can use it as a general guide when performing anaerobic conditioning. Is it helpful to meet or even try to beat your estimated maximum heart rate? Not necessarily, and here's why: Even if you're able to do so, it's not likely that you'll be able to maintain this heart rate for an extended period of time. For that reason, I often tell my athletes to stay within the ballpark (i.e., within 10-20 bpm) of this value over a sustained period of time. So, for me, that would look like working at 166-176 bpm as opposed to trying to stay at 186 bpm. This is a general guideline, but it allows you as the athlete to better understand how anaerobic and aerobic conditioning compare. When discussing this topic with my students in the classroom, I often put up an image of the most recent first-place Boston Marathon runner to represent aerobic conditioning and an image of Usain Bolt to represent anaerobic conditioning, because he can maintain such a fast pace with consistent power output. Visualizing the two types of conditioning through this format helps most people to better understand what it should look and feel like. The reason we calculate max heart rate is to give us an idea of where our heart rate should be in different types of conditioning. Max heart rate is one of the many tools that can help us navigate conditioning exercises while aiming to be as precise as possible.

For best results, include some form of anaerobic conditioning one to two days per week for an average of 8 to 15 minutes per bout. Similar to aerobic conditioning, what you do in these sessions can vary. The best part? You can choose from many types of cardio equipment to perform your anaerobic conditioning session (treadmill, elliptical, air bike, erg rower, ski erg, etc.), or from any of the outdoor options (track, field, stadium stairs, etc.). Other types of equipment in the gym can also sneak into the mix, such as sleds, dumbbells, kettlebells, medicine balls, and more. If you wish to go this route, it's easy to put together movements in a circuit fashion instead of using one piece of cardio equipment, allowing you to move around more and incorporate more variety. All of these options work well—it's your choice.

When planning an anaerobic conditioning session, aim for 8 to 15 minutes total. As with aerobic conditioning, you can manipulate overall duration of time (volume) and RPE level (intensity). Volume must decrease if intensity increases, and volume must increase if intensity decreases. Your goal should be to work at an RPE of 8 or 9 on a 10-point scale, but include rest periods. This is another key difference between anaerobic conditioning (hugely important to include time to rest and recover in between sets or rounds) and aerobic conditioning (not as important since you're not reaching levels of high intensity). To achieve an RPE of 8 or 9, you will likely be working at around 170 to 190 bpm, but the exact number depends on factors such as age, training history, and level of fitness.

Later in this book we will take a deep dive into specific conditioning session examples for both aerobic and anaerobic purposes. These routines will help you improve your conditioning while also building your overall athleticism!

CHAPTER 5

Warm-Up Exercises

A well-structured warm-up is essential for preparing the body to perform at its best, whether in training, competition, or everyday movement. An effective warm-up consists of key components that work together to enhance overall athleticism: mobility, flexibility, stability, and activation. Mobility refers to the range of motion within a joint, ensuring fluid and unrestricted movement, while flexibility focuses on the extensibility of muscles, allowing them to stretch and lengthen as needed. Both elements are crucial for efficient movement patterns, performing at a high level, and reducing the risk of injury.

In addition to mobility and flexibility, stability and activation play a vital role in improving your overall athleticism and performance. Stability ensures that joints can maintain control and resist unwanted movement, which is essential for balance and coordination in dynamic sports and activities. Activation, on the other hand, involves engaging specific muscles to "wake them up" before higher-intensity exercises, which helps to improve neuromuscular efficiency. Together, these four components create a comprehensive warm-up routine that primes the body for movement, enhances performance, and reduces injury risk.

STATIC STRETCHING VERSUS DYNAMIC STRETCHING

As kids, many of us were taught to stretch before practices and games. This usually consisted of the entire team setting up in multiple lines or even in a big circle. A few of the players from the team would typically walk the entire team through a series of stretches where we were all stationary with little to no movement. A classic example is when we would all stand with our feet roughly hip-width apart and then reach down toward our toes with our hands. We were instructed to get as low as possible and remain there for a short period of time to feel a stretch in our hamstrings on the backside of our upper legs. This is a static stretch—one that requires little to no movement or motion, and is usually held for 20 to 30 seconds on average. Static stretching certainly has a time and place in athletic performance. However, we have learned over the years that dynamic stretching is the true game changer in athletic performance and quality of movement.

Dynamic stretching, the direct opposite of static stretching, requires motion. The beauty of dynamic stretching is that it mimics the movements that will occur in sports and training. It is important to use dynamic stretching strategies in your warm-up to truly reap the benefits of your athletic endeavors. An example of a dynamic stretch is skipping. Traditionally, skipping involves setting up in lines as a team and then traveling forward for a prescribed distance. For example, you might perform skips over a distance of 20 yards in a warm-up. The way that I have always simplified static stretching and dynamic stretching in my mind is as simple as this: The *S* in *static* stands for *stationary* and the *D* in *dynamic* stands for *distance*. This certainly isn't bulletproof, but it works well the majority of the time.

When creating a warm-up routine as part of an overall training program, I have become a big fan of starting off with a few static stretches at most and then using the rest of the warm-up to focus on dynamic stretches. In some cases, we may not even include any static stretches at all depending on the athlete, the goal, or the theme of the training program. True static stretching is much more suited for the recovery component of the overall training program, which occurs at the very end when you are cooling down. During the cool-down, you've already trained and explored various ranges of motion in your body, plus your body is warm. For these reasons, you'll be able to experience greater ranges of motion when performing static stretching in the cool-down as opposed to the warm-up when your body is not warmed up yet. This concept has made the rounds in the worlds of athletic performance and strength and conditioning over the last couple of decades, and coaches have begun to tap into meaningful movement within the warm-up routine through a small amount of static stretching followed up by a larger amount of dynamic stretching prior to intense physical activity (e.g., training session, sport practice, or sport competition).

When it comes to meaningful movement, the warm-up is an opportunity to explore various ranges of motion (more on that specifically in the next section!) in a variety of movement planes. There are three distinct planes of movement that we can use. The sagittal plane consists of movements that occur while remaining in place (i.e., up and down as in squats) or linearly (i.e., forward as in forward lunges or backward as in reverse lunges). The frontal plane consists of movements that occur laterally and side-to-side (i.e., lateral squats and lateral shuffles). Lastly, the transverse plane of movement covers all types of movements that force your body to rotate and twist (i.e., medicine ball rotational wall chest passes or baseball swings). For the purposes of athleticism, the warm-up should allow you to explore all three planes of movement to develop movement quality over time. While warm-up movements are typically performed with only body weight or light resistance, they still mimic the patterns used in the main workout. This makes the warm-up not just a preparation tool, but also an opportunity to refine movement quality and restore both joint and tissue health through mobility and flexibility work.

MOBILITY AND FLEXIBILITY

Mobility and flexibility are intertwined with regard to range of motion and freedom of movement in each area of the human body. However, although these two elements of fitness go hand in hand, it's important to understand where they differ so that you train them accordingly in your warm-up. The term *mobility* refers to the freedom of movement or range of motion in a joint. Essentially, each joint in the human body has a certain degree of motion. Let's use the leg as an example. When you go down into a squat, your knee joints are expressing range of motion while flexing or bending. Now, this is where flexibility comes into the picture: *Flexibility* refers to the extensibility of a given tissue or muscle. In the example of the squat, your quadriceps muscles in the front of your thighs are extending. When considering any type of movement or exercise, always think about which joints are involved from a mobility standpoint, in addition to which muscle or muscles are involved from a flexibility standpoint. The best part about both mobility and flexibility is that they can be improved through consistent training, which is why incorporating both of these in the warm-up is crucial for anyone aiming to increase their overall athleticism.

STABILITY AND ACTIVATION

Athletes who possess an adequate amount of stability are able to remain balanced on the field, on the court, and on any type of surface or environment they perform on. The same can be said for athletes looking to maintain fitness and health outside of traditional competition by way of recreational athletics, training, and other physical activities. Stability is the ability of a given joint to maintain a position by restricting movement. In a situation in which an athlete is attempting to remain stable or still, this ability requires a concerted effort of the muscles and tissues around a joint working in tandem to create stability. For example, stand on one foot with the other knee bent and held up at roughly waist height. Attempt to hold this position for 30 seconds. This is a quick and easy way to test your ability to remain stable on one leg. Now let's increase the overall stability and balance challenge by adding in what we refer to as "perturbations"—disturbances of motion or state of equilibrium. Continue attempting to balance and stabilize on one leg, but have someone stand to the side and continually give a gentle nudge at shoulder level with minimal pressure for the entire 30 seconds. This would undoubtedly increase the overall stability and balance challenge of the pose. Through exercises like this, you can increase or decrease your stability by manipulating internal forces (i.e., your body weight) and external forces (e.g., perturbations from someone, perpendicular resistance from a band). Including exercises within the warm-up that challenge your stability, whether in your lower body, trunk, or upper body, is a sure-fire way to increase your overall athleticism in sports and in life.

Activation, often associated with exercises that are included at the very beginning of a typical warm-up routine, works in conjunction with stability. Activation exercises typically isolate a certain area of the body to essentially turn it on, wake it up, and alert it that it's time to get to work. Although this is a very loose definition of activation, I always refer back to it since it is easy not only to explain but also to understand. Consider a scenario at the very beginning of your warm-up. You're about to perform a bridge exercise, beginning by lying flat on your back with both knees bent, both feet flat, and the palms of both hands touching the floor by the side of each pocket. From here, while maintaining a straight line from your knees all the way up to your shoulders, raise your hips until they create a bridge. You'll feel the muscles behind your thighs (hamstrings) and glutes working to get up into this position and then working on the way back down to the floor. The hips are being challenged to remain stable during this bridging motion, in addition to the muscles and tissues around the hips (in this case, the hamstrings and glutes) activating. These types of isolation drills are ideal for the beginning of the warm-up to begin activating and waking up certain areas of the body that will be trained later in the workout with higher intensities and speeds. In this case, since we have now warmed up the hips, glutes, and hamstrings, a strength training exercise that challenges the same areas (e.g., trap bar deadlift) would be a great fit to use in the workout.

BAND CAT-COW

If you're having trouble with any sort of extension in the middle and upper back area of your spine, here is a great drill to use in your warm-up to address these issues.

HOW TO PERFORM

- Start by holding a long resistance band in the crease of each hand, with the band looped around your mid-to-upper back area. You can always adjust the exact placement of the band based on comfort. It is recommended to use a band with light to medium resistance.
- Now make your way down to the floor in an all-fours position, which requires your hands to be directly under your shoulders and your knees to be directly under your hips.
- From here, the only motion that should occur will be in your mid-to-upper back area (thoracic spine) as a way to increase the overall mobility in that region. In a slow and controlled manner, arch your back and then perform the exact opposite by hollowing out your abdomen.

PERFORMANCE TIPS FOR SUCCESS

- Use this exercise to increase overall mobility in the middle and upper areas of your spine, otherwise known as the *thoracic spine*, which is often a culprit for athletes lacking overhead range of motion.
- The key here is to use a slow and controlled pace to capture the benefit of spinal mobility in thoracic extension and flexion.

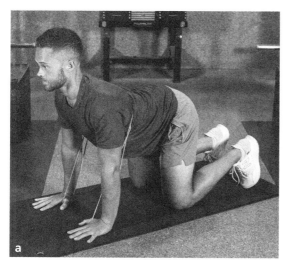 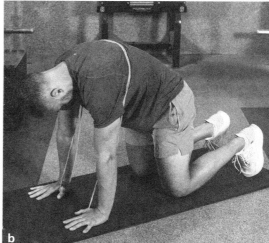

Figure 5.1 Band cat-cow: *(a)* cow and *(b)* cat.

HEELS-UP SINGLE-LEG BRIDGE ISOMETRIC WITH KNEE DRIVE ISOMETRIC

Here is a more-bang-for-your-buck isometric exercise you can perform in the warm-up that challenges your hip flexors, glutes, hamstrings, and a small but powerful muscle in the calf area of your lower leg known as the *soleus muscle*.

HOW TO PERFORM

- Set yourself up on the floor with your back flat, knees bent, and feet flat.
- Raise your hips and maintain the bridge hold position.
- Inch your heels back just a touch closer toward your butt.
- Finally, raise one knee up toward your chest and raise the heel of the foot that remains in contact with the floor.
- Hold this position for the prescribed amount of time on that side. Switch sides and repeat.

PERFORMANCE TIPS FOR SUCCESS

- The goal of this exercise is to strengthen the hip flexors, glutes, hamstrings, and soleus through an isometric (hold) position that also challenges your stability.
- It is crucial to really drive the toes of the stationary foot down into the floor, and also to drive the heel of that same foot up as high as possible. This will help to strengthen the calf muscle known as the soleus.

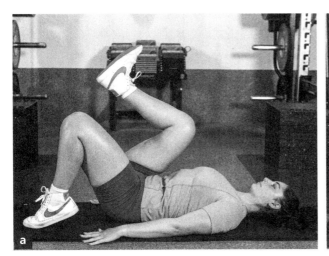 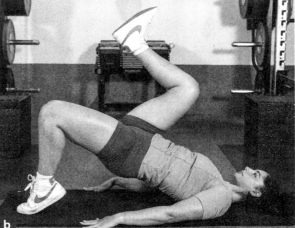

Figure 5.2 Heels-up single-leg bridge isometric with knee drive isometric: *(a)* knee drive and *(b)* bridge.

CATCHER ROCKBACK ISOMETRIC WITH REACH AND ROTATE

I'm a big fan of warm-up exercises that target the upper and lower body at the same time, which is exactly what you achieve when performing this movement.

HOW TO PERFORM

- Start on the floor facing down with your left knee down, right leg straight to your right side, and right foot flat.
- Ensure that your left knee and right foot are in a straight line.
- Place both hands in front of you on the floor and use them to help push your hips back. Once in this position, remain there for the entire set.
- Take your right hand, reach underneath your left arm as far as you can, and then take your right hand and rotate all the way up toward the ceiling on the right side. Make sure that your eyes follow where your right hand moves to get the most out of this exercise.
- Perform all reps on the right side, switch sides, and repeat.

PERFORMANCE TIPS FOR SUCCESS

- This warm-up exercise will not only increase hip joint mobility and adductor muscle flexibility but also improve thoracic spine mobility.
- An important aspect here is to really allow your eyes to follow the moving hand during each rep, which directly affects mobility and flexibility in your upper body.

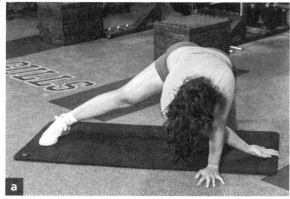
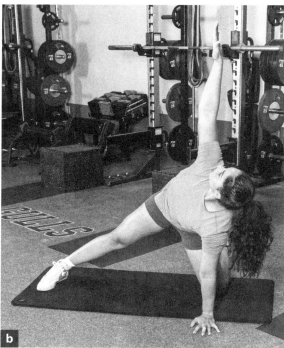

Figure 5.3 Catcher rockback isometric with reach and rotate: *(a)* catcher rockback and *(b)* reach and rotate.

FLOOR BENT-KNEE COPENHAGEN PLANK

Most people ignore the muscles of the inner thigh and groin region, otherwise known as the *adductor muscles*. When you do that, you lose out on a key area that can help strengthen and support the hip and knee, which are key for high-performing athletes. Use this exercise to develop strong and healthy adductors.

HOW TO PERFORM

- Set yourself up on the floor by lying on your right side.
- Bend your right knee to roughly 90 degrees so that your right foot is out in front of you.
- Bend your left knee to roughly 90 degrees so that your left foot is behind you.
- Now place your (bottom) right elbow directly under your right shoulder and raise your right side and hip away from the floor as if you were performing a traditional side plank.
- When doing so, reach your top (left) hand up toward the ceiling with a clenched fist for added stability, in addition to pressing the inside of your left knee down into either the floor or a pad for comfort.
- Hold this position for the prescribed amount of time. Switch sides and repeat.

PERFORMANCE TIPS FOR SUCCESS

- The best athletes in the world understand the importance of building body armor in every part of their body. This is the type of exercise that doesn't seem like it's doing much, but in reality, is a game changer for hip and knee durability. That is why it is important to dial in your intent when performing this exercise.
- It's important to really think about the muscles you are using—in this case, the inner thigh (groin) region—to effectively strengthen the area.

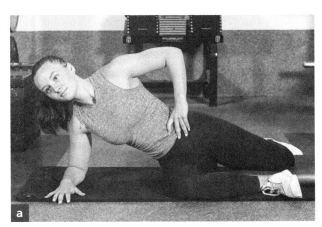

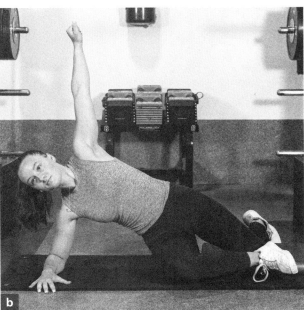

Figure 5.4 Floor bent-knee Copenhagen plank: *(a)* side plank and *(b)* lift hand.

ALTERNATING SPIDERMAN

Use this more-bang-for-your-buck warm-up exercise as a catch-all movement that allows you to target multiple joints and muscles quickly and efficiently. If you're ever in a pinch for time and in need of a quick warm-up exercise, this always seems to get the job done!

HOW TO PERFORM

- Start with your body in the top of a push-up position.
- Hike your right foot up toward the front and place it on the floor just outside your right hand.
- Leaving your left hand down on the floor, rotate your right hand up toward the ceiling and follow it with your eyes so that your entire spine rotates as well.
- Return your right hand to the floor and then repeat the sequence on the other side.
- Complete the prescribed number of reps per side in this alternating fashion.

PERFORMANCE TIPS FOR SUCCESS

- This is one of my go-to warm-up movements that targets mobility and flexibility in the entire body. You should feel like you're accessing an increased range of motion during each rep.
- When performing this warm-up movement, be sure to rotate as much as possible with your upper body and reach as high as you can with your arm. This will enhance your overall mobility and flexibility.

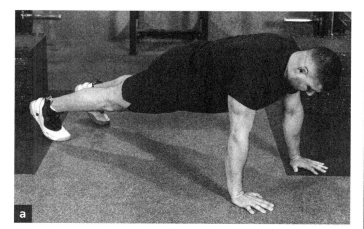

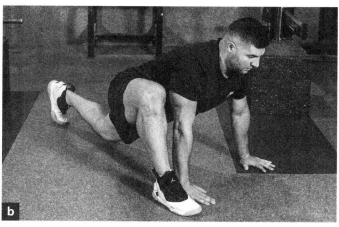

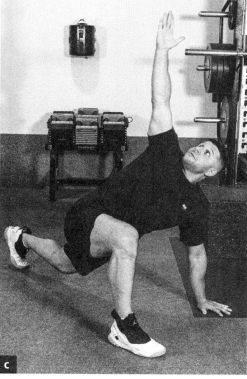

Figure 5.5 Alternating Spiderman: (a) starting push-up position, (b) right foot outside right hand, and (c) left hand on floor, right hand up.

SPLIT SQUAT ISO

An isometric (hold) exercise gives you the opportunity to develop strength and stability in specific positions that will transfer to sports and recreational activities. Use this exercise to strengthen the knees and quadriceps.

HOW TO PERFORM

- Take a knee down on the floor.
- Make sure that the front foot remains flat and that only the toes of the rear foot remain in contact with the floor.
- Ensure that your legs remain roughly hip-width apart for added stability.
- Now raise your rear knee up off the floor so that it's hovering by a couple of inches.
- With a tall torso, hold this position for the prescribed amount of time, switch sides, and repeat.

PERFORMANCE TIPS FOR SUCCESS

- The split squat position is one that we see in a variety of sports, athletic endeavors, and physical activities, which is why it's important to perform in your training program.
- When performing this warm-up exercise, fight hard to maintain the isometric (hold) position—it is much more challenging than it seems.

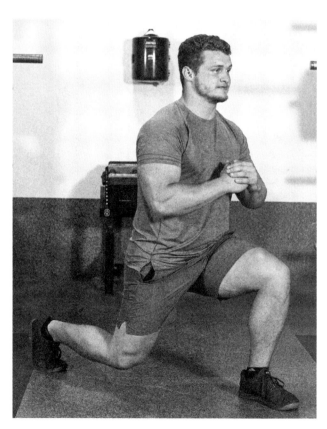

Figure 5.6 Split squat iso.

SQUAT RACK KANG SQUAT

Generally speaking, the bodyweight version of the Kang squat allows you to improve hip mobility, ankle mobility, adductor flexibility, and hamstring flexibility. However, with your hands supported on the squat rack, you'll be able to explore deeper ranges of motion.

HOW TO PERFORM

- With your feet on the floor at roughly hip-width apart, hold on to a squat rack directly in front of you and use it as support.
- Hinge your hips back behind you (imagine you're attempting to close a door with your butt).
- Squat down the remainder of the way to the bottom position.
- Perform the hip hinge motion again and, finally, stand all the way back up. Completing all these steps equals one rep. Complete the prescribed number of reps.

PERFORMANCE TIPS FOR SUCCESS

- With this warm-up exercise, you'll be able to improve lower body mobility in your hip and ankle joints, in addition to flexibility in your adductors and hamstrings.
- Use your hands for support as much as needed so that you truly reap the mobility and flexibility benefits here!

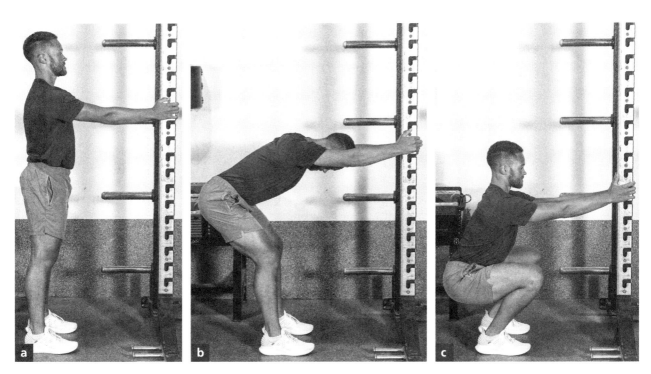

Figure 5.7 Squat rack Kang squat: *(a)* start position, *(b)* hinge hips back, and *(c)* squat down.

EXTENSIVE POGO HOP

Pogo hops are among the lowest-hanging fruit in the development of athleticism, since this exercise allows your calves and ankles to produce and absorb force. You'll be able to improve both force production (jumping) and force absorption (landing) through the ankle joints and calf muscles.

HOW TO PERFORM

- When you're performing any type of pogo hop with an extensive intent, the ultimate goal is to develop rhythm and coordination with the movement through low impact and high volume.
- The purpose is to increase capacity of the calf muscles and ankle joints, in addition to improving technique through low ground-reaction forces and low speeds.
- Make sure that your entire body remains stiff with little to no bend in the hips, knees, or ankles.
- Use the extensive approach with the pogo hop by hopping in an up-and-down motion through the toes of both feet while allowing the ankles to do the majority of the work.

PERFORMANCE TIPS FOR SUCCESS

- The most important performance tip is this: Use a relaxed pace and tempo.
- It's not important to achieve maximum height with this warm-up exercise.

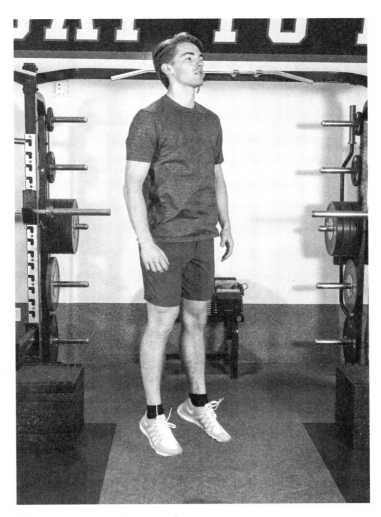

Figure 5.8 Extensive pogo hop.

DROP SQUAT TO STICK

The athletic skills of force absorption and deceleration are often overlooked in training for athletic performance yet are just as important as their direct counterparts (force production and acceleration). This exercise helps you become a more well-rounded athlete by developing deceleration skills.

HOW TO PERFORM

- Stand tall with your feet roughly hip-width apart.
- Reach both hands up high toward the ceiling while simultaneously raising both heels off the floor. Rapidly drop down as fast as you can into the bottom position of a squat.
- Your hands should end up behind you at the bottom, where you will hold that position for a moment (i.e., 1 to 2 seconds).
- The objective here is to stop on a dime (i.e., freeze your body) and absorb all that force, which will improve your ability to decelerate in sports and athletics.

PERFORMANCE TIPS FOR SUCCESS

- This warm-up exercise will help improve your ability to stop on a dime and absorb force, helping you to become a more resilient athlete.
- The most important component here is to drop down as fast as possible. When you do this, you make it much more challenging for your body to decelerate, which is the exact type of challenge we're looking for.

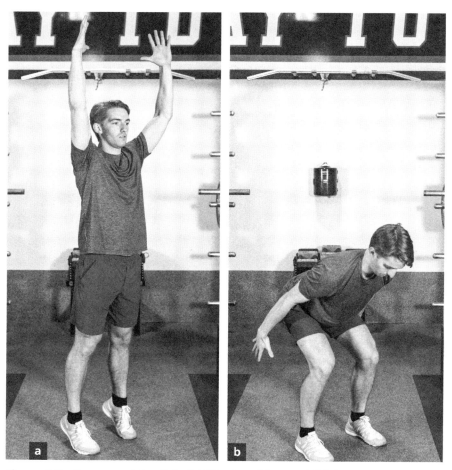

Figure 5.9 Drop squat to stick: *(a)* lifted position and *(b)* drop to squat.

LINEAR SKIP

Skipping is one of the foundational movements in elite athleticism. If you can master a basic exercise like this one, you'll be able to build off it and improve your overall athletic skills.

HOW TO PERFORM

- The key here is to move in a fluid yet robotic fashion while traveling forward (linearly) and staying tall in your torso.
- This exercise helps you build good mechanics for sprinting with regard to your arms and legs.
- The goal of sprinting is to sustain a high level of efficiency, which is what we're chasing in this exercise.
- Move your arms opposite from the motion occurring in your legs. If your left knee is up, your right arm should be up, and vice versa.
- Follow this entire sequence for the prescribed reps or distance.

PERFORMANCE TIPS FOR SUCCESS

- This is one of the best warm-up exercises to help you improve in fundamental sprinting mechanics by developing the ability to strike the ground with force as you travel up and forward.
- When performing this exercise, avoid the temptation to jump; instead, strike the foot down hard and remain tall, which will propel your body up and forward.

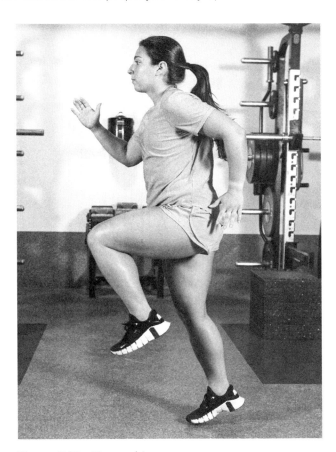

Figure 5.10 Linear skip.

LONG BRIDGE ISO

Durable hamstrings are a hallmark trait of strong and healthy athletes, so be sure to engage them when performing this hamstring-focused exercise.

HOW TO PERFORM

- Lie flat on your back on the floor with both legs long and roughly hip-width apart.
- Make sure that your palms are also flat on the floor at the sides of your pockets.
- Slightly bend both knees at roughly 5 to 10 degrees of flexion, drive both heels down into the floor, and raise your butt off the floor.
- You'll notice that your hips won't be able to raise too high above the floor, but you'll immediately feels your hamstrings working hard. That's exactly what we want.
- Hold this position for the prescribed amount of time.

PERFORMANCE TIPS FOR SUCCESS

- Here is an excellent way to bulletproof your hamstrings through an isometric (hold) strengthening exercise in a long position.
- When performing this exercise, drive both heels down hard as your hips rise up to truly challenge your hamstring muscles.

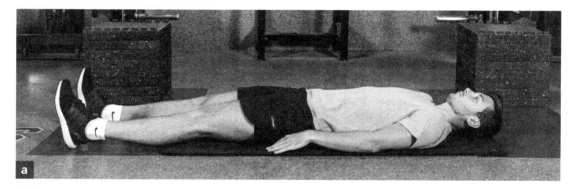

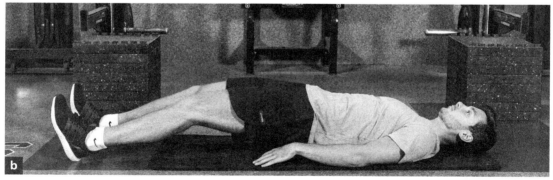

Figure 5.11 Long bridge iso: *(a)* start position and *(b)* bridge.

Warm-Up Exercises 53

WALL PRESS WITH ALTERNATING DEAD BUG

This exercise falls under the anti-extension trunk strength category, which enables you to develop a strong and stable core—a foundational characteristic of long-term health and performance.

HOW TO PERFORM

- Lie flat on your back on the floor with a wall directly behind you by just a few inches.
- Press both hands directly back into the wall, which will help to create stability in the trunk.
- Raise both knees up directly above both hips.
- Straighten one leg out and down toward the floor and then raise it back to the starting position with a bent knee. Pause for a moment, then repeat this sequence with the other leg.
- Complete all prescribed reps in this alternating format.

PERFORMANCE TIPS FOR SUCCESS

- You'll be able to develop a strong and stable core with this trunk-strengthening exercise. Focus on avoiding any sort of low back arch or ribcage flare.
- Really think about the muscles you are using—in this case, the core and abdominal region—to truly strengthen these areas.

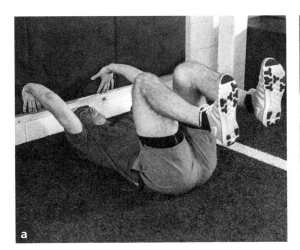
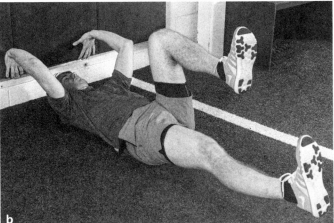
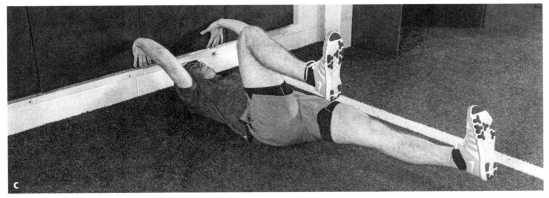

Figure 5.12 Wall press with alternating dead bug: *(a)* lift knees, *(b-c)* alternate legs.

WALL STORK

Athletes will dominate life and sports when they master single-leg strength and stability, which is exactly what you'll build when performing this unique exercise.

HOW TO PERFORM

- Position your body very close to a wall on your right.
- Keeping your feet together on the floor, sink down low toward the floor by bending both knees and hips—this will feel like a narrow squat.
- Balance on your left foot and lift your right foot just slightly off the floor.
- Press the outside of your right knee laterally into the wall.
- Hold that position for the prescribed amount of time, switch sides, and repeat.

PERFORMANCE TIPS FOR SUCCESS

- Develop single-leg strength and stability while strengthening your glutes and lateral hip muscles when performing this exercise.
- Really press the knee closest to the wall directly into it. The outside aspect of that knee should be in contact with the wall the entire time.

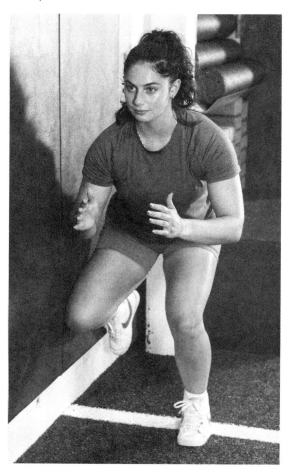

Figure 5.13 Wall stork.

WALL SINGLE-LEG HEEL RAISE ISO

You'll benefit from this exercise by improving muscular strength and endurance in your lower leg and calf muscles, an often-neglected area of the body for athletes in all walks of life. This exercise, in particular, targets the gastrocnemius muscle of the lower leg.

HOW TO PERFORM

- Stand in front of a wall with both arms straight and both hands pressed forward into the wall at shoulder height.
- Take a couple of steps back so that your body, from head to heels, is at a 45-degree angle to the wall when viewed from the side.
- From here, raise your left knee up toward your chest while your right foot remains flat on the floor.
- Keep a tall body from head to heels and the toes of your left foot pointing up.
- Without letting any other part of your body move, raise your right heel as high as possible up and away from the floor without letting your right ankle roll out to either side.
- Once you've reached this high point, hold this position for the prescribed amount of time.
- When you're done, switch sides and repeat.

PERFORMANCE TIPS FOR SUCCESS

- When performing this exercise, you'll build muscular strength and endurance in your calves, in addition to improving the strength and durability of your Achilles tendon.
- Focus on raising your heel as high as possible while avoiding any sort of rolling motion at the ankle.

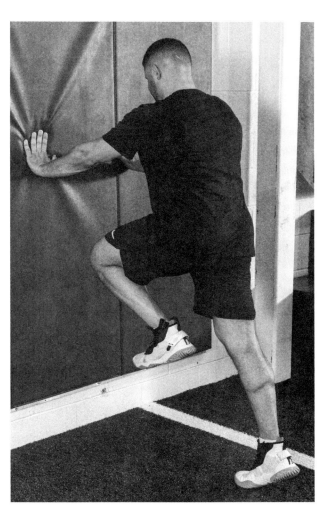

Figure 5.14 Wall single-leg heel raise iso.

ALTERNATING YOGA PLEX

This warm-up exercise is one of my favorite catch-all movements that targets your entire body from a mobility and flexibility standpoint.

HOW TO PERFORM

- Place both hands on a box or bench at roughly knee height.
- Step both feet back behind you so that your body is in the top position of a push-up.
- Step your left foot forward, place it flat on the floor, and bend your left knee.
- Allow the right knee to rest on the floor and the left hand to rest on the box or bench.
- Starting from the front, while keeping your left hand on the box or bench, raise your right arm up and around toward the back in a circular motion while your eyes, head, and neck follow.
- Make sure to finish this circular motion all the way through and return to the starting position in front.
- Step back out into the top of a push-up position, switch sides, and repeat.

PERFORMANCE TIPS FOR SUCCESS

- This warm-up exercise is one of the best for improving full-body mobility and flexibility.
- Where most athletes go wrong is lacking intent and purpose when performing this movement. Be sure to really dial in the finer details of creating the circular motion and following with your eyes, head, and neck.

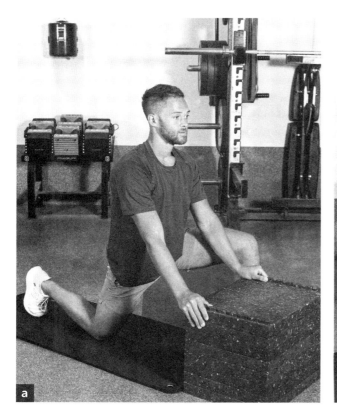 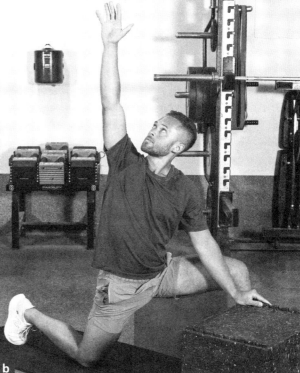

Figure 5.15 Alternating yoga plex: *(a)* start position and *(b)* finish position.

STATIONARY INCHWORM

This full-body warm-up exercise is an excellent choice to improve mobility and flexibility in your lower and upper body.

HOW TO PERFORM

- Set yourself up in the top of a push-up position.
- Keep both arms and both legs straight the entire time.
- Begin to slowly inch your toes forward toward your hands while raising your hips up toward the sky.
- Once you have moved as far forward as possible while keeping both arms and legs straight, inch your toes back to the starting position.
- Continue this sequence for all the prescribed reps.

PERFORMANCE TIPS FOR SUCCESS

- Add this warm-up exercise into the rotation anytime you're feeling stiff in your hamstrings, back, or shoulders.
- When performing this movement, be sure to keep both arms and both legs as straight as possible to achieve more range of motion in the lower body and upper body.

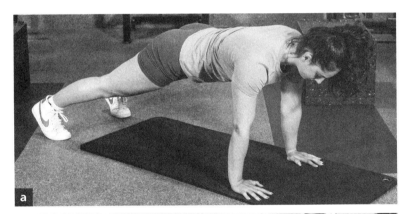

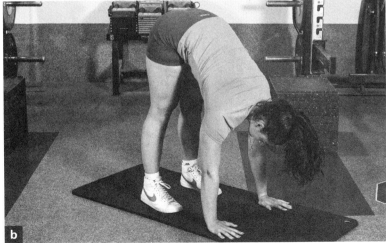

Figure 5.16 Stationary inchworm: *(a)* start position and *(b)* hips raised.

HINGE TO SQUAT

With this warm-up exercise, improve hip joint mobility, ankle joint mobility, hamstring muscle flexibility, and groin muscle flexibility.

HOW TO PERFORM

- Stand with your feet roughly hip-width apart.
- Sit your hips back into the hip hinge pattern, reach down toward your feet with your hands, and clasp your fingers underneath your toes.
- Keeping your arms between your knees, pull your butt down into the bottom of a squat position.
- From here, keep your chest proud, spine tall, and outside aspect of your elbows driving laterally into the inside of your knees.
- Bring your butt back up toward the starting position and then bring your head and upper body along with it until you reach the top.

PERFORMANCE TIPS FOR SUCCESS

- The key here is to really clasp your fingers underneath your toes and pull your butt down into position. If you can't reach down that far, you can instead clasp the front of your shins with both hands.
- When performing this exercise, really think about the muscles you are using—the quadriceps, hamstrings, and inner thigh (groin) muscles—to truly strengthen these areas.

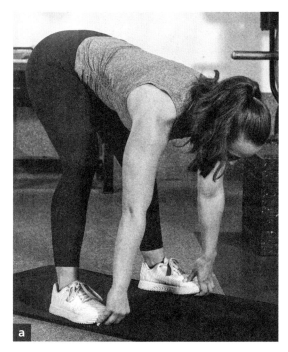 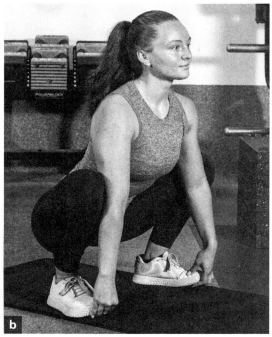

Figure 5.17 Hinge to squat: *(a)* hip hinge and reach toward feet and *(b)* pull butt down into squat position.

WALL LINEAR SINGLE EXCHANGE

This is a classic warm-up exercise to help you develop sprinting mechanics and athletic skills.

HOW TO PERFORM

- Stand in front of a wall with both arms straight and both hands pressed forward into the wall at shoulder height.
- Now take a couple of steps back so that your body, from head to heels, is at a 45-degree angle with respect to the wall when viewed from the side.
- Prop both heels up off the floor and raise your right knee up toward your chest.
- Keep a tall body from head to heels and keep the toes of your right foot pointing up.
- Without letting any other part of your body move, switch the positions of your legs in a rapid and explosive manner.
- Perform all reps in this alternating fashion until complete.

PERFORMANCE TIPS FOR SUCCESS

- With this movement, you'll develop the ability to rapidly switch leg positions, an explosive action that occurs in sprinting and running.
- Really home in on how quickly you can switch the positions of your legs. The goal is to do this as fast as possible during each rep.

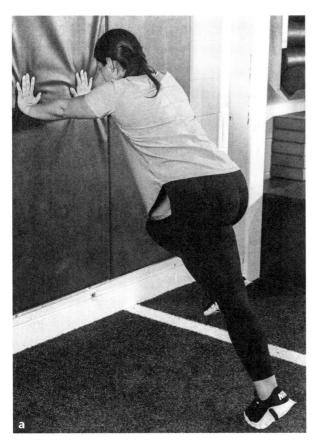 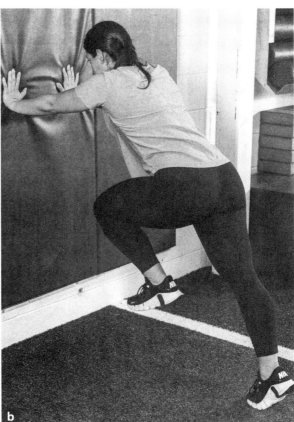

Figure 5.18 Wall linear single exchange: *(a)* right knee up and *(b)* left knee up.

STATIONARY HAMSTRING SCOOP

Develop mobility in your hips and flexibility in your hamstrings when performing this dynamic warm-up exercise while also improving your hip hinge movement pattern.

HOW TO PERFORM

- Stand with your feet roughly hip-width apart.
- Slightly step your right foot forward to the point at which the heel of your right foot is in line with the toes of your left foot.
- Drive your right heel down into the floor, point the toes of your right foot up toward the ceiling, hinge your hips back, and perform a scooping motion with your arms.
- Come back up to the top, switch sides, and repeat.
- Continue alternating sides in this stationary position until all reps are complete.

PERFORMANCE TIPS FOR SUCCESS

- One of the biggest mistakes athletes make when performing this warm-up exercise is forgetting to hinge the hips directly back. When done correctly, this will allow you to improve hip joint mobility and hamstring flexibility.
- When performing this exercise, really think about the muscles you are using—the hamstrings—to truly strengthen the area.

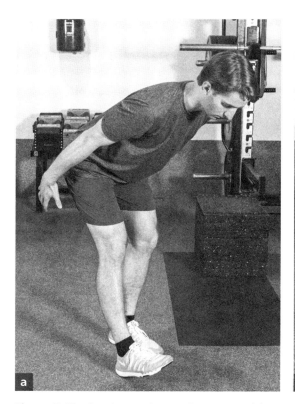
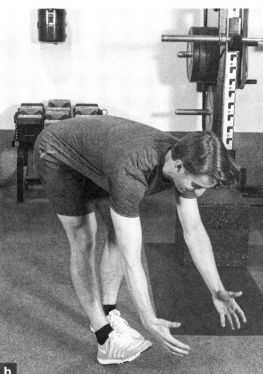

Figure 5.19 Stationary hamstring scoop: *(a)* step right foot forward and *(b)* scoop.

Warm-Up Exercises **61**

WALKING ALTERNATING SPIDERMAN

This exercise adds a dynamic element to the traditional stationary version of the alternating Spiderman—you're moving across a distance while still targeting full-body mobility and flexibility.

HOW TO PERFORM

- Start out with your body in the top of a push-up position.
- Hike your right foot up toward the front and place it on the floor just outside your right hand.
- Leaving your left hand down on the floor, rotate your right hand up toward the ceiling and follow it with your eyes so that your entire spine rotates as well.
- Stay low and crawl forward so that you're able to hike your left foot up toward the front and place it on the floor just outside your left hand.
- Complete the same sequence on the other side.

PERFORMANCE TIPS FOR SUCCESS

- When performing this warm-up exercise, be mindful of foot positioning on the floor. You want to ensure that your base is wide enough to allow you to achieve maximum mobility and flexibility.
- It's important to really think about the muscles you are using—the quadriceps, hip flexors, hamstrings, and groin (inner thigh) muscles—to truly strengthen these areas.

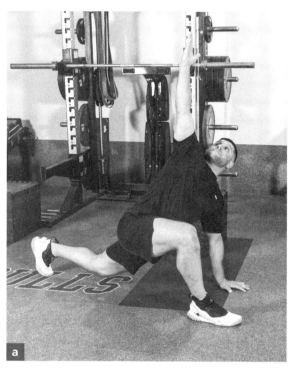
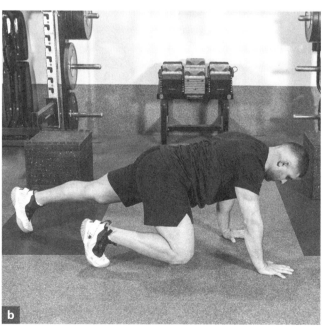
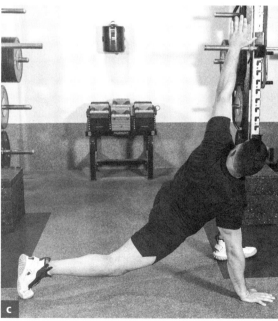

Figure 5.20 Walking alternating Spiderman: *(a)* right foot forward, right hand up, *(b)* crawl forward, and *(c)* left foot forward, left hand up.

LATERAL SHUFFLE WITH ARM SWING

Here's a classic dynamic warm-up exercise that takes place in the frontal plane of movement, allowing you to move from side to side.

HOW TO PERFORM

- Set yourself up in a wide athletic stance with both hips and knees bent.
- Allow the toes of your feet to aim forward. You may notice that the lead foot will tend to rotate out slightly, which can be beneficial for some athletes as long as it does not become excessive.
- Perform a lateral shuffle to one side while simultaneously swinging your arms in an outward and inward motion.
- Complete all reps or yards in one direction, switch sides, and repeat.

PERFORMANCE TIPS FOR SUCCESS

- A key that most people miss is to perform the arm swing simultaneously with the lateral shuffle. This sequencing can be challenging to coordinate, but is well worth it in terms of boosting your overall athleticism.
- It's important to really think about the muscles you are using—the groin (inner thigh) region, lateral hip muscles, and shoulders—to truly strengthen these areas.

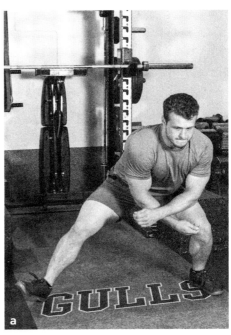
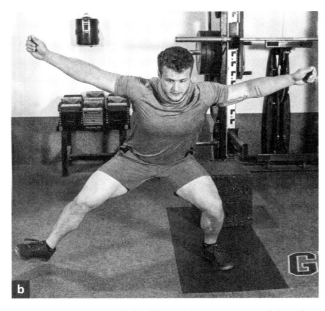
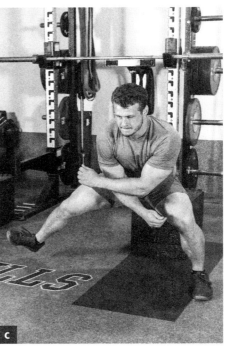

Figure 5.21 Lateral shuffle with arm swing: *(a)* wide athletic stance, *(b-c)* shuffle laterally while swinging arms, and land on other side.

BACKPEDAL

Remember back in the 1990s when Deion Sanders played defensive back and cornerback in the NFL while backpedaling his way to multiple interceptions? That's what we're working on here: the backpedaling part. Backpedaling is a classic skill in athleticism that improves balance, stability, and coordination, in addition to working your hamstring muscles during locomotion in reverse.

HOW TO PERFORM

- Place your feet hip-width apart on the floor, sit your hips down and back, and lean your chest forward slightly.
- Avoid standing up, getting tall, or letting your weight shift too far behind you.
- Keep your chest forward slightly the entire time and your hips down and back, which will allow you to evenly balance your weight during the backpedaling motion.
- From here, begin to run backward; allow your arms to become involved the way they would if you were running forward.

PERFORMANCE TIPS FOR SUCCESS

- Not only does this dynamic warm-up exercise improve your ability to backpedal, it also challenges your ability to remain stable and balanced as you coordinate your body.
- Really dial in the body position and posture while pedaling backward. When done correctly, this will allow you to remain balanced as you propel in reverse.

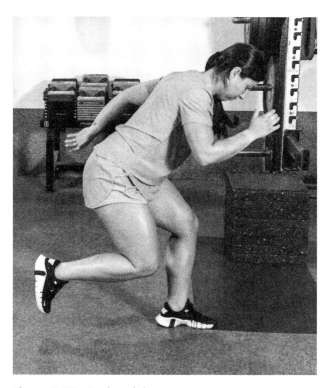

Figure 5.22 Backpedal.

CAT-COW

Improving spinal mobility is a key component of any warm-up routine to ensure that you're loosened up and ready once the training session starts. Use this exercise to increase the overall mobility of your entire spine from your head to your hips.

HOW TO PERFORM

- Start by making your way down to the floor in a quadruped (all fours) position, with your hands directly under your shoulders and your knees directly under your hips.
- From here, the only motion that should occur is in your mid-to-upper back area (thoracic spine) to increase the overall mobility in that region.
- In a slow and controlled manner, arch your back and then perform the exact opposite by hollowing out your abdomen.

PERFORMANCE TIPS FOR SUCCESS

- Although this warm-up exercise looks simple on paper, it creates a challenge if not performed at the proper pace. Be sure to move your spine at a slow and controlled pace throughout each rep to really reap the benefits.
- It's important to think about the muscles you are using—all of the muscles that run up and down the spine, such as the erector spinae and multifidus—to truly strengthen these areas.

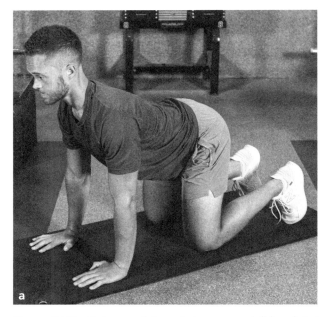 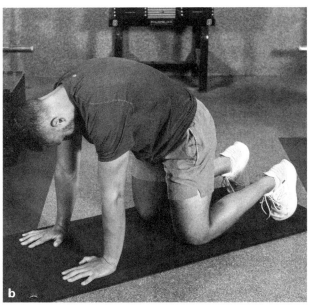

Figure 5.23 Cat-cow: *(a)* sag into cow and *(b)* arch into cat.

SINGLE-LEG BRIDGE ISOMETRIC WITH BENT-KNEE LEG WHIP

Here's a big-time hip and spine stability drill that also challenges your core muscles to work in an anti-rotation fashion.

HOW TO PERFORM

- Lie on the floor with your back flat, knees bent, and feet flat.
- Drive your left knee up toward your chest.
- With your right foot remaining in contact with the floor, raise your hips into a bridge and hold for the entire duration.
- This is the challenging part. Fight hard to create as much stability in your hips and spine as possible in an effort to avoid letting your spine rotate.
- With your left knee remaining bent (it should look like an L), slowly lower it toward the left side and then return to the starting position. This is much more challenging than it seems.
- Perform all reps on the left side, switch sides, and repeat.

PERFORMANCE TIPS FOR SUCCESS

- You'll develop anti-rotation core strength, spinal stability, and hip stability with this warm-up exercise.
- Allow motion to occur only in the leg traveling out toward the side. Fight hard to keep the non-moving hip as still as possible to improve stability in that area.

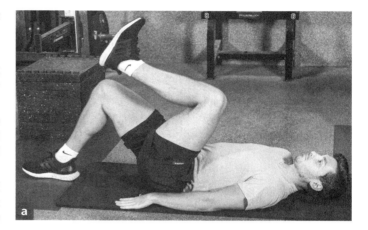

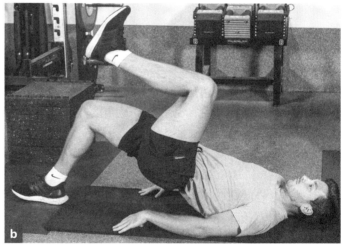

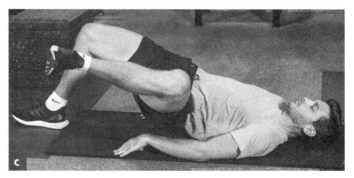

Figure 5.24 Single-leg bridge isometric with bent-knee leg whip: *(a)* lift left knee toward chest, *(b)* raise hips into a bridge, and *(c)* lower left knee to left side.

CATCHER ROCKBACK

This exercise provides the benefits of hip joint mobility and adductor muscle flexibility, which are helpful additions to any warm-up routine.

HOW TO PERFORM

- Start on the floor with your left knee down, right leg straight, and right foot flat.
- Keep a straight line from your left knee all the way to your right foot.
- Place both hands in front of you on the floor.
- Use your hands to help push your hips back and then pull them forward to return to the starting position.
- Perform all reps on the right side, switch sides, and repeat.

PERFORMANCE TIPS FOR SUCCESS

- This warm-up exercise will help you improve hip joint mobility and adductor muscle flexibility.
- Be sure to keep your foot flat on the floor with the toes aiming forward. Avoid any motion or change of position in the foot.

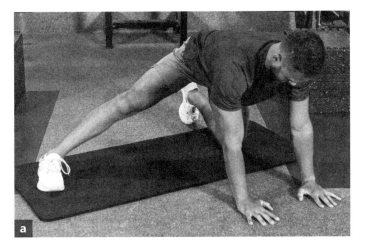
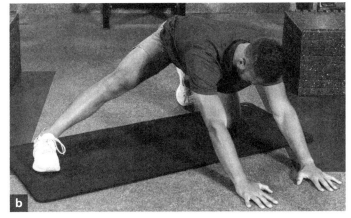
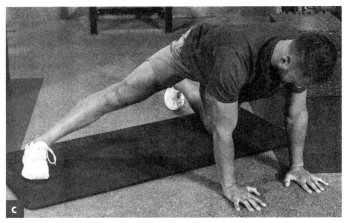

Figure 5.25 Catcher rockback: *(a)* left knee down, right leg straight, hands on floor, *(b)* push hips back, and *(c)* pull hips forward.

ELEVATED BENT-KNEE COPENHAGEN PLANK

The best athletes in the world understand the importance of building body armor in every aspect of their body. This is the type of exercise that doesn't seem like it's doing much, but is truly a game changer for hip and knee durability.

HOW TO PERFORM

- Set yourself up on the floor lying on your right side.
- Bend your right knee to roughly 90 degrees so that your right foot is out in front of you.
- Bend your left knee to roughly 90 degrees so that your left foot is behind you.
- Elevate the inside aspect of your left knee onto a box or bench for an added stability challenge.
- Place your (bottom) right elbow directly under your right shoulder and raise your right side and hip away from the floor as if you were performing a traditional side plank.
- Reach your top (left) hand up toward the ceiling with a clenched fist.
- Hold this position for the prescribed amount of time. Switch sides and repeat.

PERFORMANCE TIPS FOR SUCCESS

- Most people ignore the muscles of the inner thigh and groin region, otherwise known as the adductor muscles. When you do that, you lose out on a key area that can help strengthen and support the hip and knee, which are all key players in high-performing athletes. Use this exercise to develop strong and healthy adductors.
- Really drive your hips up and away from the floor to maximize the overall benefits.

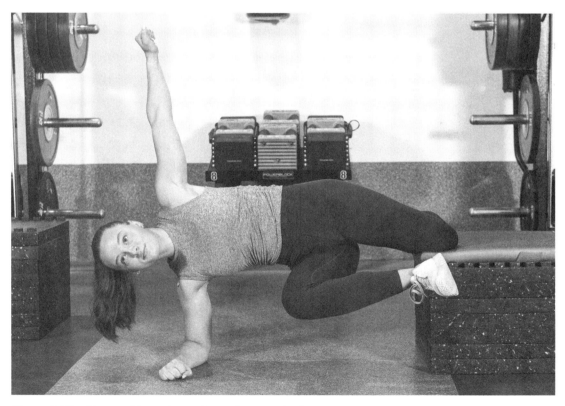

Figure 5.26 Elevated bent-knee Copenhagen plank.

ALTERNATING SPIDERMAN TO YOGA PIKE

Use this warm-up exercise as a catch-all movement that allows you to efficiently target multiple joints and muscles in your lower and upper body.

HOW TO PERFORM

- Start with your body in the top of a push-up position.
- Hike your right foot up toward the front and place it on the floor just outside your right hand.
- Leaving your left hand down on the floor, rotate your right hand up toward the ceiling and follow it with your eyes so that your entire spine rotates as well.
- Return your right hand to the floor and repeat this exact same sequence on the other side.
- Perform a downward-dog motion, otherwise known as a yoga pike, driving your hands down and away into the floor and your hips up toward the sky.
- Attempt to get both heels close to the floor as well.
- That entire sequence equals one rep. Complete all of the prescribed reps.

PERFORMANCE TIPS FOR SUCCESS

- By performing this exercise, you'll improve mobility and flexibility in your entire body.
- Move through each segment of the exercise deliberately and with intent.

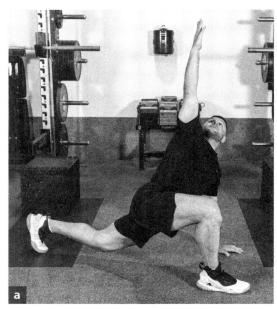
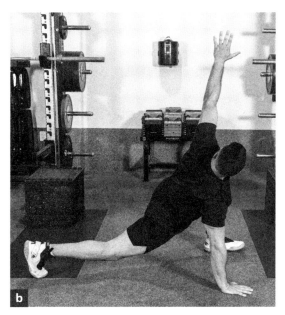
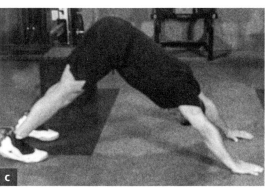

Figure 5.27 Alternating Spiderman to yoga pike: *(a)* Spiderman pose with right foot forward, *(b)* Spiderman pose with left foot forward, and *(c)* yoga pike (downward dog).

HEELS-UP SPLIT SQUAT ISOMETRIC

An isometric (hold) exercise gives you the opportunity to develop strength and stability in specific positions that will transfer to sports and recreational activities. Use this exercise to strengthen the knees, quadriceps, ankles, and calves.

HOW TO PERFORM

- Start by taking a knee down on the floor. Keep your front foot flat and only the toes of the rear foot in contact with the floor.
- Keep your legs roughly hip-width apart for added stability.
- Raise your rear knee off the floor so that it's hovering by a few inches, and raise the heel of your front foot without letting your ankle roll out to either side.
- With a tall torso, hold this position for the prescribed amount of time, switch sides, and repeat.

PERFORMANCE TIPS FOR SUCCESS

- The split squat position is one we see in a variety of sports, athletic endeavors, and physical activities—it's important to perform it to make sure you're durable in your knees and ankles.
- When performing this exercise, avoid any rotation of the ankle toward either side. Focus on keeping the ankle straight as the heel remains above the floor.

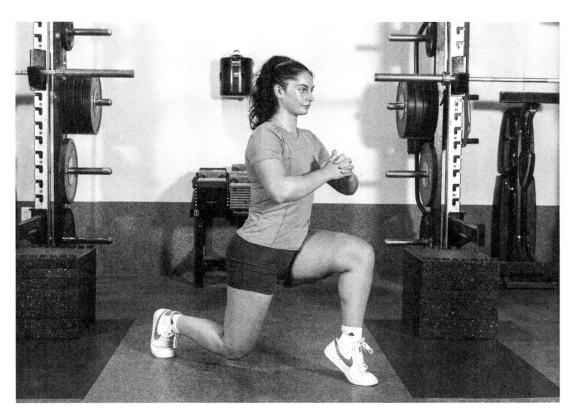

Figure 5.28 Heels-up split squat isometric.

MB HUG KANG SQUAT

The body weight version of the Kang squat allows you to improve hip mobility, ankle mobility, adductor flexibility, and hamstring flexibility. With an added medicine ball hug, you'll be able to explore a greater range of motion.

HOW TO PERFORM

- Set up with your feet on the floor roughly hip-width apart.
- Hug a large-diameter medicine ball or Dynamax medicine ball tight to your chest. The medicine ball should be large enough that you feel like you're almost hugging another person.
- Hugging the medicine ball tight to your chest, hinge your hips back behind you (imagine you're attempting to close a door with your butt).
- Squat down the remainder of the way to the bottom position.
- Perform the hip hinge motion again, and finally, stand back up to the top.
- That equals one rep. Complete all of the prescribed reps.

PERFORMANCE TIPS FOR SUCCESS

- Perform this exercise to improve lower-body mobility in your hip and ankle joints, in addition to flexibility in your adductors and hamstrings.
- Be sure to move through each section of the warm-up exercise with precision and intent. This may not seem important, but it can be a game changer for your overall health and performance.

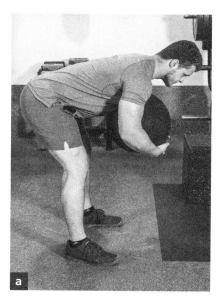 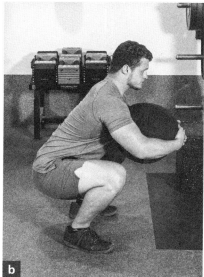 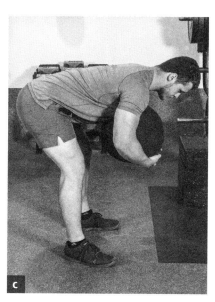

Figure 5.29 MB hug Kang squat: *(a)* hug medicine ball and hip hinge back, *(b)* squat to bottom position, and *(c)* hip hinge again.

EXTENSIVE SINGLE-LEG POGO HOP

Pogo hops are among the lowest-hanging fruit in developing athleticism, since this exercise allows your calves and ankles to produce and absorb force.

HOW TO PERFORM

- When you perform any type of pogo hop with an extensive intent (i.e., feeling fluid at a low intensity), the ultimate goal is to develop rhythm and coordination through low impact and high volume.
- The purpose is to increase capacity of the calf muscles and ankle joints, in addition to improving technique through low ground-reaction forces and low speeds.
- Stand tall with your feet hip-width apart on the floor.
- Bend your left knee and remove your left foot from the floor. With the right foot, begin by using an extensive approach while performing the pogo hop in an up-and-down motion, allowing only the right ankle to do the work. Each hop should feel fluid and bouncy.
- Keep your body stiff. Your entire body should be straight, with only the single ankle joint moving up and down while the other foot remains completely off the floor.
- Once all reps are complete on the right leg, switch sides and repeat.

PERFORMANCE TIPS FOR SUCCESS

- With this exercise, you'll be able to improve both force production (jumping) and force absorption (landing) through the ankle joints and calf muscles.
- It is important to view this exercise as using the ankle to perform the up-and-down motion. Avoid making this a jumping exercise where the knees take over. Instead, think of the knees as simply being along for the ride while the ankles take the lead.

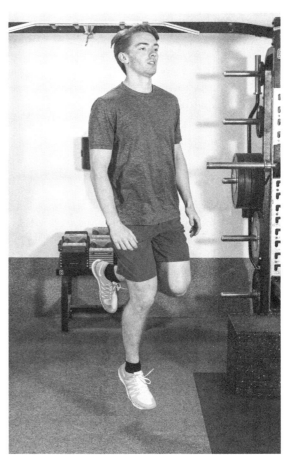

Figure 5.30 Extensive single-leg pogo hop.

DROP REVERSE LUNGE TO STICK

The athletic skills of force absorption and deceleration are often overlooked in training for athletic performance yet are just as important as their direct counterparts (force production and acceleration). This exercise helps you become a more well-rounded athlete by developing deceleration skills.

HOW TO PERFORM

- Stand tall with your feet roughly hip-width apart.
- You'll begin by standing tall with hands and heels lifted and finish in a reverse lunge position.
- Reach both hands toward the ceiling while simultaneously raising both heels off the floor, then drop down as fast as you can into the bottom position of a reverse lunge.
- Your hands should end up behind you at the bottom, where you'll hold that position for a moment.
- The goal here is to stop on a dime (i.e., freeze your body) and absorb all of that force, which will improve your ability to decelerate in sports and athletics.
- Complete all reps on one side, switch sides, and repeat.

PERFORMANCE TIPS FOR SUCCESS

- With this exercise, you'll improve your ability to absorb force, which will help you to become a more durable and resilient athlete.
- Focus on dropping down as fast as possible. When you do this, you'll make the deceleration (slowing down) aspect even more of a challenge.

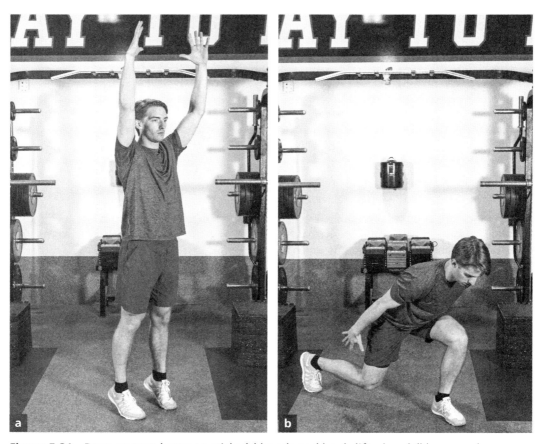

Figure 5.31 Drop reverse lunge to stick: *(a)* hands and heels lifted and *(b)* reverse lunge.

LATERAL SKIP

Skipping is a foundational movement in elite athleticism. If you can master a basic exercise like this one, you'll be able to build off it and improve your overall athletic skills.

HOW TO PERFORM

- The key here is to move in a fluid yet robotic fashion while traveling to the side (laterally).
- This exercise helps you build good mechanics for all types of frontal plane movements in sports, such as lateral shuffling, lateral running, sprinting after direction changes, and angled sprinting.
- Remain as efficient as possible with your movement.
- Avoid the temptation to jump; instead, strike the rear foot down hard and remain tall, which will propel your body up and away from the floor in the direction you're traveling (laterally).
- Make sure to move your arms opposite from the motion occurring in your legs. If your left knee is up, your right arm should be up, and vice versa.
- Follow this sequence for the prescribed number of reps or amount of distance in one direction, switch sides, and repeat.

PERFORMANCE TIPS FOR SUCCESS

- In this exercise, you'll improve in fundamental frontal plane mechanics by developing the ability to strike the ground with force as you travel up and away laterally.
- Avoid rotating the hips and avoid crossing the legs over. Keep your hips at or slightly outside of hip-width apart.

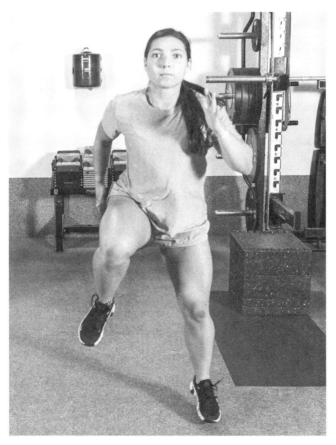

Figure 5.32 Lateral skip.

SINGLE-LEG LONG BRIDGE ISOMETRIC WITH KNEE DRIVE ISOMETRIC

Bulletproof your hamstrings with this isometric (hold) exercise to strengthen them in a long position, in addition to benefiting from the isometric position of the hip flexor muscle on the leg that is bent and up toward your chest.

HOW TO PERFORM

- Lie flat on your back with both legs long roughly hip-width apart and your palms flat on the floor at your pockets.
- Slightly bend both knees at roughly 5-10 degrees of flexion, drive both heels down into the floor, and raise your butt off the floor.
- Drive one knee up toward your chest with the toes of that foot aiming up toward your head.
- You'll notice that your hips won't be able to raise very high above the floor, but that you'll immediately feel your hamstrings working hard. That's exactly what we want.
- Hold this position for the prescribed amount of time, switch sides, and repeat.

PERFORMANCE TIPS FOR SUCCESS

- Durable hamstrings and hip flexors are hallmark characteristics of strong and healthy athletes who sprint and run on a routine basis—perform this warm-up exercise to improve in these areas over time.
- When performing this exercise, drive your heel down hard as your hips rise up to truly challenge your hamstring muscles.

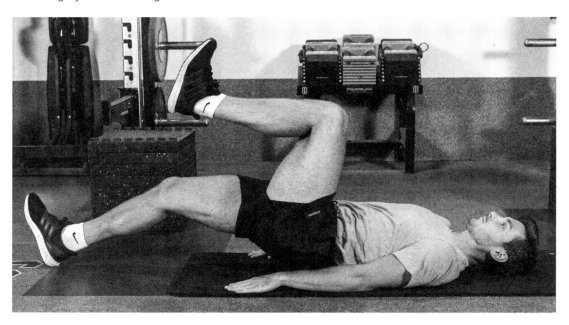

Figure 5.33 Single-leg long bridge isometric with knee drive isometric.

CROSS-CONNECT DEAD BUG (OPPOSITE SIDE)

The ability to stabilize your spine and core muscles is a foundational characteristic of athletes from all walks of life, and is what we're aiming to achieve with this movement.

HOW TO PERFORM

- Start by lying flat on your back on the floor.
- Position both knees above your hips and keep both arms straight above your chest so that your fingers are reaching up toward the ceiling.
- Now bring your left elbow and your right knee together so that they meet in the middle. If you're unable to get your elbow and knee close enough to touch, use a yoga block in between to make it work.
- The last component is to reach your right arm straight out behind your head and straighten out your left leg in front of you.
- Maintain that isometric (hold) position for the prescribed amount of time, switch sides, and repeat.

PERFORMANCE TIPS FOR SUCCESS

- Challenge your core strength and stability with this unique exercise that works on maintaining an isometric (hold) position.
- Focus on making a strong connection with the opposite elbow and knee; drive them into each other to challenge your core muscles.

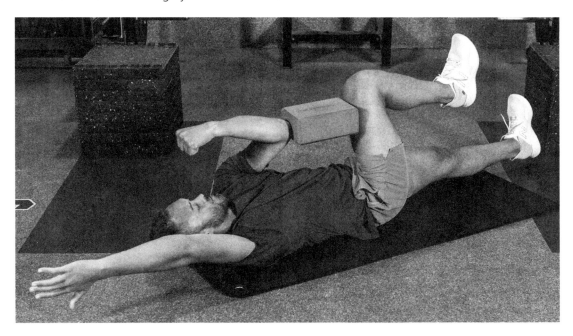

Figure 5.34 Cross-connect dead bug (opposite side).

MINI-BAND STORK

Athletes will dominate life and sports when they master single-leg strength and stability, which is what you'll develop when performing this exercise.

HOW TO PERFORM

- Place a mini-band around both legs just above both knees.
- Keeping your feet together on the floor, sink down low toward the floor by bending your knees and hips.
- From here, balance on one foot and lift the other foot just slightly off the floor.
- Raise the freestanding leg out toward the side as far as you can go without allowing the rest of your body to move.
- Hold that position for the prescribed amount of time, switch sides, and repeat.

PERFORMANCE TIPS FOR SUCCESS

- Develop single-leg strength and stability while strengthening your glutes and lateral hip muscles with this exercise.

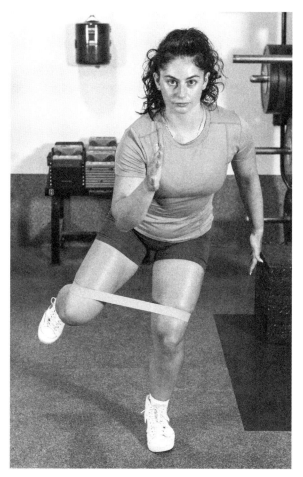

Figure 5.35 Mini-band stork.

WALL BENT-KNEE SINGLE-LEG HEEL RAISE ISOMETRIC

You'll benefit from this exercise by improving muscular strength and endurance in your lower leg and calf muscles, an often-neglected area of the body. This exercise, in particular, targets the soleus muscle of the lower leg.

HOW TO PERFORM

- Stand in front of a wall at arm's length, bend both knees slightly, and lower roughly a quarter of the way down into a squat.
- Keep both arms straight with your hands pressed forward into the wall at shoulder height.
- Take a couple of small steps back so that your body, from head to heels, is at a 45-degree angle to the wall when viewed from the side.
- From here, bend your right knee so that your right foot is behind you and off the floor. Keep your left foot flat on the floor.
- Without letting any other part of your body move, raise your left heel as high as possible up and away from the floor without letting your left ankle roll out to either side.
- Once you've reached this high point, hold this position for the prescribed amount of time. When you're done, switch sides and repeat.

PERFORMANCE TIPS FOR SUCCESS

- This warm-up exercise will help improve the muscular strength and endurance in your calves, in addition to improving the strength and durability of your Achilles tendon.
- Focus on raising your heel as high as possible while avoiding any rolling motion at the ankle.

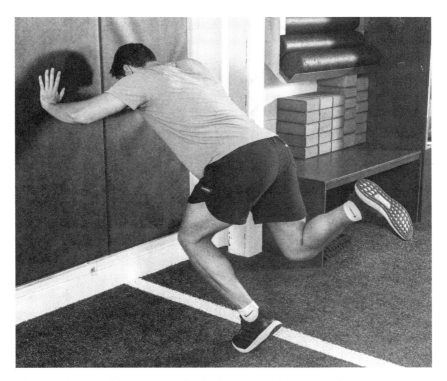

Figure 5.36   Wall bent-knee single-leg heel raise isometric.

ALTERNATING YOGA PLEX TO YOGA PIKE

This is a great catch-all warm-up exercise that targets your entire body from a mobility and flexibility standpoint. Improve full-body mobility and flexibility, in addition to coordination from step to step.

HOW TO PERFORM

- Place your hands on a box or bench at roughly knee height.
- Step both feet back behind you so that your body is in the top position of a push-up.
- Step your left foot forward, place it flat on the floor, and bend your left knee.
- Allow the right knee to rest on the floor.
- Starting from the front, raise your right arm up and around toward the back in a circular motion while your eyes, head, and neck follow. Perform this circular motion all the way through and return to the starting position.
- Step back out into the top of a push-up position and perform the same sequence on the opposite side.
- Step back out to the top of a push-up position again and perform a downward-dog motion, otherwise known as a yoga pike.
- Drive your hands down into the floor and push your hips up toward the sky.
- At the same time, attempt to get both heels close to the floor.
- That entire sequence equals one rep. Complete the prescribed number of reps.

PERFORMANCE TIPS FOR SUCCESS

- The way most athletes go wrong is lacking intent and purpose when performing this exercise. Be sure to dial in the finer details of creating the circular motion and have your eyes, head, and neck follow along throughout this pattern.
- It's important to really think about the muscles you are using—the quadriceps, hamstrings, groin (inner thigh), and shoulder muscles—to truly strengthen these areas.

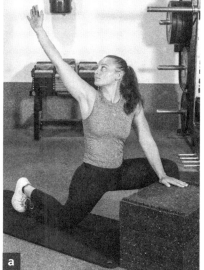 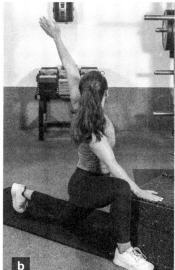 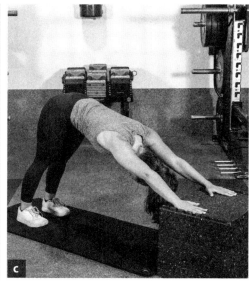

Figure 5.37 Alternating yoga plex to yoga pike: *(a)* left foot forward, right arm circle, *(b)* right foot forward, left arm circle, and *(c)* yoga pike (downward dog).

WALKING INCHWORM

This full-body warm-up exercise is an excellent choice to improve mobility and flexibility in your lower and upper body.

HOW TO PERFORM

- Set yourself up in the top of a push-up position.
- Keep both arms and both legs straight the entire time.
- Slowly inch your toes forward toward your hands while raising your hips toward the sky.
- Once you've moved as far forward as possible while keeping both arms and legs straight, stop the motion in your ankles and then begin that same exact motion with your hands.
- Continue this sequence for all of the prescribed reps or yards.

PERFORMANCE TIPS FOR SUCCESS

- Add this warm-up exercise into the rotation any time you're feeling stiff in your hamstrings, back, or shoulders.
- Keep both arms and both legs straight to enhance your overall range of motion.

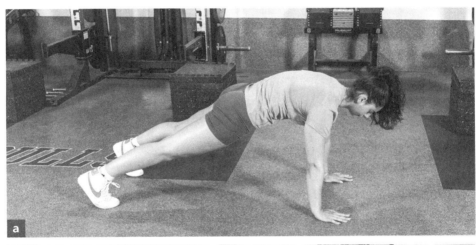
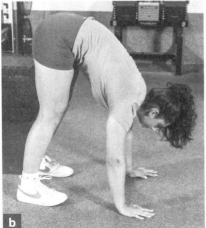
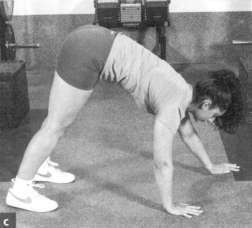

Figure 5.38 Walking inchworm: *(a)* push-up position, *(b)* inch toes toward hands, hips lifted, and *(c)* inch hands forward to return to push-up position.

HINGE TO SQUAT WITH ALTERNATING ROTATION

This exercise allows you to warm up the hamstrings, quadriceps, adductors (inner thigh muscles), ankles, shoulders, and mid-to-upper back region (thoracic spine). Being able to address all these areas with one movement is always a plus!

HOW TO PERFORM

- Stand with your feet slightly wider than hip-width apart.
- Slightly bend your hips and knees while reaching your hands down toward your feet. If you're able to do so, clamp your fingers underneath your toes. If you can't get down that far, clasp the front of your lower legs just above your feet instead.
- Keep your arms between your legs as you pull your butt down and hold the bottom position of the squat with a proud chest. Make sure that I can see the logo on your shirt when you're holding that bottom position.
- Rotate your hand up toward the right and follow it with your eyes.
- Return to the bottom position and complete that sequence on the left side.
- Shoot your hips up and stand back up into the starting position.
- That equals one rep. Complete the prescribed number of reps.

PERFORMANCE TIPS FOR SUCCESS

- In this exercise, you'll improve full-body joint mobility and tissue flexibility. Be sure to move through each step of the sequence at a fluid and controlled pace.
- It's important to really think about the muscles you are using—the quadriceps, hamstrings, groin (inner thigh) region, and shoulders—to truly strengthen these areas.

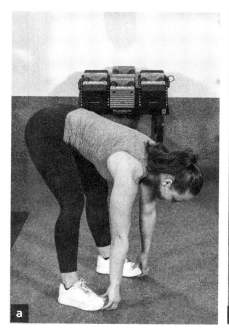
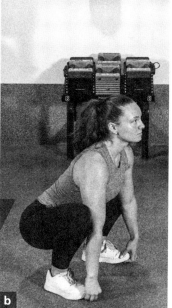
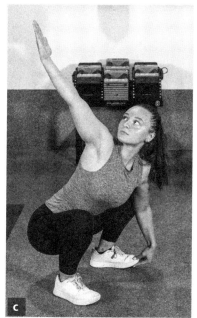

Figure 5.39 Hinge to squat with alternating rotation: *(a)* hip hinge with fingers under toes, *(b)* squat to bottom position, and *(c)* rotate hand up to right side.

WALL LINEAR DOUBLE EXCHANGE

The wall linear double exchange is a classic warm-up exercise to help you develop sprinting mechanics and athletic skills. This exercise will also help you improve the ability to rapidly switch leg positions, an explosive action that occurs in sprinting and running.

HOW TO PERFORM

- Stand in front of a wall with both arms straight and both hands pressed forward into the wall at shoulder height.
- Take a couple of steps back so that your body, from head to heels, is at a 45-degree angle to the wall when viewed from the side.
- From here, prop both heels up off the floor and raise your right knee up toward your chest.
- Keep a tall body from head to heels and keep the toes of your right foot pointing up.
- Without letting any other part of your body move, switch the positions of your legs in a rapid and explosive manner, then switch them back to their starting position again in a rapid and explosive manner.
- There should be no pause or downtime between these two rapid actions of the lower body.

PERFORMANCE TIPS FOR SUCCESS

- One primary coaching tip: Move as fast as possible during each leg action. This sounds easy, but is surprisingly challenging. It helps you develop elite speed and quickness when applied in training.
- When performing this exercise, think about how powerful and bouncy your feet are when you're sprinting. Apply that same level of power and bounciness with your feet when performing this drill for maximum gains in athleticism!

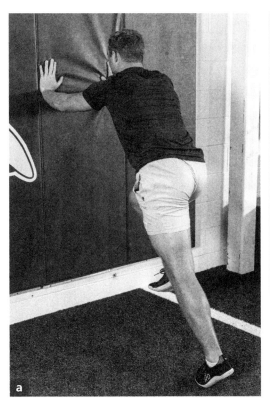 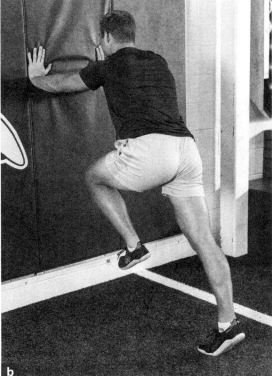

Figure 5.40 Wall linear double exchange: *(a)* start position and *(b)* lift knee.

WALKING ALTERNATING HAMSTRING SCOOP

Develop mobility in your hips and flexibility in your hamstrings by performing this dynamic warm-up exercise.

HOW TO PERFORM

- Stand with your feet roughly hip-width apart.
- Now slightly step your right foot forward so the heel of your right foot is in line with the toes of your left foot.
- Drive your right heel down into the floor, point the toes of your right foot up toward the ceiling, hinge your hips back, and perform a scooping motion with your arms.
- Come back up to the top, take a slight step forward with your left foot, and complete the same sequence on the other side.
- Continue alternating sides until all reps are complete.

PERFORMANCE TIPS FOR SUCCESS

- This warm-up exercise promotes hip joint mobility and hamstring flexibility.
- When performing the exercise, really hinge your hips back to enhance your overall hamstring flexibility and hip mobility.

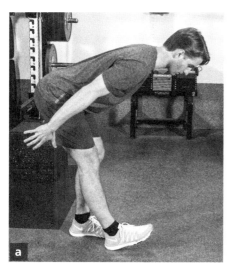 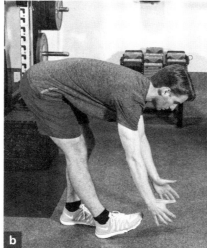 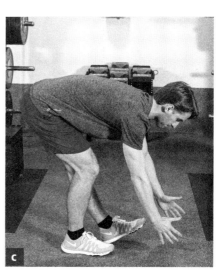

Figure 5.41 Walking alternating hamstring scoop: *(a)* start position, *(b)* right foot, and *(c)* left foot.

Warm-Up Exercises 83

WALKING ALTERNATING SPIDERMAN TO REACH AND ROTATE

This exercise takes the traditional stationary version of the alternating Spiderman and adds a dynamic element—you're moving across a distance while still targeting full-body mobility and flexibility. You're also building rotational mobility through your thoracic spine and shoulders with the reach and rotate element.

HOW TO PERFORM

- Start with your body in the top of a push-up position.
- Hike your right foot up toward the front and place it on the floor just outside your right hand.
- Leaving your left hand on the floor, reach your right hand out toward the left side and allow your entire spine and head to turn with it.
- Rotate your right hand up toward the ceiling and follow it with your eyes so that your entire spine rotates as well.
- Return your right hand to the ground, stay low, and crawl forward so that you're able to hike your left foot up toward the front and place it on the floor just outside your left hand.
- Complete the same sequence on the other side.

PERFORMANCE TIPS FOR SUCCESS

- As an athlete, you need full-body mobility and flexibility, which is exactly what you'll get by performing this exercise.
- Keep an eye on your pace and move fluidly without rushing through any component.

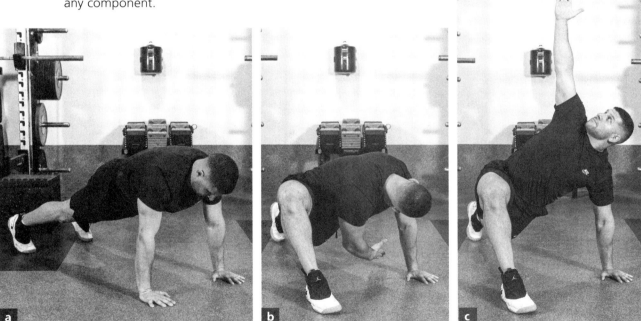

Figure 5.42 Walking alternating Spiderman to reach and rotate: *(a)* start position, *(b)* right foot forward, and *(c)* right hand up to ceiling.

DOUBLE LATERAL SHUFFLE WITH ALTERNATING LATERAL SQUAT

This exercise combines dynamic movement with coordination, mobility, and flexibility in the lower body. The bonus is that you'll be able to move within the frontal plane (side-to-side) to prepare your hip joints and groin muscles for athletic skill development.

HOW TO PERFORM

- Position your body in an athletic stance, with a slight bend in your knees and hips, active hands down by your sides ready to move, chest aiming forward, and eyes alert.
- From here, begin to shuffle laterally toward your left.
- Once you have completed two lateral shuffles to the left, sink down into a lateral squat on your left side and then again on your right side.
- That entire sequence equals one rep.
- Complete all of the prescribed reps or yards on one side, switch sides, and repeat.

PERFORMANCE TIPS FOR SUCCESS

- Performing this exercise will improve your dynamic movement and coordination in the frontal plane of motion, in addition to improving hip joint mobility and groin muscle flexibility.
- It's important to really think about the muscles you are using—the groin (inner thigh) region and shoulders—to truly strengthen these areas.

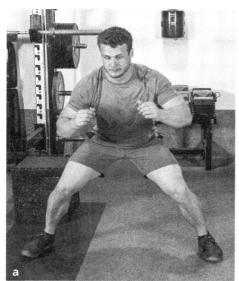 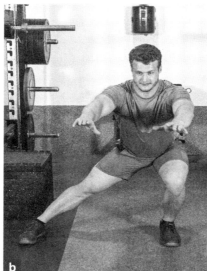 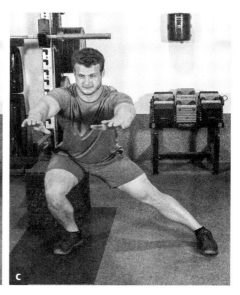

Figure 5.43 Double lateral shuffle with alternating lateral squat: *(a)* shuffle laterally, *(b)* lateral squat to left side, and *(c)* lateral squat to right side.

BACKWARD REACH RUN

Forward running and sprinting are among the most common movements in sports, life, and athletics. However, well-rounded athletes have a large movement menu, meaning that they are proficient movers in all planes of motion and a variety of directions.

HOW TO PERFORM

- Place your feet hip-width apart on the floor, sit your hips down and back, and lean your chest forward slightly.
- Avoid standing up or getting tall. Keep your chest forward slightly the entire time and, once you begin the running component, keep your hips down and behind your head.
- All of this will allow you to evenly balance your weight during the backward running motion.
- From here, begin to run backward and reach your foot back behind you during each rep.
- This will likely feel unnatural, so take your time by working at lower speeds until you've grasped the concept.
- Lastly, allow your arms to become involved in the same way they would if you were running forward.
- Perform for the prescribed amount of distance.

PERFORMANCE TIPS FOR SUCCESS

- This warm-up exercise will improve your ability to run backward, in addition to enhancing your ability to reach your leg back while evenly distributing your entire body weight. These are pieces of the athleticism puzzle and will improve your overall health and performance.
- It's important to really think about the muscles you are using—the hamstrings and glutes—to truly strengthen these areas.

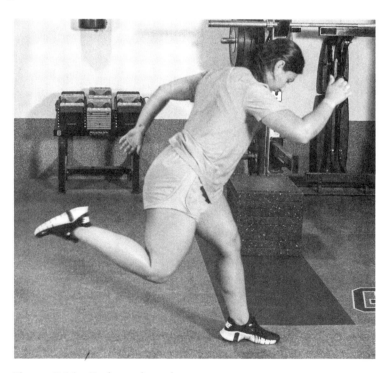

Figure 5.44 Backward reach run.

SEGMENTAL CAT-COW

Increase mobility in your entire spine with a strong emphasis on a slow pace by moving through one segment at a time.

HOW TO PERFORM

- Think of your spine as a series of little segments from your hips to your head.
- With that in mind, the goal is to move at a pace equivalent to a snail attempting to travel uphill on a river of molasses. Slow. *Really* slow. Move deliberately from one segment to the next segment, which takes a ton of focus.
- Start by making your way down to the floor in a quadruped position, with your hands directly under your shoulders and your knees directly under your hips.
- From here, the only motion that should occur is in your mid-to-upper back area (thoracic spine) to increase the overall mobility in that region.
- Create a large arch in your spine from your head all the way down toward your hips.
- In a slow and controlled manner, hollow out your spine one segment at a time from your head to your hips.

PERFORMANCE TIPS FOR SUCCESS

- Use this warm-up exercise to loosen up your entire spine prior to your training session.
- Move at a slower pace than you think you need to. Motion at each segment of your spine must be slow and deliberate to reap the benefits.

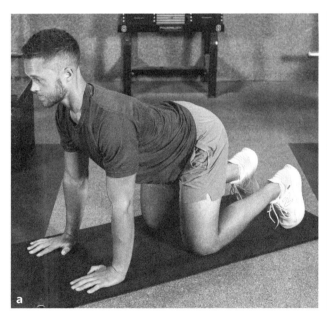 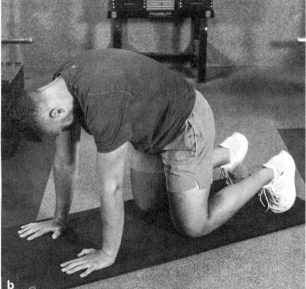

Figure 5.45 Segmental cat-cow: *(a)* cow and *(b)* cat.

BRIDGE ISOMETRIC WITH ALTERNATING REACH

Develop stability in your hips, strength in your hamstrings and glutes, and mobility through your thoracic (mid-to-upper) spine and shoulders.

HOW TO PERFORM

- Lie down on the floor with your back flat and knees bent, feet flat on the floor.
- Raise your hips into a bridge and hold them there.
- Bend both elbows, drive your left elbow down into the floor next to your left ribcage, and reach up and over with your right arm toward the opposite (left) side as far as you can. Then return the arm to its starting position.
- Continue performing this motion in an alternating fashion until all reps are complete.

PERFORMANCE TIPS FOR SUCCESS

- Here you will improve lower body stability and upper body mobility. Reach up and over as far as you can to improve thoracic (mid-to-upper) spine mobility.
- When performing this exercise, it's important to really think about the muscles you are using—the hamstrings, glutes, and shoulders—to truly strengthen these areas.

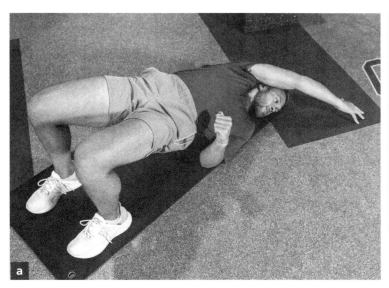
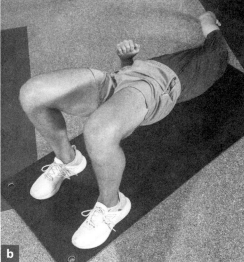

Figure 5.46 Bridge isometric with alternating reach: *(a)* right hand reach and *(b)* left hand reach.

CATCHER ROCKBACK WITH TOE TURN

As with the traditional catcher rockback warm-up exercise, you'll be able to improve hip mobility and adductor flexibility. However, with the addition of the toe turn, you'll be able to do so in a greater range of motion.

HOW TO PERFORM

- Start on the floor with your left knee down, right leg straight, and right foot flat.
- Keep a straight line from your left knee all the way to your right foot.
- Place both hands in front of you on the floor.
- Use your hands to help push your hips back. Allow the right foot to rotate up and back at the same time.
- Return the hips forward to the starting position while rotating the right foot down and forward.
- Perform all reps on the right side, switch sides, and repeat.

PERFORMANCE TIPS FOR SUCCESS

- This is a great warm-up exercise that helps you improve hip joint mobility and adductor muscle flexibility.
- Keep the motion fluid and controlled and avoid flying through your reps too quickly.

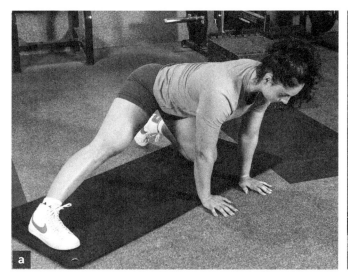 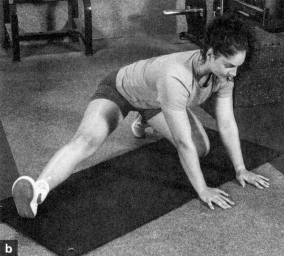

Figure 5.47 Catcher rockback with toe turn: *(a)* start position and *(b)* push hips back.

FLOOR BENT-KNEE COPENHAGEN PLANK WITH LIFTOFF

Most people ignore the muscles of the inner thigh and groin region, otherwise known as the adductor muscles. When you do that, you lose out on an area that can strengthen and support the hip and knee—key for high-performing athletes. Use this exercise to develop strong and healthy adductors.

HOW TO PERFORM

- Set yourself up on the floor by lying on your right side.
- Bend your right knee to roughly 90 degrees so that your right foot is out in front of you, but keep it rested on the floor for now.
- Bend your left knee to roughly 90 degrees so that your left foot is behind you.
- Place your (bottom) right elbow directly under your right shoulder and raise your right side and hip away from the floor as if you were performing a traditional side plank. Reach your top (left) hand up toward the ceiling with a clenched fist for added stability, pressing the inside of your left knee down into either the floor or a pad for comfort.
- Lift your right knee up and off the floor as high as you can go, then lower it back down.
- Complete all liftoff reps based on what the training program calls for, switch sides, and repeat.

PERFORMANCE TIPS FOR SUCCESS

- The best athletes in the world understand the importance of building body armor in every aspect of their body. This type of exercise doesn't seem like it's doing much, but is truly a game changer for hip and knee durability.
- Move with precision and intent to squeeze the most value out of the exercise.

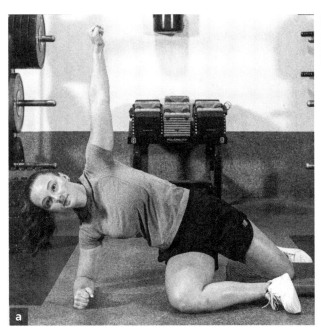 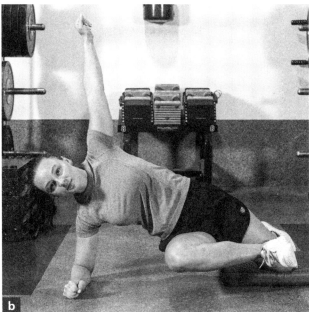

Figure 5.48 Floor bent-knee Copenhagen plank with liftoff: *(a)* Copenhagen plank and *(b)* lift knee.

ALTERNATING SPIDERMAN TO STATIONARY INCHWORM

This exercise helps you target every aspect of your body from head to toe from a mobility and flexibility standpoint.

HOW TO PERFORM

- Start with your body in the top of a push-up position.
- Hike your right foot up toward the front and place it on the floor just outside your right hand.
- Leaving your left hand on the floor, rotate your right hand up toward the ceiling and follow it with your eyes so that your entire spine rotates as well.
- Return your right hand to the floor and repeat this sequence on the other side.
- Keeping both arms and both legs straight, slowly inch your toes forward toward your hands while raising your hips toward the sky.
- Once you have moved as far forward as possible while continuing to keep both arms and legs straight, inch your toes back to the starting position.
- This entire sequence equals one rep. Complete all the prescribed reps.

PERFORMANCE TIPS FOR SUCCESS

- This is an excellent full-body warm-up exercise that will prepare you for an upcoming training session.
- Dial in the finer details to squeeze out every ounce of value!

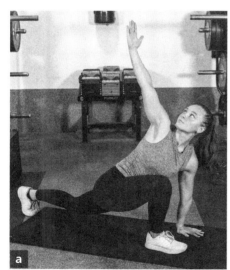 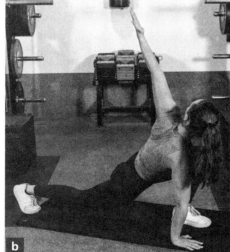 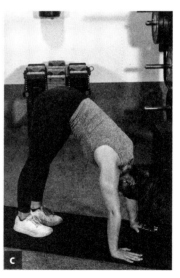

Figure 5.49 Alternating Spiderman to stationary inchworm: *(a)* Spiderman on right side, *(b)* Spiderman on left side, and *(c)* inchworm.

Warm-Up Exercises **91**

REAR FOOT ELEVATED SPLIT SQUAT ISOMETRIC

An isometric (hold) exercise gives you the opportunity to develop strength and stability in specific positions that will transfer to sports and recreational activities. Use this exercise to strengthen the knees and quadriceps, in addition to improving hip joint mobility, hip flexor flexibility, and quadriceps flexibility.

HOW TO PERFORM

- Take a knee down on the floor.
- Keep the front foot flat and only the toes of the rear foot in contact with the floor.
- Ensure that your legs remain roughly hip-width apart for added stability.
- Elevate your rear knee off the floor so that it's hovering by a few inches and the laces of that foot are resting on a sturdy surface at roughly knee height (e.g., bench, split squat bench).
- With a tall torso, hold this position for the prescribed amount of time, switch sides, and repeat.

PERFORMANCE TIPS FOR SUCCESS

- When performing this warm-up exercise, focus on the position you are holding and fight hard to maintain it. This exercise will strengthen your knees and quadriceps, in addition to improving your hip joint mobility, hip flexor flexibility, and quadriceps flexibility.
- Really think about the muscles you are using—the quadriceps, hip flexors, hamstrings, and glutes—to truly strengthen these areas.

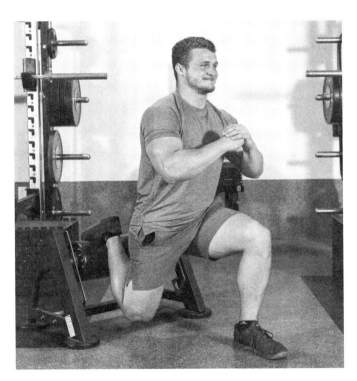

Figure 5.50 Rear foot elevated split squat isometric.

KB GOBLET KANG SQUAT

The body weight version of the Kang squat allows you to improve hip mobility, ankle mobility, adductor flexibility, and hamstring flexibility. With a kettlebell added into the mix, you'll be able to get even lower with more range of motion.

HOW TO PERFORM

- With your feet on the floor roughly hip-width apart, hold a kettlebell tight to your chest with both hands as if you're holding a large bowl.
- Keeping the kettlebell in this position the entire time, hinge your hips back behind you (imagine you're attempting to close a door with your butt).
- Squat down the remainder of the way to the bottom position.
- Perform the hip hinge motion again, and then finally, stand back up to the top.

PERFORMANCE TIPS FOR SUCCESS

- By performing this catch-all warm-up exercise, you'll improve lower-body mobility in your hip and ankle joints, in addition to flexibility in your adductor and hamstring muscles.
- It's important to really think about the muscles you are using—the quadriceps, hamstrings, and groin (inner thigh) muscles—to truly strengthen these areas.

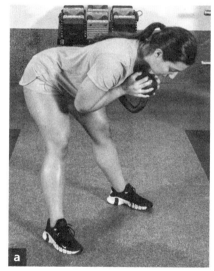 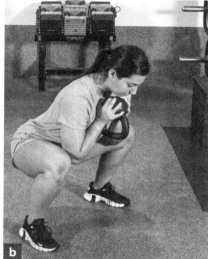 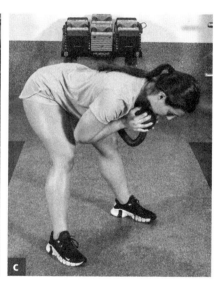

Figure 5.51 KB goblet Kang squat: *(a)* start position, *(b)* squat, and *(c)* hip hinge.

INTENSIVE POGO HOP

Pogo hops are among the lowest-hanging fruit in the development of athleticism, since this exercise allows your calves and ankles to produce and absorb force.

HOW TO PERFORM

- When you perform any type of pogo hop with an intensive intent (i.e., generating force at a high intensity), the goal is to use maximal effort and develop power through high impact and low volume.
- The purpose of this exercise is to increase force output of the calf muscles and ankle joints, in addition to becoming more explosive through high ground-reaction forces and high speeds.
- Stand tall with your feet hip-width apart on the floor.
- Keep your entire body stiff and straight, and allow only your ankle joints to move up and down.
- With both feet, use the intensive approach while performing the pogo hop in an up-and-down motion for maximum height for the prescribed number of reps or amount of time.

PERFORMANCE TIPS FOR SUCCESS

- When you perform this warm-up exercise, you'll improve both force production (jumping) and force absorption (landing) through the ankle joints and calf muscles.
- Really think about the muscles you are using—the calves—to truly strengthen this area.

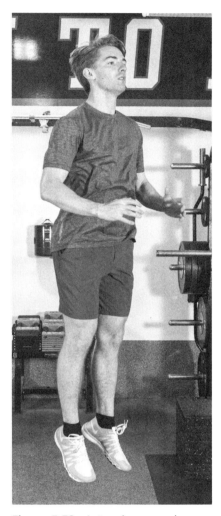

Figure 5.52 Intensive pogo hop.

DROP SKATER SQUAT TO STICK

The athletic skills of force absorption and deceleration are often overlooked in training for athletic performance yet are just as important as their direct counterparts (force production and acceleration). This exercise helps you become a more well-rounded athlete by developing deceleration skills.

HOW TO PERFORM

- Stand tall on one foot. In this movement, you'll begin on one leg and finish on one leg.
- Reach both hands up high toward the ceiling while simultaneously raising your bottom heel off the floor, then rapidly drop down as fast as you can into the bottom position of a skater squat.
- Your hands should end up behind you at the bottom, where you will deliberately hold that position for a moment.
- The goal here is to stop on a dime (i.e., freeze your body) and absorb all of that force, which will improve your ability to decelerate in sports and athletics.

PERFORMANCE TIPS FOR SUCCESS

- Here you'll work hard to improve the ability to absorb force, which will help you to become a more durable and resilient athlete.

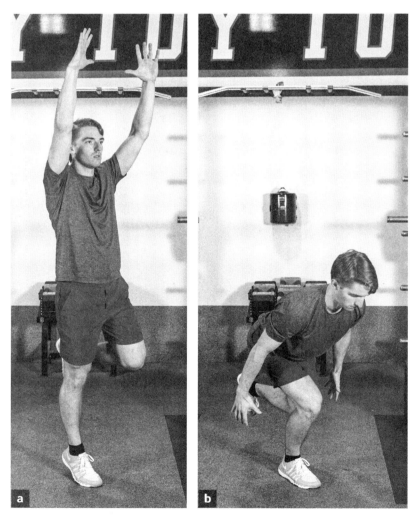

Figure 5.53 Drop skater squat to stick: *(a)* start position and *(b)* skater squat.

LATERAL CROSSOVER SKIP

Skipping is a foundational movement in elite athleticism. If you can master a basic exercise like this one, you'll be able to build off it and improve your overall athletic skills. The added benefit here is that you'll be able to skip during the lower-body crossover motion, which occurs in a variety of sport-related movements.

HOW TO PERFORM

- The key here is to move in a fluid yet robotic fashion while traveling to the side (laterally) during a crossover skip.
- This exercise helps you build good mechanics for any type of lower-body crossover motion that occurs in competitive athletics and recreational sports.
- Remain as efficient as possible with your movement.
- When going through the lateral crossover skip, avoid the temptation to jump, and instead, cross the rear leg over in front of the lead leg, strike the rear foot down hard, and remain tall. This sequence will propel your body up and away from the floor in the direction you're traveling.
- Move your arms opposite from the motion occurring in your legs. If your left knee is up, your right arm should be up, and vice versa.
- Follow this entire sequence for the prescribed number of reps or distance in one direction, switch sides, and repeat.

PERFORMANCE TIPS FOR SUCCESS

- This warm-up exercise will help you improve in fundamental frontal plane mechanics by developing the ability to strike the ground with force as you travel up and away laterally while also enhancing your ability to cross over with your legs.
- When performing this exercise, really think about the muscles you are using—the lateral hips, glutes, and groin (inner thigh) region—to truly strengthen these areas.

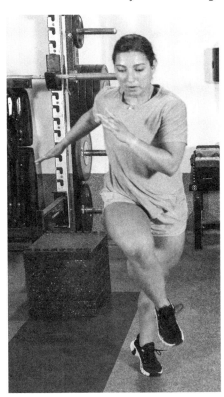

Figure 5.54 Lateral crossover skip.

SINGLE-LEG LONG BRIDGE ISOMETRIC WITH POWER SWITCH

Hamstring and hip flexor muscles that can work in a quick and explosive manner set you up for success in sports, athletics, and life. Lock in with this warm-up exercise to excel in these areas.

HOW TO PERFORM

- Lie flat on your back with both legs long at roughly hip-width apart and your palms flat on the floor at the sides of your pockets.
- Slightly bend both knees at roughly 5 to 10 degrees of knee flexion, drive both heels down into the floor, and raise your butt up off the floor. Then drive one knee up toward your chest with the toes of that foot aiming up toward your head.
- You'll notice that your hips won't be able to raise very high above the floor, but you'll immediately feel your hamstrings working hard. That's exactly what we want.
- The final step is to perform a rapid power switch in which your legs explosively switch positions while the rest of your body remains relatively still.
- This is much more challenging than it seems, so ease into it and, once you're feeling primed and ready, go full throttle.

PERFORMANCE TIPS FOR SUCCESS

- By performing this warm-up exercise, you'll develop a strong and powerful lower body, especially in the hamstrings and hip flexors.
- Focus on how fast and powerfully you can move your lower body. Imagine how fast and powerful you feel with your lower body when you're sprinting. Use that same level of intent with your lower body in this exercise to improve your overall athleticism!

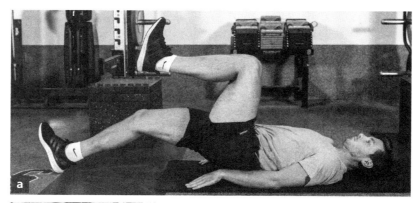

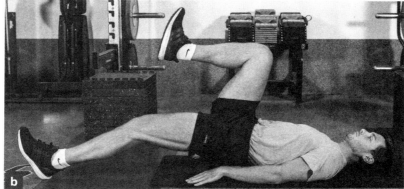

Figure 5.55 Single-leg long bridge isometric with power switch: *(a)* left knee and *(b)* right knee.

WALL PRESS WITH SINGLE-LEG LOWER

This movement falls under the anti-extension core strength category, which enables you to develop a strong and stable mid-section. You'll also benefit from hip flexor strengthening.

HOW TO PERFORM

- Lie flat on your back on the floor with a wall directly behind you by just a few inches.
- Press both hands directly back into the wall to create stability in the trunk.
- From here, raise both legs straight up above your hips so that the bottoms of both feet are aiming up toward the ceiling.
- Lower one leg down toward the floor. At the bottom, avoid actually touching the floor, and instead, just lower down until you're close to it.
- Raise the leg back up to the top position.
- Complete all reps on one side, switch sides, and repeat.

PERFORMANCE TIPS FOR SUCCESS

- You'll develop a strong and stable trunk with this core-strengthening exercise.
- Avoid any sort of low back arch or ribcage flare.

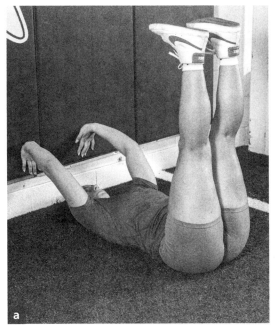 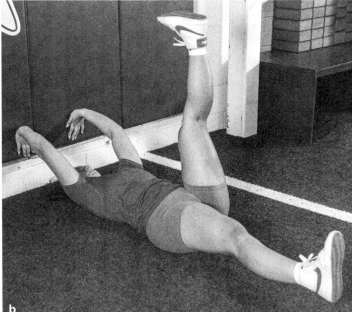

Figure 5.56 Wall press with single-leg lower: *(a)* legs up and *(b)* lower one leg.

MINI-BAND STORK WITH CLAM LIFT

Athletes will dominate life and sports when they master single-leg strength and stability, which is what you'll build when you perform this exercise.

HOW TO PERFORM

- Place a mini-band around both legs just above both knees.
- Keeping your feet together on the floor, sink down toward the floor by bending your knees and hips.
- From here, balance on one foot and lift the other foot just slightly off the floor.
- Raise the freestanding leg out toward the side as far as you can go without allowing the rest of your body to move. Once you can't go any further, return that leg to the starting position.
- Perform all reps on one side, switch sides, and repeat.

PERFORMANCE TIPS FOR SUCCESS

- By performing this exercise, you'll be developing single-leg strength and stability while also strengthening your glutes and lateral hip muscles.
- Really think about the muscles you are using—the quadriceps, lateral hips, and glutes—to truly strengthen these areas.

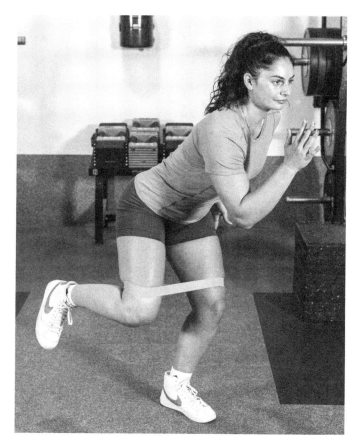

Figure 5.57 Mini-band stork with clam lift.

TEMPO WALL HEEL RAISE (3 SECONDS UP/3 SECONDS ISO/3 SECONDS DOWN)

Develop strength in your calves and ankles with this warm-up exercise, which will aid in your sprinting and multidirectional abilities.

HOW TO PERFORM

- Stand in front of a wall at a slight angle with both arms long, both hands on the wall, and both feet roughly hip-width apart.
- From there, raise your heels up for a 3-second count (concentric), hold the top position for a 3-second count (isometric), and lastly, lower your heels down toward the floor for a 3-second count (eccentric).
- That's one rep. Complete all of the prescribed reps.

PERFORMANCE TIPS FOR SUCCESS

- Most people completely skip calf training and wonder why they run (literally) into lower leg, ankle, and foot issues. As an athlete looking to stay sharp and powerful, you should always keep some sort of calf training like this drill in your warm-up routine.
- When performing this exercise, really think about the muscles you are using—the calves—to truly strengthen this area.

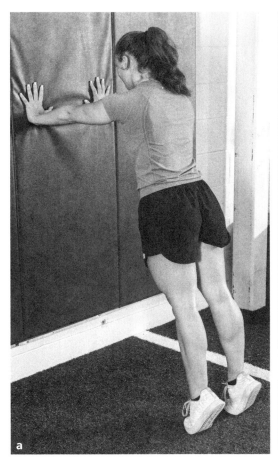
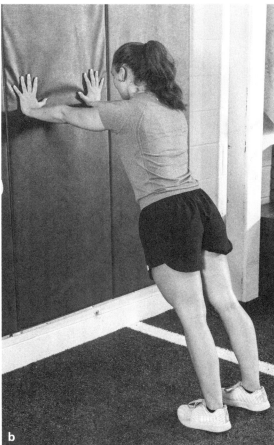

Figure 5.58 Tempo wall heel raise: *(a)* heels up and *(b)* heels down.

HAND-SUPPORTED ALTERNATING REVERSE LUNGE WITH SINGLE-ARM OVERHEAD REACH

Performing this full-body exercise will help to warm up your upper and lower body prior to strength training and sport participation.

HOW TO PERFORM

- Set both hands on a box between knee and hip height for support.
- While standing in front of the box with your feet a few inches from it, step your right foot back into the reverse lunge pattern while reaching your right hand straight up toward the ceiling.
- Return to the top position and perform that exact same sequence on the left side.
- Complete all of the prescribed reps in this alternating sequence.

PERFORMANCE TIPS FOR SUCCESS

- Not only will this movement help with balance, stability, and coordination, it's also a great way to add more extension in your hips, back, and shoulders—be sure to reach up as high as possible during each rep.
- It's important to really think about the muscles you are using—the quadriceps, hamstrings, glutes, and shoulders—to truly strengthen these areas.

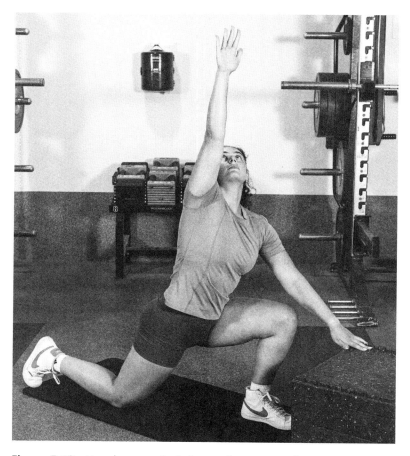

Figure 5.59 Hand-supported alternating reverse lunge with single-arm overhead reach.

Warm-Up Exercises **101**

WALKING INCHWORM TO PUSH-UP

Warm up your hamstrings, calves, core muscles, and shoulders with this combo lower- and upper-body exercise.

HOW TO PERFORM

- Maintain straight arms and legs the entire time here.
- Start out in the top position of a push-up, then inch your toes up toward your fingers.
- Once you reach a point where your knees want to bend, stop there and begin inching your fingers out in front of you until you're back in the top position of a push-up.
- Perform one push-up with perfect technique, avoiding any sort of arch in your back or sagging in your hips.
- That equals one rep. Complete all of the prescribed reps.

PERFORMANCE TIPS FOR SUCCESS

- This advanced warm-up exercise targets your lower and upper body in one movement. Move with intent and precision throughout each component of the exercise for maximum results.
- It's important to really think about the muscles you are using—the hamstrings, glutes, core, and shoulders—to truly strengthen these areas.

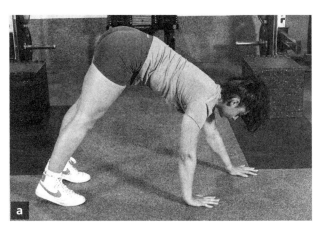
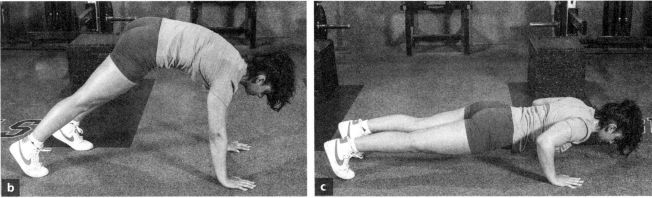

Figure 5.60 Walking inchworm to push-up: *(a)* inch toes forward, *(b)* inch fingers forward, and *(c)* push-up.

HINGE TO SQUAT ISOMETRIC WITH ALTERNATING ROTATION

This exercise allows you to warm up the hamstrings, quadriceps, adductors (inner thigh muscles), ankles, shoulders, and mid-to-upper back region (thoracic spine). Being able to address all of these areas with one movement is always a plus in training!

HOW TO PERFORM

- Stand with your feet slightly wider than hip-width apart.
- Slightly bend your hips and knees while reaching your hands down toward your feet.
- If you're able to do so, clamp your fingers underneath your toes. If you can't get down that far, clasp the front aspect of your lower legs just above your feet instead.
- Keep your arms in between your legs as you pull your butt down and hold the bottom position of the squat with a proud chest. Make sure that I can see the logo on your shirt when you're holding that bottom position.
- Now rotate your hand up toward the right side and have your eyes follow your hand in the right direction.
- Return to the bottom position and complete the same sequence on the left side.
- Remaining in the bottom position, complete all of the prescribed reps per side.

PERFORMANCE TIPS FOR SUCCESS

- By performing this warm-up exercise, you'll develop full-body joint mobility and tissue flexibility.
- It's important to really think about the muscles you are using—the quadriceps, hamstrings, glutes, groin (inner thigh) region, and shoulders—to truly strengthen these areas.

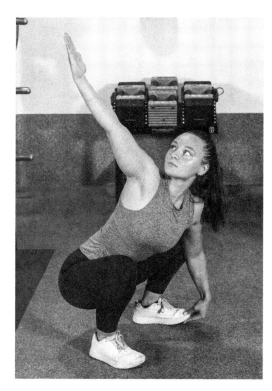

Figure 5.61 Hinge to squat isometric with alternating rotation.

WALL PRESS SINGLE-LEG RDL WITH POWER DRIVE

Athletes tend to skip some of the basic learning steps when it comes to sprinting and acceleration. These mechanics are often the culprit for improper technique and form in sprinting. Use this warm-up exercise to sharpen your first-step speed and sprinting mechanics and become a more powerful athlete.

HOW TO PERFORM

- Start with both hands in front of you placed on a wall.
- Keep a slight bend in your right knee while your right foot remains flat on the floor.
- Leave enough room for your upper body and head to drop down forward as you simultaneously reach your left foot directly behind you.
- Immediately drive your left foot forward and up toward the wall with power and explosiveness.
- Raise the right heel off the floor at the same time.

PERFORMANCE TIPS FOR SUCCESS

- The key here is to move fast! Quickness and explosiveness are traits of some of the best athletes in the world.
- By moving fast, you'll develop the ability to be powerful and explosive with the first step of any sort of sprint or acceleration that you'll encounter in sports and in life.

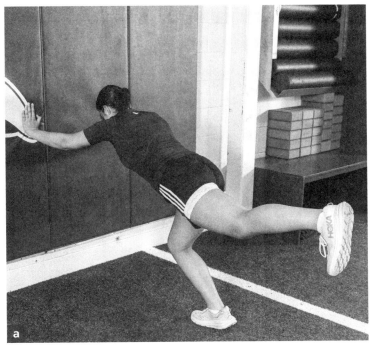
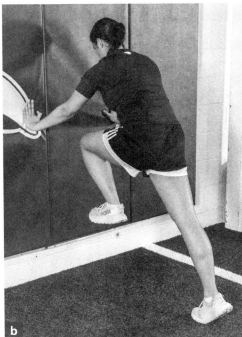

Figure 5.62 Wall press single-leg RDL with power drive: *(a)* single-leg RDL and *(b)* drive leg forward.

REVERSE WALKING SINGLE-LEG RDL

Single-leg strength and stability are characteristics of some of the best athletes in the world—perform this drill and you can reap the same benefits!

HOW TO PERFORM

- Stand tall with both feet roughly hip-width apart.
- Leaving your right foot on the floor with a slight bend in your right knee, reach your left foot back behind you and simultaneously lower your chest.
- From a side view, your entire body from the top of your head to the bottom of your left heel should be parallel with the floor.
- Return to the top position and reach your left foot slightly behind you; this is the reverse walking component.
- Switch sides and repeat that entire sequence.

PERFORMANCE TIPS FOR SUCCESS

- When you perform it correctly with precision and intent, you'll be able to feel this warm-up exercise in the hamstrings and glutes. It will challenge your single-leg stability while also warming up the posterior chain of your lower body.
- Really think about the muscles you are using—the hamstrings and glutes—to truly strengthen these areas.

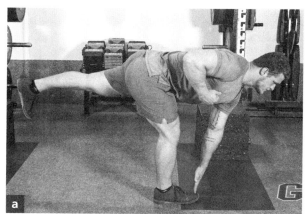 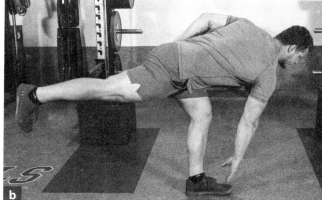

Figure 5.63 Reverse walking single-leg RDL.

Warm-Up Exercises **105**

WALKING ALTERNATING SPIDERMAN TO YOGA PUSH-UP

Use this warm-up exercise as a catch-all movement that efficiently targets multiple joints and muscles in the body.

HOW TO PERFORM

- Start out with your body in the top of a push-up position.
- Hike your left foot up toward the front and place it on the floor just outside your right hand.
- Leaving your right hand down on the floor, rotate your left hand up toward the ceiling and follow it with your eyes so that your entire spine rotates as well.
- Return your hand to the floor and then repeat the sequence on the other side.
- Lower your body down into the bottom portion of a push-up and then simultaneously perform all of the following: Push your body back up toward the ceiling, drive your hips up high, shoot your head forward toward the floor and through your arms, and lower your heels as close to the floor as possible.
- This entire sequence is known as a downward dog.
- That entire sequence is one rep. Complete all of the prescribed reps.

PERFORMANCE TIPS FOR SUCCESS

- This is the ultimate full-body mobility and flexibility exercise that belongs in every warm-up routine!
- Perform this entire warm-up exercise at a fluid and controlled pace to reap all of the benefits.

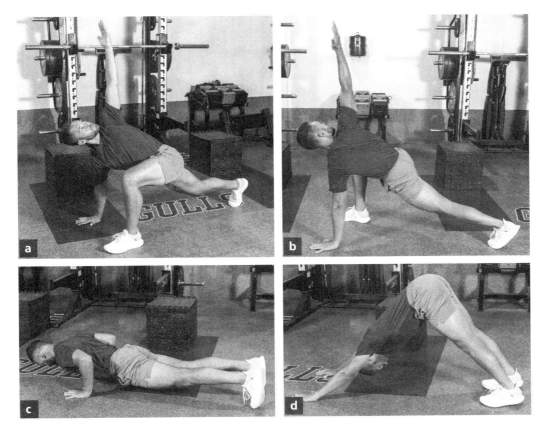

Figure 5.64 Walking alternating Spiderman to yoga push-up: *(a)* Spiderman on left side, *(b)* Spiderman on right side, *(c)* lower into push-up position, and *(d)* downward dog.

5-YARD LATERAL SHUFFLE TO TURN AND 10-YARD SPRINT

The primary quality gained from performing this exercise is the ability to quickly and efficiently change directions from lateral shuffling to sprinting, a movement that occurs frequently in sports and athletics.

HOW TO PERFORM

- Start out in an athletic stance with both knees bent, both hips bent, and a slight forward lean in your trunk.
- Lateral shuffle to the left for 5 yards, immediately turn your hips in the opposite direction of your shuffle (right), and sprint for 10 yards.
- Complete the same sequence on the other side.
- That's one rep per side. Perform all the prescribed reps and sets.

PERFORMANCE TIPS FOR SUCCESS

- When performed correctly, this warm-up exercise will help you learn how to rapidly change directions from shuffling to turning your hips and sprinting in tight spaces.
- In this exercise, think about how a running back would shuffle to the side when trying to avoid getting tackled by a linebacker, and then once evaded, begin sprinting toward the end zone.

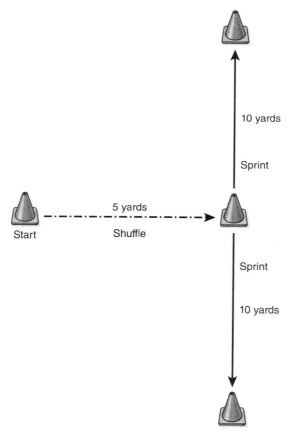

Figure 5.65 5-yard lateral shuffle to turn and 10-yard sprint.

5-YARD BACKPEDAL TO TURN AND 10-YARD SPRINT

The primary quality gained from performing this exercise is the ability to quickly and efficiently change directions from backpedaling to sprinting, a movement that occurs frequently in sports and athletics.

HOW TO PERFORM

- Start out in an athletic stance with both knees bent, both hips bent, and a slight forward lean in your trunk.
- Now backpedal for 5 yards, immediately turn your hips around to continue moving your body in the same direction, and sprint for 10 yards.
- Complete this sequence on the other side.
- That's one rep per side. Perform all of the prescribed reps and sets.

PERFORMANCE TIPS FOR SUCCESS

- When performed correctly, this warm-up exercise will help you learn how to rapidly change directions from backpedaling to turning your hips and sprinting in small spaces.
- In this exercise, think about how a cornerback would backpedal when the wide receiver jumps off of the line of scrimmage after the whistle is blown and the play is live, then use their hips to rapidly change directions and continue sprinting. Use that same type of intent by rapidly turning the hips and sprinting.

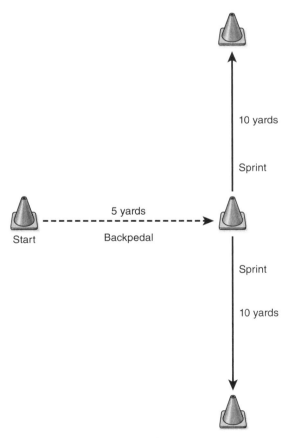

Figure 5.66 5-yard backpedal to turn and 10-yard sprint.

CHAPTER 6

Strength Exercises

When it comes to strength training and resistance exercise, simple is always best. The strength exercises in this book were included to help you cover all the bases of human movement and athletic development. You'll be exposed to all the following movement patterns and exercise types: bilateral squat, unilateral squat, bilateral hip hinge, unilateral hip hinge, bilateral upper body horizontal push, unilateral upper body horizontal push, bilateral upper body horizontal pull, unilateral upper body horizontal pull, bilateral upper body vertical push, unilateral upper body vertical push, bilateral upper body vertical pull, unilateral upper body vertical pull, anti-rotation core strengthening, anti-extension core strengthening, anti-flexion core strengthening, anti-side bend (anti-lateral flexion) core strengthening, locomotion, and carrying. You'll also be exposed to a variety of training equipment, such as dumbbells, barbells, kettlebells, long resistance bands, mini-bands, medicine balls, cable pulley machines, sliders, sleds, physioballs, suspension straps, and more.

Although this book includes a wide variety of exercises and equipment, the key to using them in your training is strategic balance. I use an evidence-based approach to strength training coupled with in-the-trenches coaching and lifting experience spanning two decades. The strength training exercises you'll perform will help you reach your goals through a consistent approach that is sustainable for many years down the road. We've left no stone unturned selecting the best strength training exercises to help you achieve your maximal level of athleticism, and enjoy the training process!

KB GOBLET SQUAT WITH 3-SECOND ISOMETRIC

Perform this exercise to strengthen your lower body, especially your quadriceps, knees, and hips, in addition to mastering the bottom position of a squat with the 3-second isometric hold.

HOW TO PERFORM

- Stand tall with your feet roughly hip-width apart.
- Hold a kettlebell tightly to your chest with both hands as if you were holding a bowl.
- Keeping both feet flat and your spine straight, sink down into the bottom position of a squat.
- Once there, ensure that you have a proud chest so that I could see the logo on the front of your shirt if I were standing in front of you.
- Maintain that bottom isometric (hold) position for 3 seconds, then stand back up to the top position.

PERFORMANCE TIPS FOR SUCCESS

- The squat is a foundational movement pattern in life and athletic performance, which is why we've included it in this training program.
- When performing this exercise, really commit to the 3-second isometric hold at the bottom of each rep for maximum results.

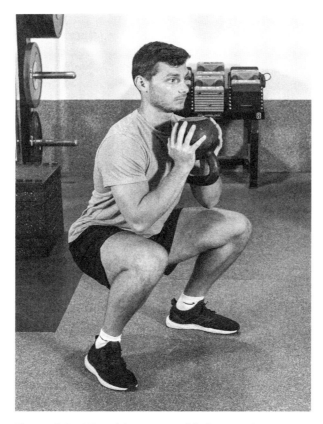

Figure 6.1 KB goblet squat with 3-second isometric.

BAND TALL-KNEELING PALLOF PRESS ISOMETRIC

Improve your core strength in an anti-rotation movement where the muscles in your midsection have to stabilize against a rotational force, in addition to improving shoulder strength.

HOW TO PERFORM

- Position yourself on the floor on both knees at roughly hip-width apart.
- Place a pad under both knees for comfort. Ensure that the toes of both feet are aiming directly down into the floor.
- Anchor a long resistance band around a squat rack or cable column at roughly chest height on your left side. The band should be resistant enough to make this exercise moderately challenging to very challenging.
- Place the band inside your hands and interlock your fingers together.
- Start out with enough resistance from the band that it provides a challenge, but not so much that you're unable to remain stable.
- Press your arms out straight in front of your upper chest and shoulders and maintain that long position for the prescribed amount of time. Switch sides and repeat.

PERFORMANCE TIPS FOR SUCCESS

- This is a classic exercise to improve your overall anti-rotation core strength and stability.
- Be sure to hold a strong and stable position with both arms straight when performing this exercise. Trust me: It's easier said than done!

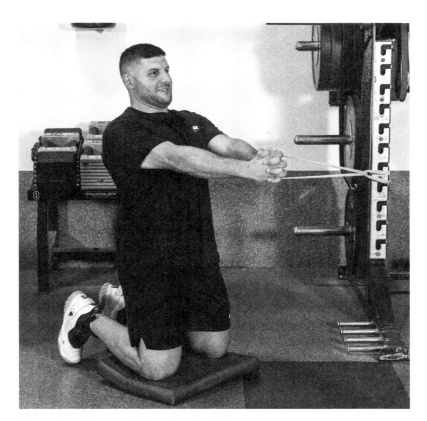

Figure 6.2 Band tall-kneeling Pallof press isometric.

DB ROMANIAN DEADLIFT (RDL)

Challenge hamstring muscle strength and flexibility with this classic lower-body exercise, in addition to improving hip joint mobility.

HOW TO PERFORM

- Stand with your feet roughly hip-width apart.
- Hold a pair of dumbbells in front of your hips and keep a tall spine from start to finish (i.e., avoid arching your low back or flaring your rib cage).
- The goal here is to keep the dumbbells close to your body throughout the entire range of motion within each rep.
- Start by sitting your hips back into the hip hinge pattern with a slight bend in your knees.
- In terms of how low to go, ensure that the dumbbells end up between the spot just below your knees and mid-shin.
- Aside from the slight knee bend, all the other motion should occur at your hips.
- Once you're in the bottom position, retrace the movement back up to the top.

PERFORMANCE TIPS FOR SUCCESS

- Strong and flexible hamstrings developed from performing this exercise will allow you to become more proficient in a variety of athletic skills, such as sprinting, jumping, and cutting.
- When performing this exercise, allow the hips to initiate the majority of the movement while the knees bend only slightly.

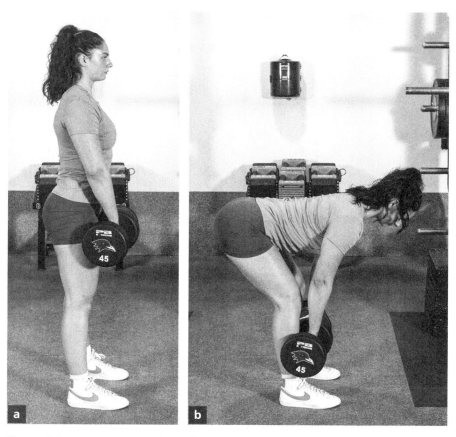

Figure 6.3 DB Romanian deadlift (RDL): *(a)* start position and *(b)* hip hinge.

Strength Exercises **113**

KB HALF-KNEELING SHOULDER PRESS WITH 3-SECOND ISOMETRIC

Improve shoulder strength and stability, hip and trunk stability, and strength in the top position of an overhead press via the 3-second isometric hold.

HOW TO PERFORM

- Take a knee on top of a pad with your right knee and make sure that the toes of your right foot are aiming directly down into the floor.
- Place your left foot flat on the floor in front of you with your left knee up.
- Your hips should be roughly hip-width apart.
- Hold a kettlebell in each hand so that your knuckles are aiming up toward the ceiling.
- Press that kettlebells up into the overhead position so that your arms are straight, and hold them there for 3 seconds.
- Lower them back down to the bottom position.
- Ensure that your core muscles are engaged the entire time by avoiding a low back arch or rib cage flare.

PERFORMANCE TIPS FOR SUCCESS

- This exercise provides a variety of benefits that support your overall athletic abilities, including shoulder strength, shoulder stability, hip stability, trunk stability, and overhead positional strength.
- A key to performing this exercise is to really squeeze the kettlebell and reach up during the shoulder press motion while avoiding a low back arch or rib cage flare.

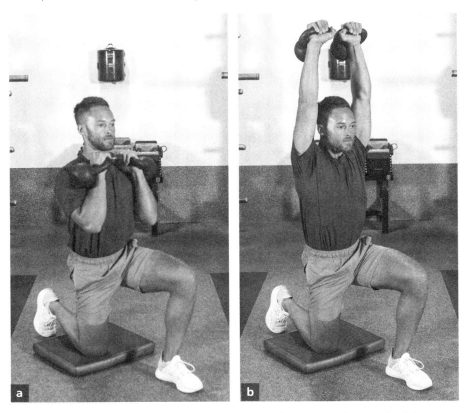

Figure 6.4 KB half-kneeling shoulder press with 3-second isometric: *(a)* start position and *(b)* shoulder press.

SUSPENSION SKATER SQUAT WITH 3-SECOND ISOMETRIC

Knee strength and durability are key components of athleticism, as are strong quadriceps muscles in your legs. These are the primary benefits you'll receive from performing this exercise.

HOW TO PERFORM

- Hold suspension straps with both hands in front of you and use the handles as support.
- Place your left foot flat on the floor and bend your right knee so that your right heel is almost touching your right glute.
- Begin your descent to the floor, allowing your chest to travel slightly forward, your left knee to bend forward and past the toes of your left foot, and your right leg to shift slightly behind you.
- Once you reach the bottom position just above the floor, maintain that isometric hold for a total of 3 seconds, then return to the top.

PERFORMANCE TIPS FOR SUCCESS

- Strong and durable knees and quadriceps are the key qualities developed by performing this exercise.
- It is important to commit to the 3-second hold at the bottom of each rep for maximum results.

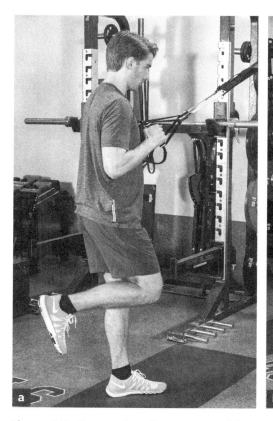
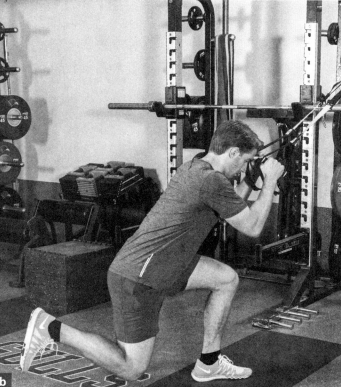

Figure 6.5 Suspension skater squat with 3-second isometric: *(a)* start position and *(b)* squat.

DB STANDING HAMMER CURL

Most people view biceps training only as a way to build muscle in your biceps, without ever considering the benefits it has for developing durable elbow joints, durable wrist joints, and strong forearms. When you perform this curl properly, you'll make gains in all of these areas.

HOW TO PERFORM

- Stand with your feet roughly hip-width apart.
- Hold a pair of dumbbells in both hands down by the sides of your body.
- Use a hammer grip with your thumbs at the top.
- Keeping your upper arms and elbows as close to the sides of your body as possible, begin to perform the hammer curl with both hands in a slow and controlled fashion.
- Once you've reached the top position without letting anything else move, lower both dumbbells back down to the bottom position.

PERFORMANCE TIPS FOR SUCCESS

- Athletes need strong arms and durable wrist and elbow joints, which is why we've included this direct arm training exercise in the program.
- Performing this exercise will not only strengthen the previously mentioned areas, but improve grip strength, an often-overlooked area for athletes.

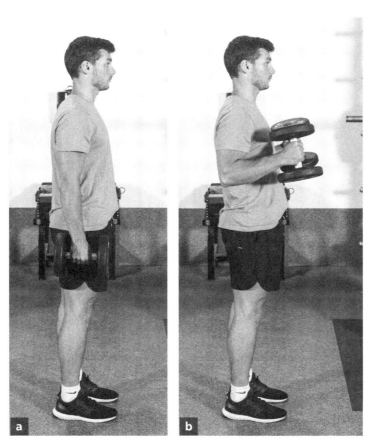

Figure 6.6 DB standing hammer curl: *(a)* start position and *(b)* hammer curl.

DB BENCH PRESS WITH 3-SECOND ISOMETRIC (TOP)

Bench pressing isn't just for powerlifters and individuals seeking maximal strength. It's also a great exercise for athletes looking to develop upper body horizontal pushing strength.

HOW TO PERFORM

- Lie flat on your back on a bench and place your feet on the floor on either side of the bench.
- Drive both feet directly down into the floor when performing this exercise to create leg drive, hip stability, and trunk stability.
- Holding a pair of dumbbells with your knuckles aiming up toward the ceiling, create a 45-degree angle with your elbows to allow for a strong bench press.
- Press both dumbbells up into the top position with your arms straight.
- Maintain that top isometric (hold) position for 3 seconds, then lower the dumbbells back down to the starting position.

PERFORMANCE TIPS FOR SUCCESS

- The addition of the 3-second isometric hold at the top of each rep ensures that you'll take your time, use proper technique, and develop shoulder stability in the top position. This is key to reaping the benefits of the exercise.
- Really root your feet down into the floor to help stabilize the hips and core muscles, which will make the upper body pressing action much stronger.

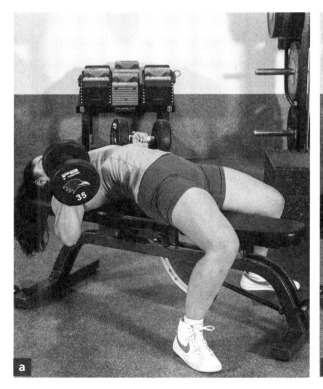
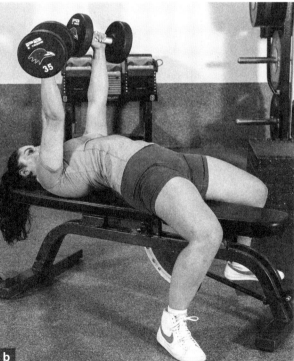

Figure 6.7 DB bench press with 3-second isometric (top): *(a)* start position and *(b)* bench press.

Strength Exercises 117

BENT-KNEE STAR PLANK WITH TOP LEG LONG

This exercise allows you to make gains in many areas, specifically your hips, shoulders, and core muscles.

HOW TO PERFORM

- Lie on your right side on the floor, bend both knees, and stack your legs. Keep your back flush with your heels rather than placing your heels behind your back.
- Place your right elbow directly under your right shoulder.
- From here, reach your top hand straight up toward the ceiling with a clenched fist and rise into the star plank position with both knees bent, but separated.
- Once you're at the top, straighten your left leg.
- Hold this position for the prescribed amount of time, switch sides, and repeat.

PERFORMANCE TIPS FOR SUCCESS

- By performing this exercise, you'll benefit from developing strength and stability in your shoulders, core, and hips, in addition to improving anti-side bend core strength.
- A pro tip is to think about driving the bottom hip up and away from the floor as hard as possible to truly challenge these muscles.

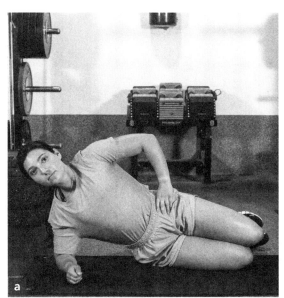
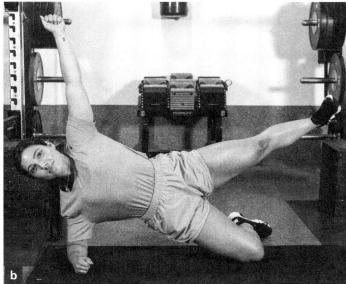

Figure 6.8 Bent-knee star plank with top leg long: *(a)* star plank position and *(b)* lifted leg.

DB CHEST-SUPPORTED ROW

Not only will you develop grip strength with this exercise, you'll improve your overall back strength, which is pivotal for health and performance.

HOW TO PERFORM

- Start by setting up a bench in the incline position somewhere between 33 and 45 degrees based on comfort.
- Place a pair of dumbbells on the floor at the front (head) of the bench.
- Place your feet on the floor at the back (foot) of the bench and rest the entire front side of your body on the bench.
- Pressing your feet down and away into the floor and keeping both legs long, grab dumbbells with your hands and perform a rowing motion up toward the ceiling.
- During this rowing motion, ensure that the inside aspect of your elbows and upper arms remain as close to the sides of your body as possible.
- Once you've reached the top, slowly lower both dumbbells to the bottom position.

PERFORMANCE TIPS FOR SUCCESS

- By performing this exercise consistently, you'll improve your back strength and grip strength.
- A pro tip is to really drive the toes of both feet down into the floor while keeping both legs straight, which will add stability in the lower body for a better base of support.

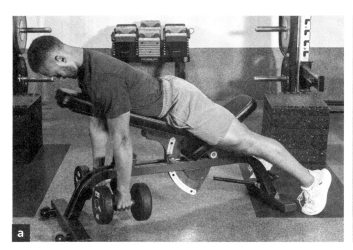 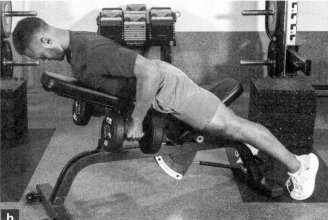

Figure 6.9 DB chest-supported row: *(a)* start position and *(b)* row.

KB SINGLE-ARM OFFSET LATERAL SQUAT WITH 1-SECOND ISOMETRIC

This frontal plane of motion (side-to-side) exercise is a great way to strengthen the inner thigh muscles (adductors) in your legs, which will help you during cutting, turning, sprinting, and other athletic movements.

HOW TO PERFORM

- Hold a kettlebell in your left hand.
- Assume a wide stance with both feet flat on the floor and the toes of both feet aimed forward.
- Allow your hips to hinge back while simultaneously lateral squatting down toward your right side. In this bottom position, your left leg should remain straight, your right knee should bend, and your torso should remain straight from head to hips with a slight forward lean.
- Maintain this bottom isometric (hold) position for 1 second, then return to the top position.
- Complete all reps, switch sides, and repeat.

PERFORMANCE TIPS FOR SUCCESS

- Here you'll be able to develop lower-body strength in your adductor muscles, quadriceps, and glutes.
- Be sure to fully commit to the 1-second isometric (hold) at the bottom of each rep.

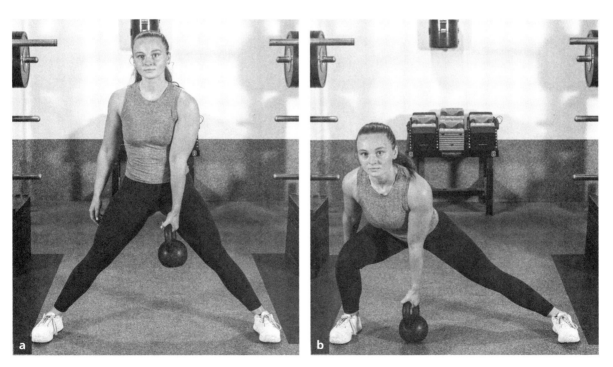

Figure 6.10 KB single-arm offset lateral squat with 1-second isometric: *(a)* start position and *(b)* lateral squat.

KB GOBLET CARRY

Core strength, upper back strength, and upper back endurance are all important skills that the best athletes in the world possess. Now it's your turn to start developing these skills!

HOW TO PERFORM

- Hold a kettlebell tight to your chest with both hands as if you were holding a large bowl.
- Keeping a tall spine and avoiding letting the kettlebell pull you forward, walk (carry) for the prescribed distance or reps.
- The key here is to keep a strong and sturdy upper back and core in order to resist the anterior pulling force created by the kettlebell held in front of you.

PERFORMANCE TIPS FOR SUCCESS

- Here is an excellent exercise to develop anti-flexion core strength, in addition to upper back strength and endurance.
- A key is to avoid letting the weight pull your chest down toward the floor. Avoid slouching by keeping a tall spine and proud chest.

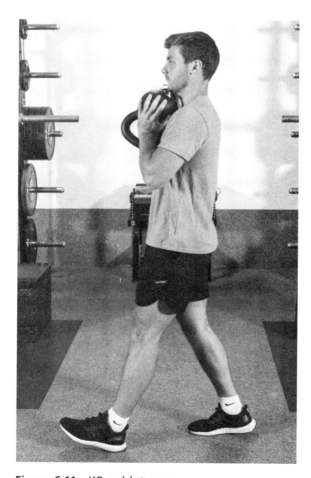

Figure 6.11 KB goblet carry.

Strength Exercises **121**

BAND TALL-KNEELING PULL-APART

Strengthen your upper back and shoulders with this exercise, while challenging your core muscles to work in an anti-extension fashion based on the tall kneeling position.

HOW TO PERFORM

- Place both knees on a pad on the floor roughly hip-width apart, aiming the toes of both feet directly down into the floor.
- Hold a long resistance band with both hands directly in front of your upper chest and shoulders.
- Keeping both arms long the entire time, begin to pull the band apart so that your hands travel backward.
- Once you've reached your end point, bring the band back to the starting position.

PERFORMANCE TIPS FOR SUCCESS

- When performing this exercise, make sure only your arms move and keep the rest of your body still.
- With proper technique, the band pull-apart is an excellent exercise choice for not only improving shoulder strength but also increasing the strength of the postural muscles in your upper back.

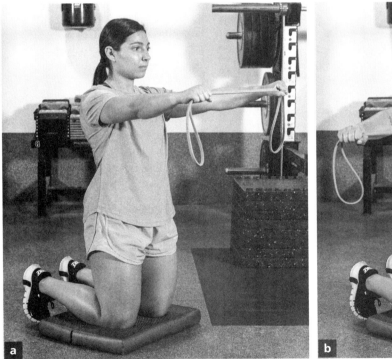 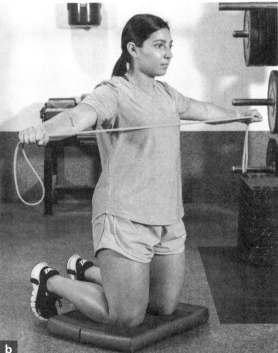

Figure 6.12 Band tall-kneeling pull-apart: *(a)* start position and *(b)* pull band apart.

TRAP BAR DEADLIFT

The deadlift is a foundational movement that helps you develop complete lower-body strength and power while increasing your overall grip strength. The benefit of using the trap bar for the deadlift is that is requires slightly more knee bend than the conventional barbell deadlift exercise, and reduces the shearing forces on the spine to ensure a safer exercise.

HOW TO PERFORM

- Stand inside a trap bar with your feet roughly hip-width apart.
- Sit your hips back into a hip hinge and slightly bend your knees.
- Although the deadlift is technically a hip hinge movement pattern, this exercise requires a bit more of a knee bend than usual based on the height of the trap bar handles.
- Once you're in the bottom position, grab each side of the trap bar handles directly in the center and line up the tongues of your sneakers with your hands. This alignment with your hands and sneakers will position your hips and spine where we want them to allow you to be strong and powerful.
- Keeping a straight spine from head to hips with a subtle chin tuck, press both feet down into the floor as hard as possible and stand tall.
- Retrace that pattern back down to the floor.

PERFORMANCE TIPS FOR SUCCESS

- This deadlift exercise will develop a strong lower body in addition to improving grip and forearm strength.
- It's easy to see the deadlift as a hip hinge lower-body exercise focused on pulling weight up from the floor. However, a pro tip for maximum benefit is to drive both feet down hard into the floor while standing up, which will help you use more of your posterior chain (glute and hamstring) muscles.

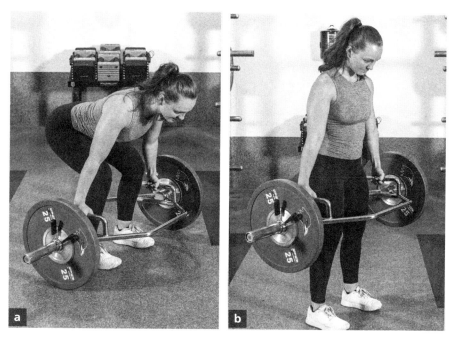

Figure 6.13 Trap bar deadlift: *(a)* start position and *(b)* lift.

Strength Exercises **123**

PHYSIOBALL PUSH–PULL

This is an anti-extension core strengthening exercise that improves the durability and resilience in your lower back muscles.

HOW TO PERFORM

- Start in a plank position with your toes on the floor, a straight body from heels to head, and both elbows in a triangle formation on the top of a physioball.
- There will likely be a circle on the top of the physioball; ensure that the triangle formation you've created with your elbows is directly on top of that and that the fingers of both hands are interlocked.
- From here, drive both elbows down into the physioball and press your chest and upper back slightly away up toward the ceiling. This is where the exercise begins.
- Slightly push the ball forward by an inch or two, then return it to the starting position.
- Do not allow any motion to occur anywhere in your body aside from your arms.

PERFORMANCE TIPS FOR SUCCESS

- It is important not to move any part of your body except your arms.
- Think about how stable and firm your body becomes when keeping it tense during a classic plank exercise on the floor. Use that same level of full-body tension here with the physioball.

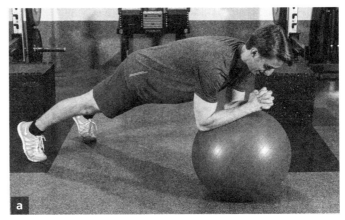

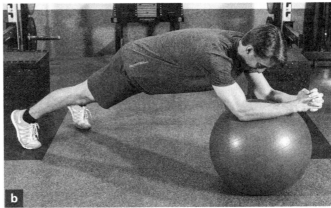

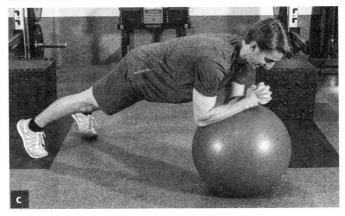

Figure 6.14 Physioball push–pull: *(a)* start position, *(b)* push the ball forward, and *(c)* pull the ball back.

TWO DB FOAM ROLLER HACK SQUAT AGAINST A WALL

Bulletproof your knees with this hack squat variation through increased quadriceps strength and increased durability in your quadriceps tendon and patella tendon.

HOW TO PERFORM

- Place a long (3-foot) foam roller against a wall and press the middle of your back into it.
- Hold a pair of dumbbells in your hands and walk your feet out away from the wall by roughly one or two feet. You may need to adjust this based on your squat pattern and comfort.
- Lower down into the squat, keeping your back in contact with the foam roller and the wall.
- Keep a tall spine and lower as far down as possible with good technique and form.
- Once you've reached your bottom position, stand back up to the top.

PERFORMANCE TIPS FOR SUCCESS

- Performing this exercise in this unique setup will allow you to target the quadriceps muscles a bit more than a traditional squat. You'll also benefit from improved strength and durability in both knee tendons (patella tendon and quadriceps tendon).
- A pro tip here is to not only drive both feet down into the floor, but also push your back into the foam roller and wall. When doing all of this, you'll create a ton of stability, helping you effectively perform this exercise.

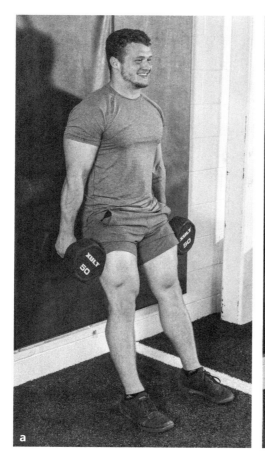
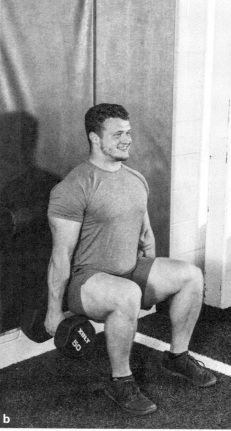

Figure 6.15 Two DB foam roller hack squat against a wall: *(a)* start position and *(b)* squat.

CABLE HALF-KNEELING HIGH ROW WITH 1-SECOND ISOMETRIC

Develop a strong upper back and mid-back with this vertical rowing exercise, while benefiting from improved hip joint mobility and hip flexor flexibility.

HOW TO PERFORM

- Set up two handles at a high anchor point on a cable column.
- Place your left knee down on a pad on the floor with the toes of your left foot aiming directly down into the floor.
- Place your right foot flat on the floor in front of you with your right knee up.
- Reach both arms up high and grab both handles.
- Row both hands down toward your chest, aiming both elbows toward your pockets.
- Maintain this bottom isometric (hold) position for 1 second, then return your hands to the top position.
- Complete all reps in this setup, switch sides, and repeat.

PERFORMANCE TIPS FOR SUCCESS

- In rowing, most athletes focus only on horizontal exercises in which your arm rows out in front of you. Performing this exercise will help you focus on a vertical rowing pattern that aids in your overall shoulder health and develops strength in your upper and mid-back.
- A pro tip is to really squeeze your shoulder blades together at the bottom of each rep during the 1-second isometric hold to challenge your upper and mid-back muscles.

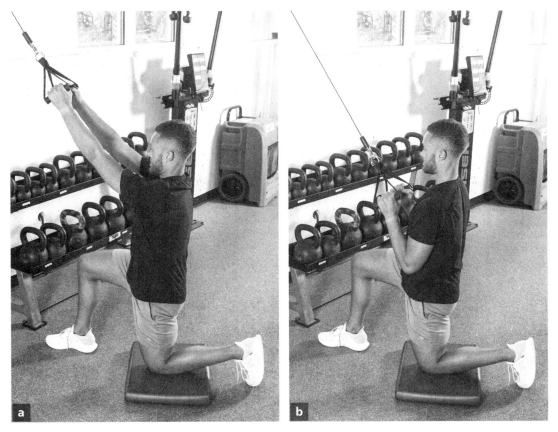

Figure 6.16 Cable half-kneeling high row with 1-second isometric: *(a)* start position and *(b)* row.

CABLE DOUBLE-ARM SINGLE-LEG ROMANIAN DEADLIFT (RDL)

Single-leg strength and stability are hallmark traits of athleticism; this exercise will get you on the fast track to success in this department.

HOW TO PERFORM

- Set up two handles at a low anchor point on a cable column.
- Grab both handles with your hands and take a few steps back.
- Keep your right foot flat on the floor with a subtle bend in your right knee.
- Now, keeping a relatively straight line from your left heel to the back of your head, hinge at the hips so that your chest lowers down to the front and your left leg raises up toward the back.
- Keep a subtle chin tuck and avoid letting the toes of your left foot rotate away toward the left. Move at a slow and controlled pace to really dial in your technique here.
- Once your body is parallel to the floor, your chest is aiming down, and your heel is aiming up, slowly reverse the pattern and return to the starting (top) position.
- Complete all reps on one side, switch sides, and repeat.

PERFORMANCE TIPS FOR SUCCESS

- Performing this exercise consistently will help you make gains in single-leg strength, single-leg stability, hamstring strength, and glute strength.
- One of the biggest pro tips here is to think about grasping the floor with your stable foot as if you were trying to grip with your toes. This will help to give you a stable foot position and allow for better balance.

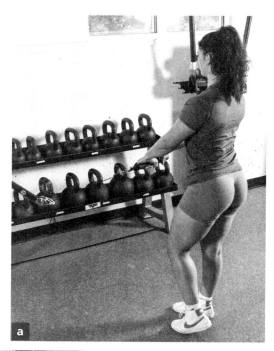

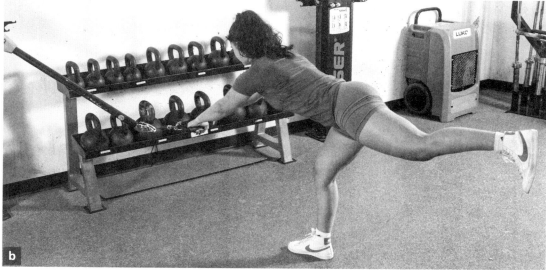

Figure 6.17 Cable double-arm single-leg Romanian deadlift (RDL): *(a)* start position and *(b)* deadlift.

BAND STANDING TRICEPS EXTENSION

Athletes need strong arms and durable wrist and elbow joints, which is why we've included this direct arm training exercise in this program for you.

HOW TO PERFORM

- Anchor a long resistance band to a pull-up bar above your head. Use a band with moderate to heavy resistance.
- Stand directly under the band anchor point, grab the long resistance band with both hands, and keep the inside aspect of your arms and elbows tight to the sides of your body.
- Straighten your arms out so that your hands travel down toward your pockets.
- Once you're there, retrace that pattern back to the top.

PERFORMANCE TIPS FOR SUCCESS

- Most athletes view direct triceps training only as a way to build muscle in the triceps, without considering the benefits it has for developing durable elbow joints, durable wrist joints, and strong forearms. When performed properly, this exercise will allow you to make gains in all of these areas.
- A pro tip here is to squeeze your triceps muscles at the bottom of each rep to get the most bang for your buck out of each rep.

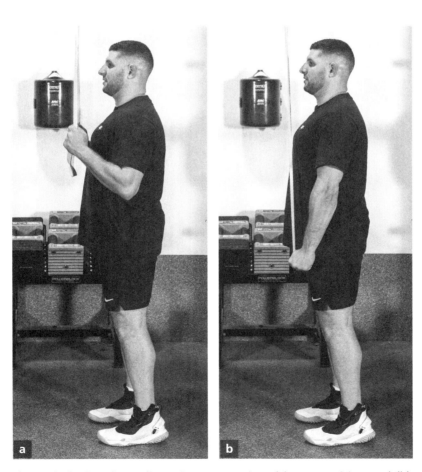

Figure 6.18 Band standing triceps extension: *(a)* start position and *(b)* extension.

DB STEP-UP

Step-ups are overlooked and underused in the world of athletic performance. However, you can receive tremendous benefits in lower-body strength and single-leg stability when performing them, which is why we've added them into the training program for you!

HOW TO PERFORM

- Position a sturdy box directly in front of both feet.
- The box should be high enough to challenge you, but not so high that you lose proper technique and form. For a general reference, use a box height between 12 and 24 inches.
- Hold a pair of dumbbells in both hands.
- Step up on to the sturdy box with your right foot so that the entire surface of the right foot is flat.
- Driving your right foot directly down into the box, stand up tall on to the box with your left foot as well.
- Now drive the right foot directly down into the box as your left foot lowers back down to the floor behind you. Notice the emphasis on the right leg doing all the work. That's important since we want only the working leg performing the work.
- Complete all reps on the right side, switch sides, and repeat.

PERFORMANCE TIPS FOR SUCCESS

- This exercise will help you improve single-leg strength and stability, in addition to developing a high level of balance.
- A pro tip is to ensure that the entire surface of the top foot is placed onto the box without any of the heel hanging off. This may not seem like a big deal, but it helps you tremendously in terms of generating force and building strength in your lower body.

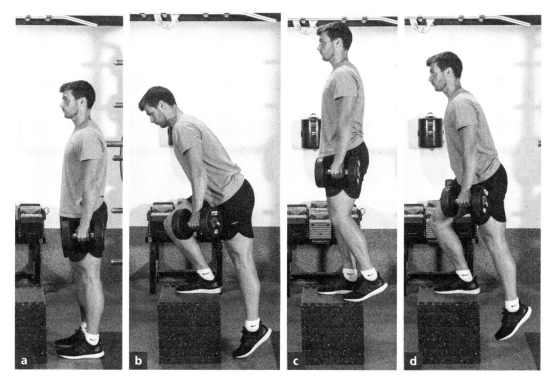

Figure 6.19 DB step-up: *(a)* start position, *(b)* step-up, *(c)* stand on box, and *(d)* step down.

DB HEELS-UP THREE-POINT ROW WITH 3-SECOND ECCENTRIC

Not only will you strengthen your upper back and mid-back muscles here, you'll also improve shoulder health with the added eccentric lowering component. Lastly, you'll benefit from the anti-extension core challenge from being in this position and the anti-rotation challenge from holding the dumbbell in one hand.

HOW TO PERFORM

- Stand in an athletic stance with a slight bend in your knees and hips.
- Slowly lower your hands down in front of you until you're able to rest them on a sturdy box or bench at roughly knee to hip height, depending on how tall you are.
- Keep your spine roughly parallel to the floor.
- Keep the heels of both feet slightly raised above the floor just enough to fit a magazine or two underneath.
- Grab a dumbbell with your left hand and row it up toward your rib cage.
- Once you're in the top position, without letting your shoulder joint stick out or your neck shrug, lower the dumbbell back down toward the floor for a 3-second count until your arm is straight again.
- Complete all reps on one side, switch sides, and repeat.

PERFORMANCE TIPS FOR SUCCESS

- This exercise is much more challenging than it looks. It will help you improve upper back strength, mid-back strength, shoulder health, and core strength in both an anti-extension and anti-rotation fashion.
- Truly focus on the 3-second eccentric (lowering) component during each rep.

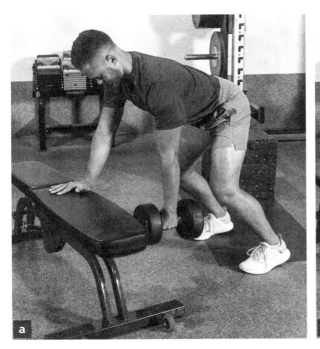 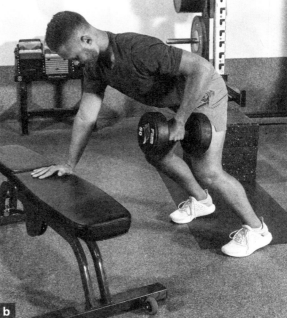

Figure 6.20 DB heels-up three-point row with 3-second eccentric: *(a)* start position and *(b)* row.

TWO DB CYCLIST SQUAT

You'll be able to get a bit deeper into your squat in this exercise as opposed to a traditional squat since your heels are propped up. As a result, you'll improve strength in your quadriceps and both tendons in your knees (patella tendon and quadriceps tendon).

HOW TO PERFORM

- Prop the heels of both feet up on a bumper weight plate.
- Use a plate between 25 and 45 pounds, roughly 2 to 4 inches high. Keep in mind that the higher the plate, the more challenging and intense the exercise will be.
- Placing the toes of both feet down into the floor, hold a pair of dumbbells in your hands down by your sides and slowly descend into a squat. Ascend back to the top position.

PERFORMANCE TIPS FOR SUCCESS

- This exercise will help you explore a deeper range of motion in the squat while also improving quadriceps strength.
- Move at a slow and controlled pace.

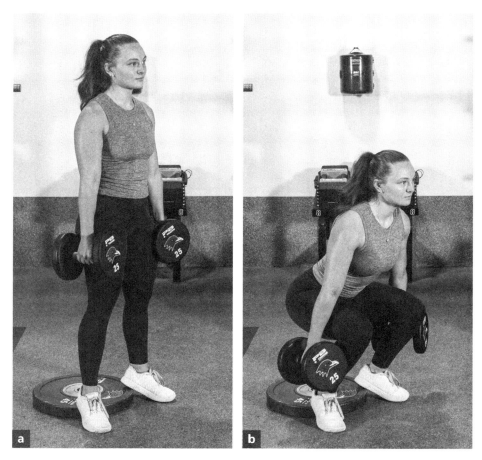

Figure 6.21 Two DB cyclist squat: *(a)* start position and *(b)* squat.

CABLE SEATED LAT PULL-DOWN WITH 3-SECOND ECCENTRIC

A strong back is common in athletes in a variety of sports and the backbone of upper body strength and power. It's time to lock in, build strength, and improve power in your upper back and mid-back areas with this exercise! An added benefit here is that you'll improve shoulder health with the added 3-second eccentric component.

HOW TO PERFORM

- Sit on a sturdy bench or box roughly 18 to 24 inches in height.
- Anchor a long bar to a high anchor point on a cable column.
- Hold the long bar just outside of shoulder width.
- Keeping a tall spine, slightly lean back without arching your back or flaring your rib cage and pull the bar down toward your upper chest.
- In a slow and controlled manner, raise the bar back to the top position for a 3-second count.

PERFORMANCE TIPS FOR SUCCESS

- The single most important component to this exercise is a dedicated approach to the 3-second eccentric (raise) movement, since that is where you'll make the most gains in muscular development due to time under tension.
- A pro tip here is to really press the toes of both feet down into the floor to create stability in your ankle and lower leg for a much more controlled movement.

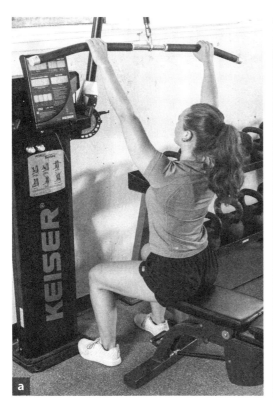
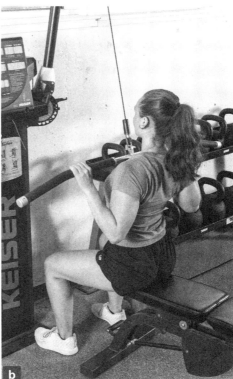

Figure 6.22 Cable seated lat pull-down with 3-second eccentric: *(a)* start position and *(b)* pull-down.

KB FRONT RACK CARRY

This exercise comes with a host of benefits, including grip strength, upper back strength, upper back endurance, balance, lower body stability, and anti-flexion core strength.

HOW TO PERFORM

- Hold two kettlebells with your hands tight to your upper chest area in the front rack position.
- Ensure that the knuckles of both hands are aiming up toward the ceiling and that you're gripping the kettlebells tightly with both hands.
- While keeping both kettlebells pressed against your upper chest the entire time, walk (carry) for the prescribed distance or number of reps.

PERFORMANCE TIPS FOR SUCCESS

- It is important to avoid letting the kettlebells pull you down or cause you to slouch. Instead, remain tall in your spine.
- Grip both kettlebells hard and keep them tight to your chest. This will create more stability in your core muscles, which will make the exercise easier to perform while maintaining good form.

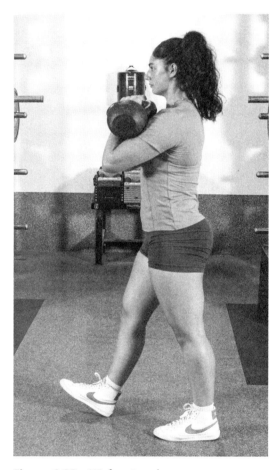

Figure 6.23 KB front rack carry.

CABLE TALL-KNEELING ROPE TRICEPS EXTENSION

Most athletes view direct triceps training only as a way to build muscle in your triceps, without considering the benefits it has for developing durable elbow joints, durable wrist joints, and strong forearms. When performed properly, you'll make gains in all of these areas.

HOW TO PERFORM

- Anchor a rope to a high point on a cable column.
- Place both knees on a pad on the floor roughly hip-width apart with the toes of both feet aiming directly down into the floor.
- Grab the rope on either side with both hands and keep the inside aspect of your arms and elbows tight to the sides of your body.
- Now simply straighten your arms out so that your hands travel down toward your pockets.
- Once you're there, retrace that pattern back to the top.

PERFORMANCE TIPS FOR SUCCESS

- Athletes need strong arms and durable wrist and elbow joints, which is why we've included this direct arm training exercise in this program for you. Performing this exercise on a consistent basis will keep your wrists and elbows healthy.
- A pro tip is to brace your core muscles hard in an effort to maintain the tall kneeling position and avoid letting the resistance pull your lower back into extension.

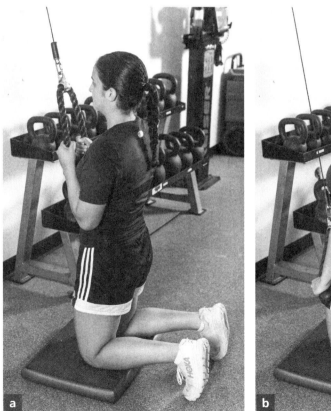 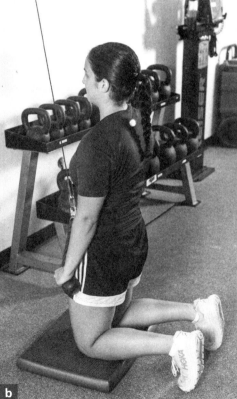

Figure 6.24 Cable tall-kneeling rope triceps extension: *(a)* start position and *(b)* extension.

WEIGHTED ECCENTRIC-ONLY NEUTRAL GRIP PULL-UP WITH 5-SECOND ECCENTRIC

Upper back strength is a major player in overall upper-body development for athletes, which is exactly why we've incorporated this foundational movement in this training program for you.

HOW TO PERFORM

- Stand on top of a sturdy bench or box roughly 18 to 24 inches in height.
- Add external load to your body (i.e., weight vest, chains, weight belt, etc.).
- The goal here is to perform only the lower portion of a neutral grip pull-up.
- Hold on to a neutral-grip pull-up bar with the knuckles of both hands facing in toward each other.
- Jump up into the top of a neutral-grip pull-up position, using assistance from your hands to get there.
- Once you're there, slowly lower from the top to the bottom position for a 5-second count.
- Feel free to reset during each rep at the bottom if you need to.

PERFORMANCE TIPS FOR SUCCESS

- Performing this exercise will help you develop upper back strength, grip strength, and shoulder health.
- To see the benefit of this exercise, it is important to commit yourself to the 5-second eccentric (lowering) movement during each rep.

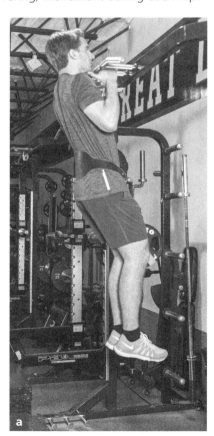 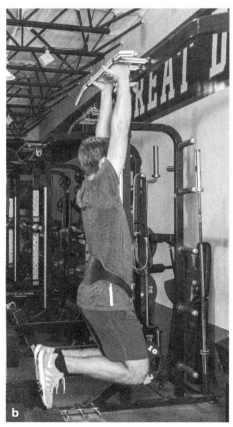

Figure 6.25 Weighted eccentric-only neutral grip pull-up with 5-second eccentric: *(a)* top position of pull-up and *(b)* lower to bottom position.

LANDMINE GOBLET LATERAL SQUAT

This frontal-plane-of-motion (side-to-side) exercise is a great way to begin strengthening the inner thigh muscles (adductors), which will help you during cutting, turning, sprinting, and other athletic movements.

HOW TO PERFORM

- Place a barbell in the landmine position on the floor with one end resting on the floor and anchored down into bumper weight plates or into a corner. Hold the other end of the barbell with both hands, interlacing your fingers around it and covering the end of the barbell. Be sure to leave about one or two inches of space between the barbell and your chest, since you'll need that space during the descent portion of each rep. This position of the hands on the landmine is known as the goblet position and is similar to how you'd hold a dumbbell or kettlebell in a dumbbell goblet lateral squat or kettlebell lateral goblet squat. If your gym doesn't have a barbell, bumper plates, or a landmine collar, simply swap in a heavy dumbbell or heavy kettlebell.
- Assume a wide stance with the toes of both feet aiming forward and both feet flat on the floor.
- Allow your hips to hinge back while simultaneously lateral squatting toward your left side.
- In this bottom position, your right leg should remain straight, your left knee should bend, and your torso should remain straight from head to hips with a slight forward lean.
- Once you've reached the bottom position, make your way back to the top with both legs straight.
- Perform all reps on one side, switch sides, and repeat.

PERFORMANCE TIPS FOR SUCCESS

- By performing this exercise, you'll build strength in your adductors, quadriceps, and glutes.
- By unlocking your lower body strength in the frontal plane, you'll benefit from improved strength in your hips and knees in addition to the surrounding muscles. A pro tip here is to keep each rep feeling smooth and ease into the bottom position, which will become easier over time.

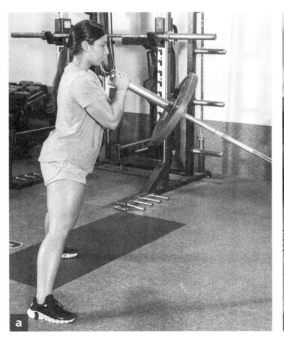 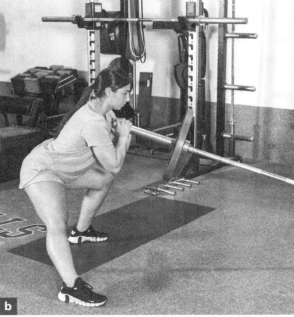

Figure 6.26 Landmine goblet lateral squat: *(a)* start position and *(b)* lateral squat.

DB CAPTAIN STANCE SINGLE-ARM SHOULDER PRESS

The benefit of the captain stance position is improving hip joint mobility and hip flexor flexibility, in addition to challenging both single-leg stability and anti-extension core strength. You'll also improve overall shoulder strength and stability when performing this exercise.

HOW TO PERFORM

- Place your left foot flat on top of a sturdy box or bench at roughly knee height.
- Keeping your right foot flat on the floor and your right leg straight, lean forward slightly.
- Grab a dumbbell in your right hand and hold it just in front of your right shoulder with your right elbow bent.
- Here's where the exercise kicks in: Squeeze the dumbbell hard with your right hand and press it up into the overhead position until your right arm is straight.
- Lower the dumbbell back to the starting position.

PERFORMANCE TIPS FOR SUCCESS

- The most important part of this exercise is to avoid a low back arch or rib cage flare.
- Make sure you're squeezing the dumbbell hard and reaching up at the same time.
- This is a full-body, more-bang-for-your-buck exercise that athletes from all walks of life will benefit from.

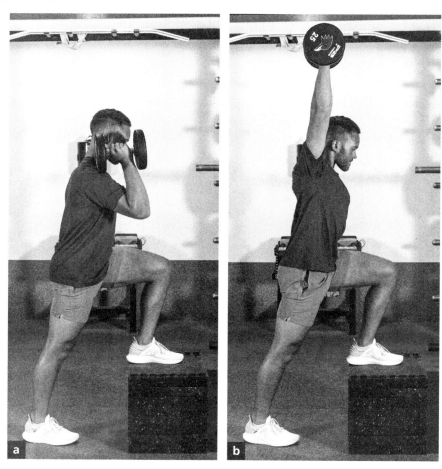

Figure 6.27 DB captain stance single-arm shoulder press: *(a)* start position and *(b)* press dumbbell up.

Strength Exercises **137**

CABLE PLANK SINGLE-ARM ROW TO TRICEPS EXTENSION

This is a full-body exercise that challenges strength and stability from head to toe. You'll benefit from this exercise by building shoulder strength and stability, core strength in an anti-extension and anti-rotation fashion, and hip stability.

HOW TO PERFORM

- Set yourself down on the floor in the classic plank position: feet roughly hip-width apart, toes of both feet pointing down into the floor, entire body straight from your heels to the back of your head, both elbows on the floor directly underneath your shoulders, and fists of both hands clenched.
- With your left hand, reach forward to grab the handle of a cable column attached to a low anchor point.
- Without letting anything else move in your body, reach your left elbow toward your left pocket, pin the inside aspect of your left elbow and upper arm to your left rib cage, and straighten your left arm.
- Now trace that exact pattern in the opposite order back to the starting position.
- Complete all reps with the left arm, switch sides, and repeat.

PERFORMANCE TIPS FOR SUCCESS

- When performing this exercise, fight hard to disallow your body from rotating or extending at the hips. Keep a strong and stable position while the arm moves.
- Maintain the plank position while the arm moves. This is easier said than done but will help you improve in full-body stability when performed correctly.

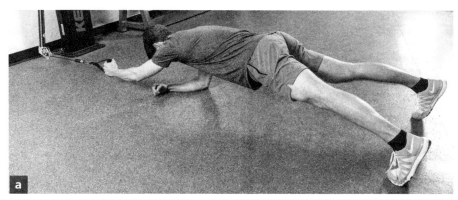

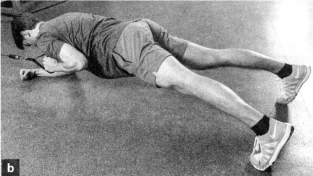
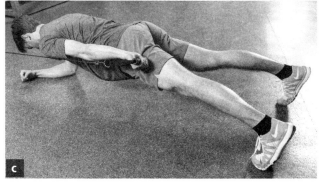

Figure 6.28 Cable plank single-arm row to triceps extension: *(a)* start position, *(b)* row, and *(c)* triceps extension.

KB SUITCASE CARRY

This exercise is much more challenging than it looks, especially when the weight becomes heavier! Perform this movement to make gains in grip strength, balance, stability, coordination, and anti–side bend core strength.

HOW TO PERFORM

- Stand tall and hold one kettlebell in your left hand.
- Avoid letting any part of the kettlebell touch the side of your body throughout this exercise.
- Clench your fist in your right hand slightly away from the side of your body, engage your core muscles, and walk forward for the prescribed distance or reps.
- Switch sides and repeat.

PERFORMANCE TIPS FOR SUCCESS

- Remain tall without letting the weight pull you down toward the side.
- Avoid letting the weight touch the side of your body, which is easier said than done. Squeeze the weight hard with your hand to maintain stability and control.

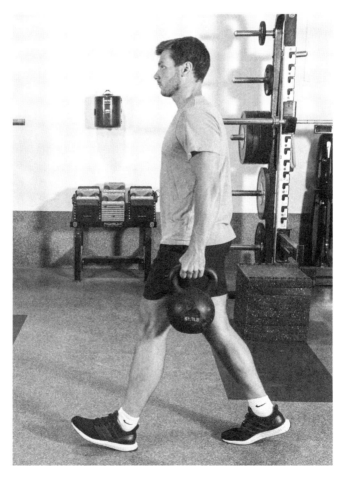

Figure 6.29 KB suitcase carry.

DB INCLINE BENCH TRAP RAISE (Y) WITH 3-SECOND ECCENTRIC

Lifting heavy weights to build your shoulders is important. However, performing shoulder health exercises at lighter loads is just as important, which is why we've incorporated this exercise into the training program.

HOW TO PERFORM

- Start by setting up a bench in the incline position somewhere between 33 and 45 degrees based on comfort.
- Place a pair of dumbbells on the floor at the front (head) of the bench.
- Place your feet on the floor at the back (foot) of the bench and rest the entire front side of your body on the bench.
- Pressing your feet down and away into the floor and keeping both legs long, grab the dumbbells with your hands.
- Hold both dumbbells with your hands so that your thumbs are closest to the ceiling and then raise them up with straight arms into a Y shape.
- Avoid shrugging your neck during this process. Allow motion to occur only at the shoulders.
- Once you've reached the top, slowly lower the dumbbells back down for a 3-second count.

PERFORMANCE TIPS FOR SUCCESS

- Shoulder health is a staple of athletic performance, but many athletes neglect or overlook this area. Don't be like them. Perform these on a consistent basis to support your overall shoulder health.
- Do not swing the dumbbells and avoid shrugging your neck. All of this is easier said than done, but super important for your success with this exercise.

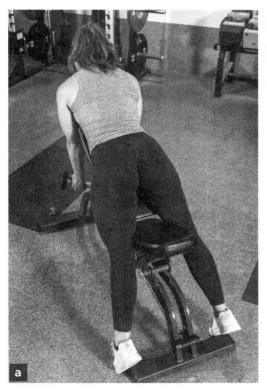
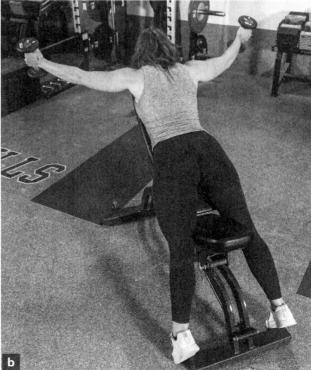

Figure 6.30 DB incline bench trap raise (Y) with 3-second eccentric: *(a)* start position and *(b)* Y position.

DB SINGLE-LEG RDL

Single-leg strength and stability are hallmark traits of athleticism, and this is the type of exercise to perform to get yourself on the fast-track to success in this department. Achieve gains in single-leg strength, single-leg stability, hamstring strength, and glute strength.

HOW TO PERFORM

- Hold a dumbbell in your left hand—a contralateral (opposite side) hold since your right foot will remain stable on the floor.
- With the right foot flat on the floor, keep a subtle bend in your right knee.
- Keeping a roughly straight line from your left heel to the back of your head, hinge at the hips so that your chest lowers to the front and your left leg raises up toward the back.
- Once your body is parallel to the floor, your chest is aiming down, and your heel is aiming up, it is then time to slowly reverse that pattern back into the starting (top) position.
- Keep a subtle chin tuck and avoid letting the toes of your left foot rotate away toward the left.
- Complete all reps on one side, switch sides, and repeat.

PERFORMANCE TIPS FOR SUCCESS

- Move at a slow and controlled pace. You really want to avoid going fast in order to dial in your technique.
- Grip the ground with your foot to provide more stability in the ankle. Think about scrunching the toes toward the heel as if you were grabbing the floor. Although this doesn't sound like it would make a difference, it will help a ton!

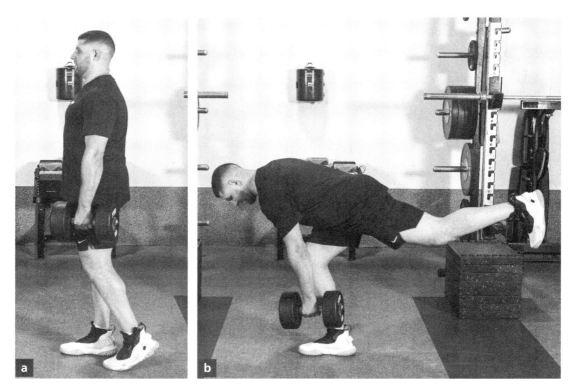

Figure 6.31 DB single-leg RDL: *(a)* start position and *(b)* Romanian deadlift position.

DB SINGLE-ARM BENCH PRESS WITH SINGLE-LEG HIP THRUST ISOMETRIC

Strong and healthy shoulders are pivotal for athletes in all walks of life. The added component of challenging your stability by only having one foot on the floor forces the hips and core to work harder while the chest and shoulders perform the horizontal pressing motion.

HOW TO PERFORM

- Position your mid-back against a sturdy bench or box with both feet flat on the floor.
- Hold a dumbbell with your left hand.
- Raise your hips into a bridge position. Bend your right knee up toward your chest and reach your right arm straight up toward the ceiling with a clenched fist for added stability. Begin to bench press the left arm up and down for the prescribed amount of reps.
- Once complete, switch to the opposite side and perform the prescribed number of reps with the right arm.
- The goal for the bench-pressing component is to create a 45-degree angle with your elbows, which will allow for a strong bench press with shoulder health in mind.

PERFORMANCE TIPS FOR SUCCESS

- When performed with proper technique and form, this exercise helps you improve chest strength, shoulder strength and stability, glute strength, and anti-rotation core strength.
- Fight to keep the bottom leg stable on the floor by driving it down hard to maximize stability in your hips and core muscles.

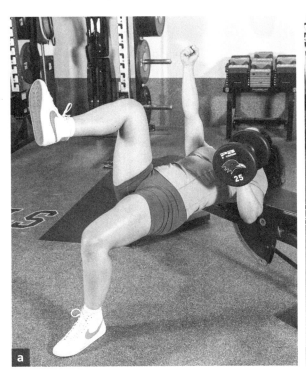 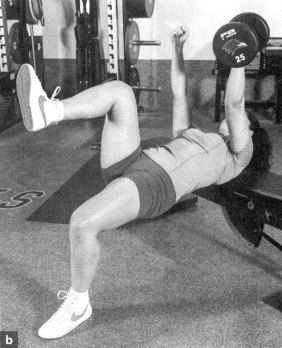

Figure 6.32 DB single-arm bench press with single-leg hip thrust isometric: *(a)* start position and *(b)* press dumbbell up.

CABLE PULL-THROUGH

The hip hinge is a foundational movement pattern in athletic performance. This exercise is a building block of your future gains in lower-body strength and power.

HOW TO PERFORM

- Anchor a rope at a low anchor point on a cable column while facing away from the cable column with the rope on the floor between your legs.
- Grab each end of the rope with each hand. Take a few steps away from the cable column to create resistance on the pulley system.
- Keeping a tall spine, a subtle chin tuck, and both arms straight, allow the rope to slowly pull your hips directly back into a hip hinge with only a subtle bend in your knees. This will occur since the cable column has resistance on it, challenging your hip hinge pattern.
- Once you've reached the bottom position with the logo on your shirt aiming down and forward by a few feet, stop downward motion and raise back up to the top.
- At the top, slightly squeeze your glutes and straighten your legs. The key word here is *slightly*.

PERFORMANCE TIPS FOR SUCCESS

- Performing this exercise consistently with good technique is a surefire way to develop a strong and powerful hip hinge movement pattern, strengthening the hamstrings and glutes.
- Use a slow and controlled pace throughout each rep to truly challenge the hip hinge patterns and your posterior chain (i.e., glute and hamstring) muscles; avoid arching your lower back or flaring your rib cage at the top of each rep.

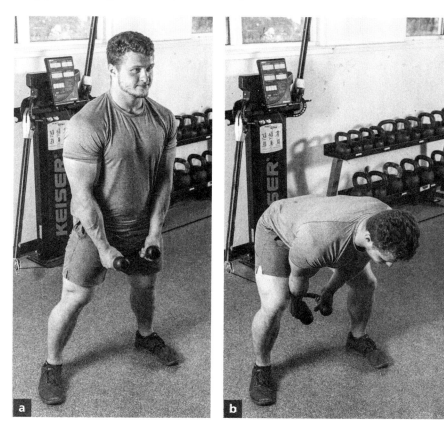

Figure 6.33 Cable pull-through: *(a)* start position and *(b)* hip hinge.

DB SEAL ROW

Having a strong mid-back is foundational to upper-body strength for all types of physical activities, athletics, and sports. Use this exercise to develop world-class mid-back strength.

HOW TO PERFORM

- Elevate a bench roughly 4 to 8 inches above the floor, depending on your height and arm length.
- Lie flat on your front side on the bench so that your kneecaps are just off of bench, not in contact with it.
- From here, create a subtle chin tuck and have a staring contest with the bench without letting your nose or face touch it.
- Grab a dumbbell in each hand and row them up toward the sides of your rib cage so that both arms are close to your body.
- Never allow your hands or the dumbbells to touch the floor during each rep.
- Avoid letting your elbows flare out to the side.
- Lower your arms back to the bottom position.

PERFORMANCE TIPS FOR SUCCESS

- A quick tip for success in this exercise is letting the arms do all the work. Really squeeze and pull up hard with your arms. When done correctly, this will help you develop mid-back strength, grip strength, and core strength.
- Think about squeezing the muscles between your shoulder blades at the top of each rep to maximize muscle gains in your upper and mid-back.

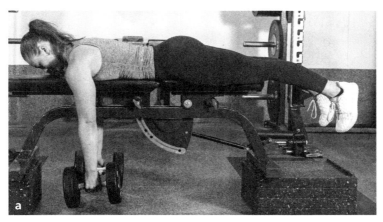

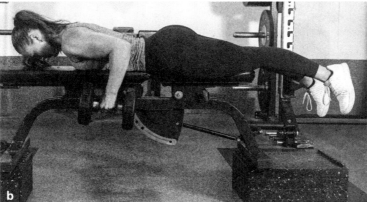

Figure 6.34 DB seal row: *(a)* start position and *(b)* row.

BAND WIDE-STANCE VERTICAL PALLOF PRESS

This exercise will help you improve overall anti-rotation core strength and shoulder strength, in addition to increasing your hip joint mobility and groin flexibility.

HOW TO PERFORM

- Anchor a band on your right-hand side to a squat rack or cable column at roughly shoulder height. The band resistance should be between moderate intensity and heavy intensity.
- Grab the band with both hands and interlock your fingers.
- Step away from the anchor point toward the left so that the band is fully stretched out.
- Assume a wide stance with the toes of both feet aimed forward, both feet flat, and both legs straight.
- Press the band straight out in front of your shoulders until both arms are straight.
- Return arms to the starting position.
- Complete all reps on one side, switch sides, and repeat.

PERFORMANCE TIPS FOR SUCCESS

- Performing this exercise will not only increase your anti-rotation core strength, shoulder strength, hip joint mobility, and groin flexibility; it will also challenge lower body stability.
- Make sure that you're pressing both hands directly out in front of your shoulders instead of allowing the band to drift up or down. This is much more challenging than it sounds.

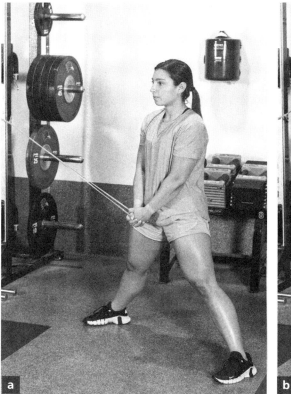 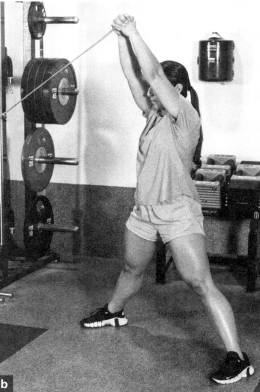

Figure 6.35 Band wide-stance vertical Pallof press: *(a)* start position and *(b)* press.

CABLE TALL-KNEELING STRAIGHT BAR BICEPS CURL

Athletes need strong arms and durable wrist and elbow joints, which is why we've included this direct arm training exercise in the program.

HOW TO PERFORM

- Anchor a straight bar to a low point on a cable column.
- Place both knees on a pad on the floor roughly hip-width apart with the toes of both feet aiming directly down into the floor.
- Grab the straight bar with both hands in an underhand grip, with hands roughly shoulder-width apart.
- Keep the inside of your arms and elbows tight to the sides of your body.
- Bend your arms so that your knuckles travel up toward your shoulders.
- Once you're there, retrace that pattern back down to the bottom.

PERFORMANCE TIPS FOR SUCCESS

- Most athletes view direct biceps training only as a way to build muscle in your biceps, without considering the benefits it has for developing durable elbow and wrist joints and strong forearms. When you perform it properly, you'll make gains in all these areas.
- Brace your core muscles hard to maintain the tall kneeling position and avoid letting the resistance pull your lower back into flexion.

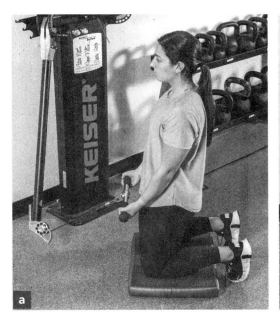 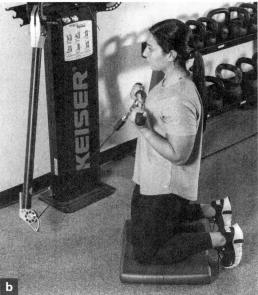

Figure 6.36 Cable tall-kneeling straight bar biceps curl: *(a)* start position and *(b)* curl.

LANDMINE SINGLE-LEG RDL (LATERAL ORIENTATION)

Single-leg strength and stability are hallmark traits of athleticism, and this is exactly the type of exercise to perform to get yourself on the fast track to success in this department. Achieve gains in single-leg strength, single-leg stability, hamstring strength, and glute strength.

HOW TO PERFORM

- Set up a barbell in the landmine position (i.e., anchored down with bumper plates, anchored into a sturdy corner, etc.).
- Hold the free end of the barbell in your left hand—a contralateral (opposite side) hold since the right foot remains stable on the floor.
- Keep your right foot flat on the floor and a subtle bend in your right knee.
- Staying in a roughly straight line from your left heel to the back of your head, hinge at the hips so that your chest lowers to the front and your left leg rises toward the back.
- Once you reach a point where your body is parallel to the floor, your chest is aiming down, and your heel is aiming up, slowly reverse that pattern back into the starting (top) position.
- Keep a subtle chin tuck and avoid letting the toes of your left foot rotate away toward the left.

PERFORMANCE TIPS FOR SUCCESS

- It's important to move at a slow and controlled pace. Avoid moving fast so you can dial in your technique.
- Grip the ground with your foot to provide more stability in the ankle. Think about scrunching the toes toward the heel as if you were grabbing the floor. This doesn't sound like it would make much of a difference, but will help a ton!

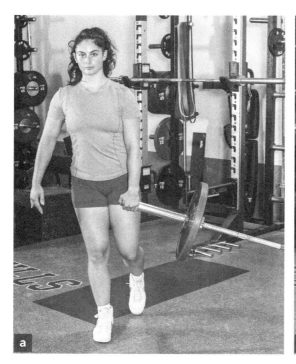 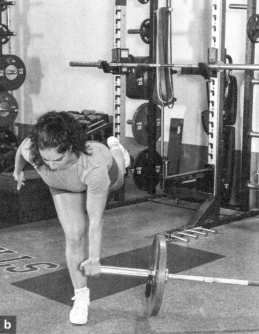

Figure 6.37 Landmine single-leg RDL (lateral orientation): *(a)* start position and *(b)* RDL.

Strength Exercises 147

DB SINGLE-ARM BENCH PRESS WITH SINGLE-ARM FIXED (TOP)

Bench pressing isn't just for powerlifters and individuals seeking maximal strength. It's also a great exercise for athletes looking to develop upper body horizontal pushing strength.

HOW TO PERFORM

- Lie flat on your back on a bench.
- Place your feet on either side of the bench on the floor.
- Drive both feet directly down into the floor to create leg drive, hip stability, and trunk stability and set a sturdy base from which to press.
- Hold a dumbbell in each hand with your knuckles aimed toward the ceiling. Start with both arms straight in the top position above your chest.
- In terms of the position of the pressing arm, the goal is to create a 45-degree angle with your elbow, which will allow for a stronger bench press.
- Without moving your right arm at all, lower your left arm toward your chest and then raise it to the top position again.
- Complete all reps in this setup, switch sides, and repeat.

PERFORMANCE TIPS FOR SUCCESS

- Perform this exercise to improve shoulder strength, shoulder stability, muscular strength in your chest, grip strength, and anti-rotation core strength.
- Keep the non-moving arm strong and stable by squeezing the dumbbell and making an effort to keep the arm straight throughout the duration of each set. This will help provide shoulder stability for easier pressing.

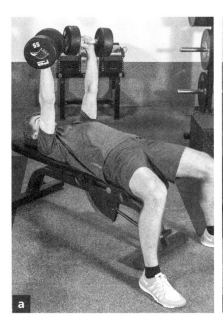 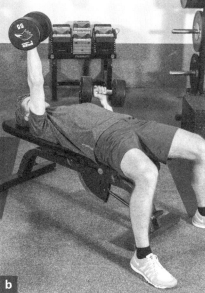 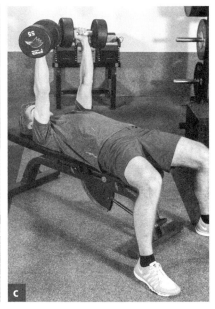

Figure 6.38 DB single-arm bench press with single-arm fixed (top position): *(a)* start position with both arms extended, *(b)* lower left arm toward chest, and *(c)* return left arm to top position.

DB NEUTRAL GRIP KICKSTAND RDL

Challenge hamstring muscle strength and flexibility plus improve hip joint mobility with this classic lower body exercise.

HOW TO PERFORM

- Stand with your feet roughly hip-width apart.
- Hold a dumbbell in each hand on either side of your legs and keep a tall spine from start to finish (i.e., avoid arching your low back or flaring your rib cage).
- Keep the dumbbells close to the sides of your body throughout each rep.
- This is where the kickstand part comes into play. Trace your left foot back so the toes of your left foot are in line with the heel of your right foot. Prop your left heel up, press your left toes down into the floor, and keep your right foot flat.
- Sit your hips back into the hip hinge pattern with a slight bend in your knees.
- Go low enough that the dumbbells end up on the sides of your legs at the spot just below your knees and near mid-shin.
- Aside from the slight knee bend, you'll want all the other motion to occur at your hips.
- Once you're in the bottom position, retrace the movement on the way back up to the top.
- Complete all reps on one side, switch sides, and repeat.

PERFORMANCE TIPS FOR SUCCESS

- Strong and flexible hamstrings developed from performing this exercise will make you more proficient in athletic skills such as sprinting, jumping, and cutting.
- Keep the entire surface of the stable foot pressing down into the floor to provide stability in your hips, with the foot of the kickstand leg there for secondary support.

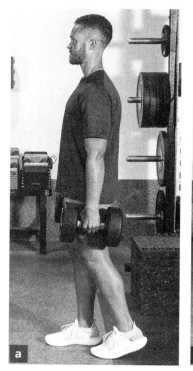 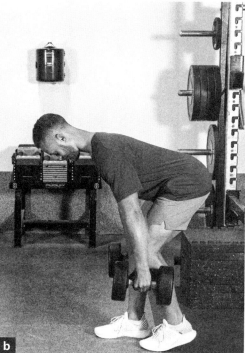

Figure 6.39 DB neutral grip kickstand RDL: *(a)* start position and *(b)* RDL.

CABLE SPLIT-STANCE SINGLE-ARM MID ROW WITH OPPOSITE HAND REACH

Challenge lower body stability and balance while strengthening your mid-back and core muscles in an anti-rotation fashion. The added component of the reach tacks on shoulder health, specifically in the shoulder blades.

HOW TO PERFORM

- Anchor one handle at mid-abdomen height on a cable column, grab it with your right hand, and take a few steps back from the column to create resistance on the pulley system.
- Position your lower body in a split stance with your left foot forward and flat on the floor and your right leg behind you with only your toes in contact with the floor.
- Stand halfway down toward the floor with both knees bent.
- At the same time, row your right arm toward your body while your left arm reaches straight forward and away from your body.
- Retrace that motion and bring both arms back to the starting position.
- Complete all reps in this setup, switch sides, and repeat.

PERFORMANCE TIPS FOR SUCCESS

- This exercise will help improve mid-back strength, lower body stability and balance, and shoulder blade health.
- Reach as far as you can straight forward during each rep to achieve maximum gains in shoulder health.

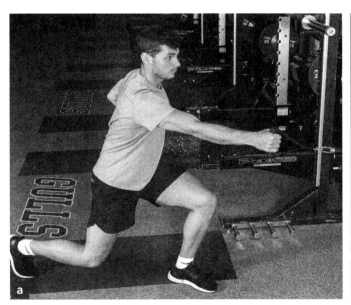
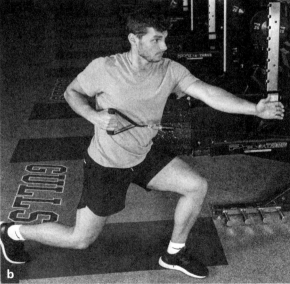

Figure 6.40 Cable split-stance single-arm mid row with opposite hand reach: *(a)* start position and *(b)* row and reach.

DB BENT-OVER LATERAL RAISE

Improve shoulder strength and health and benefit hip joint mobility and hamstring muscle flexibility while maintaining the bent-over position for this exercise.

HOW TO PERFORM

- Hold a dumbbell in each hand.
- Sit your hips back into the hip hinge pattern and slightly bend both knees.
- The logo on your t-shirt should be aimed down toward the floor and slightly forward.
- Keeping a subtle chin tuck and both arms long, raise both arms up laterally until you've reached roughly shoulder level, then lower them back to the starting position.
- The key here is to avoid any sort of swinging motion or momentum.

PERFORMANCE TIPS FOR SUCCESS

- The small muscles in and around your shoulders will make gains in strength and health when you perform this exercise.
- Focus on a slow and controlled motion during each rep.

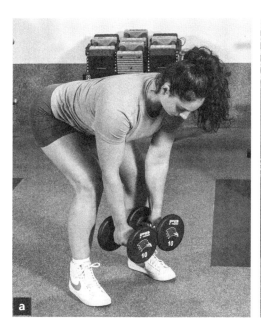
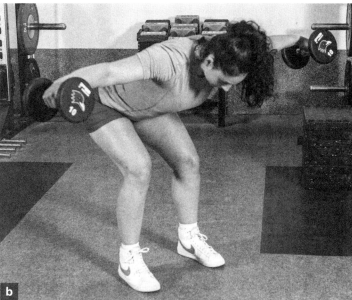

Figure 6.41 DB bent-over lateral raise: *(a)* start position and *(b)* lateral raise.

Strength Exercises **151**

AB WHEEL TALL-KNEELING ROLLOUT

This is a very challenging anti-extension core strength exercise, so be sure to really dial in technique and control your pace to make gains in this department!

HOW TO PERFORM

- Place both knees on top of a pad on the floor.
- Keep the toes of both feet aimed directly down into the floor.
- Hold both sides of an ab wheel with your hands.
- Before rolling forward, hollow out your abdomen and create a slight bend (flexion) in your mid-back. Avoid any sort of shrugging at your neck.
- Keeping both arms straight, lower your body out and forward until your nose and face are within inches of the floor. Return to the starting position.
- Avoid any sort of low back arch or rib cage flare.

PERFORMANCE TIPS FOR SUCCESS

- To avoid low back arch or rib cage flare, travel only as far forward as you can while maintaining a straight spine, then return to the start position. It may take a while to increase the overall distance you travel, so be patient with the process.
- Keep a smooth and controlled pace throughout the duration of each rep to maximize the core-strengthening benefits.

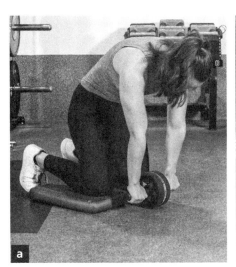
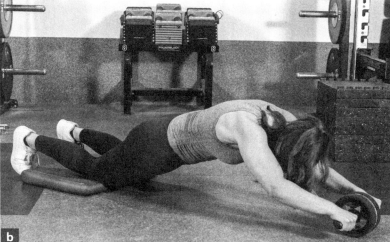

Figure 6.42 Ab wheel tall-kneeling rollout: *(a)* start position and *(b)* rollout.

BARBELL BENCH PRESS

Bench pressing isn't just for powerlifters and individuals seeking maximal strength. It's also a great exercise for athletes looking to develop upper-body horizontal pushing strength.

HOW TO PERFORM

- Lie flat on your back on a bench.
- Place your feet on either side of the bench on the floor.
- Drive both feet directly down into the floor to create leg drive, hip stability, and trunk stability and set a sturdy base from which to press.
- Hold a barbell with your hands slightly outside of shoulder-width apart. Aim your knuckles toward the ceiling. In terms of arm position, the goal is to create a 45-degree angle with your elbows, which will allow for a stronger bench press.
- Remove the barbell from the rack, position it directly above your chest, lower it until it gently touches your chest, then press it powerfully back up into the top position.
- Complete all prescribed reps.

PERFORMANCE TIPS FOR SUCCESS

- Performing this exercise with correct technique and form will allow you to improve shoulder strength, shoulder stability, muscular strength in your chest, and overall grip strength.
- Drive both feet down hard into the floor to add stability in the hips and core muscles for an easier press. This little detail goes a long way in your success with this exercise.

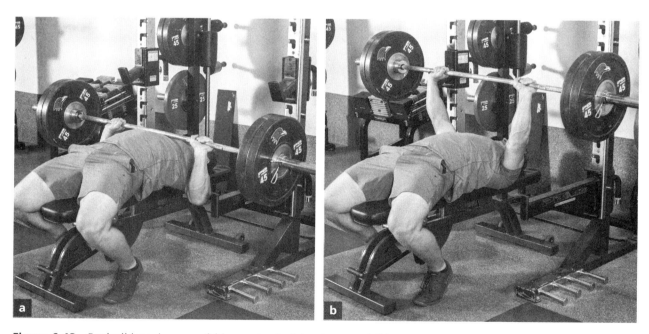

Figure 6.43 Barbell bench press: *(a)* lower barbell to chest and *(b)* press up.

DB SINGLE-ARM OFFSET BAND SLIDER LATERAL LUNGE

This challenging frontal plane of motion (side-to-side) exercise strengthens your groin muscles, in addition to providing durability to your hips and knees.

HOW TO PERFORM

- Loop a long resistance band around your right ankle and anchor the band at a low point on a sturdy object. The band resistance should be light to medium.
- Take a few steps away from the band anchor point and stand tall.
- Place a slider underneath your right foot and keep your left foot flat on the floor.
- The goal is to keep the toes of both feet aimed forward the entire time during each rep.
- Holding a dumbbell in your right hand, simultaneously bend your left knee, reach your right leg out to the right side while remaining straight, sit your hips back behind you, and keep a subtle chin tuck.
- Once you've reached the bottom position, actively pull the band back in toward your body with your right leg and stand up tall.
- Complete all reps on one side, switch sides, and repeat.

PERFORMANCE TIPS FOR SUCCESS

- Performing this exercise consistently will help you master lower-body strength in the frontal plane of motion in the groin muscles, hip joints, and knee joints.
- Think about sinking your hips down and back at the same time at the same pace. This one requires a ton of body control, so take your time and really focus on technique.

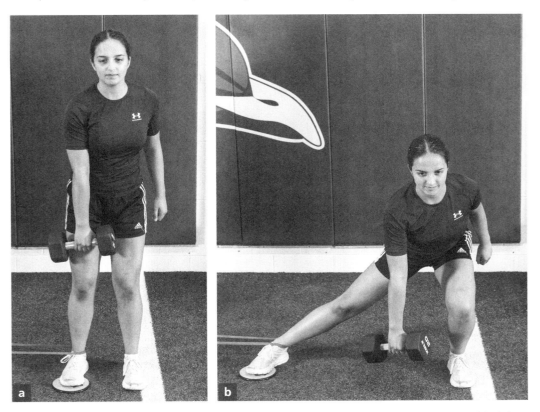

Figure 6.44 DB single-arm offset band slider lateral lunge: *(a)* start position and *(b)* slide right foot to the side.

LANDMINE STANDING VIKING SHOULDER PRESS

Here you'll be able to improve overhead pressing strength in your shoulders and anti-extension core strength.

HOW TO PERFORM

- Set up a barbell in the landmine position (i.e., anchored by bumper plates or into a corner of a wall).
- Use the Viking attachment, which allows your hands to be in a neutral grip position with the palms of both hands facing in toward each other. If you don't have access to this attachment, simply interlock the fingers of both hands at the end of the barbell closest to you and clench down tightly.
- Keep a very subtle bend in your knees and hips.
- Hold the Viking attachment on the landmine in the neutral grip position with a firm grip.
- While keeping your core muscles engaged (i.e., avoid lower back arch or rib cage flare), press both arms up into the overhead position, then lower to the starting position.

PERFORMANCE TIPS FOR SUCCESS

- Performing this exercise will help you make gains in overall shoulder strength and anti-extension core strength.
- Squeeze the handle or bar hard to increase stability in your wrists, elbows, and shoulders. Doing this will make a big difference in the strength of your overhead pressing.

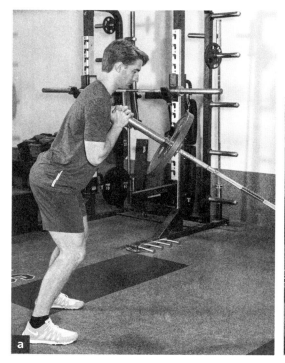 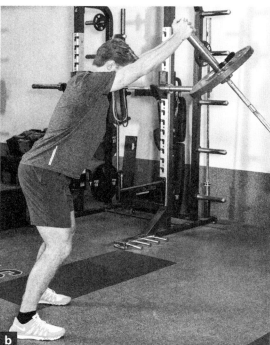

Figure 6.45 Landmine standing Viking shoulder press: *(a)* start position and *(b)* shoulder press.

BAND WIDE-STANCE CROSSBODY LONG CHOP

Improve your overall anti-rotation core strength and shoulder strength with this exercise, in addition to increasing hip joint mobility and groin flexibility.

HOW TO PERFORM

- Anchor a band on your right-hand side to a squat rack or cable column at roughly shoulder height. The band resistance should be between moderate intensity and heavy intensity.
- Grab the band with both hands at roughly shoulder-width apart and both arms straight.
- Step away from the anchor point toward the left so that the band is fully stretched out.
- Assume a wide stance with the toes of both feet aimed forward, both feet flat, and both legs straight.
- Keeping both arms straight, and without letting any other part of your body move, bring your arms and the band across your body at shoulder height from the right to the left side, and retrace that pattern back to the starting position.
- Complete all reps on one side, switch sides, and repeat.

PERFORMANCE TIPS FOR SUCCESS

- Really home in on keeping both arms straight without letting any other part of your body move.
- Squeeze your quadriceps on both legs to ensure that both legs remain straight to provide more stability in your lower body.

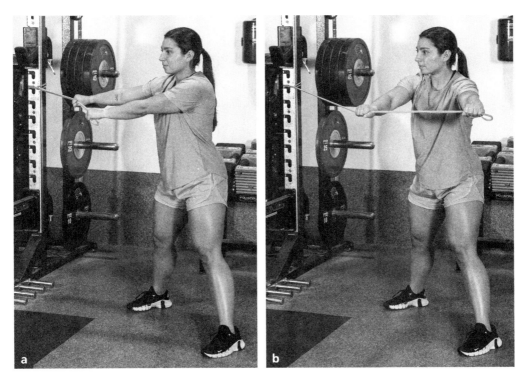

Figure 6.46 Band wide-stance crossbody long chop: *(a)* start position and *(b)* chop.

KB TOWEL STANDING HAMMER CURL

Many athletes view direct biceps training only as a way to build muscle in the biceps, without considering its benefits for developing durable elbow and wrist joints and strong forearms. When you perform this exercise properly, you'll make gains in all these areas.

HOW TO PERFORM

- Stand with your feet roughly hip-width apart.
- Loop a thick towel around the horn of a kettlebell and grab both ends of the towel. Holding the towel here on both ends will challenge your overall grip. If you don't have access to a towel, you can instead use a thick resistance band. You want the distance between your hands and the kettlebell to be around 8 to 12 inches.
- Use a hammer grip with your thumbs at the top.
- Keeping your upper arm and elbows as close to the sides of your body as possible, perform the hammer curl in a slow and controlled fashion.
- Once you've reached the top position without letting anything else move, lower the kettlebell back to the bottom position.

PERFORMANCE TIPS FOR SUCCESS

- Athletes need strong arms and durable wrist and elbow joints, which is why we've included this direct arm-training exercise in this program.
- Grip down hard on the towel or band to truly challenge your overall grip strength.

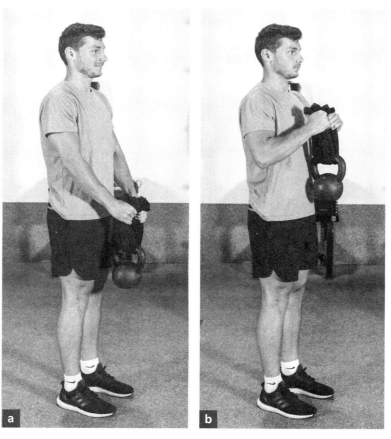

Figure 6.47 KB towel standing hammer curl: *(a)* start position and *(b)* curl.

BENT-KNEE STAR PLANK WITH CLAMSHELL

This exercise allows you to make gains in a variety of areas, namely your glutes, hips, shoulders, and core muscles.

HOW TO PERFORM

- Lie on the floor on your right side. Bend both knees to stack your legs.
- Ensure that your back is flush with your heels rather than your heels being behind your back.
- Place your right elbow directly under your right shoulder.
- From here, reach your top hand straight up toward the ceiling with a clenched fist.
- Rise up into the star plank position with both knees bent and both legs spread as wide apart as possible. Return to the bottom position while bringing your legs together again and resting your bottom hip back on the floor.
- Complete the prescribed reps on one side, switch sides, and repeat.

PERFORMANCE TIPS FOR SUCCESS

- Performing this exercise consistently will help you develop strength and stability in your shoulders, core, hips, and glutes, in addition to improving anti–side bend core strength.
- Really spread your hips apart in the top position to challenge lateral hip strength of both legs through what is known as hip abduction.

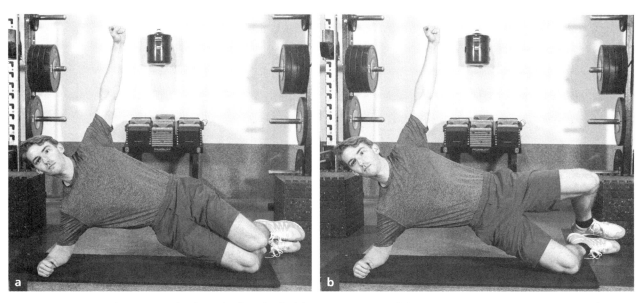

Figure 6.48 Bent-knee star plank with clamshell: *(a)* star plank and *(b)* legs spread in clamshell at top of star plank.

DB REAR FOOT–ELEVATED SPLIT SQUAT

The split squat position is one that we often see in a variety of sports and athletic endeavors; perform this exercise in your training program to remain strong and powerful in your knees, quadriceps, hips, and glutes. The rear foot–elevated variation is a true bump-up in overall intensity and is well-known as an exercise that athletes have a love–hate relationship with.

HOW TO PERFORM

- Place the laces of your right foot on top of a bench or split squat pad behind you. Keep your shoelaces in contact with the bench for added stability in your back leg.
- Stand tall with your left foot flat on the floor out in front. Hold a dumbbell in each hand.
- Lower your right knee toward the floor. Gently tap the floor with your right knee, then rise to the top position.
- Complete all reps on one side, switch sides, and repeat.

PERFORMANCE TIPS FOR SUCCESS

- Keep a tall torso throughout the duration of each rep. If staying completely upright is too much of a challenge, aim to keep a slight forward lean in the trunk instead.
- When in the bottom position, drive the front foot down hard into the floor to power yourself back up to the top during each rep.

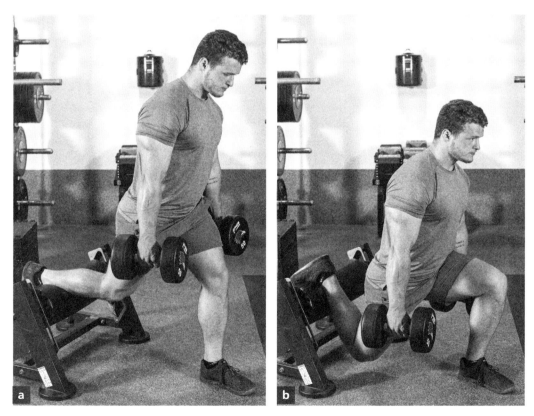

Figure 6.49 DB rear foot–elevated split squat: *(a)* top position and *(b)* knee lowered to floor.

DB SINGLE-ARM ROW

Athletes who develop good mid-back strength and shoulder strength often fare better in life, athletics, and recreational sports. We've included this exercise so that you can improve mid-back strength, shoulder strength, and grip strength.

HOW TO PERFORM

- Place your left knee on a bench with the laces of your left foot in contact with the bottom end (foot) of the bench.
- Place your left hand flat on the bench near the top end (head) of the bench.
- Keep your spine long and parallel with both the bench and the floor.
- From here, step your right foot out toward the right just enough to allow your right hand to move freely.
- Grab a dumbbell with your right hand and perform a horizontal rowing motion.
- Bring your right elbow up toward the right side of your rib cage and then lower it to the bottom position.
- Complete all reps on one side, switch sides, and repeat.

PERFORMANCE TIPS FOR SUCCESS

- Avoid any excessive motion at your shoulders or shrugging at your neck
- Maintain a smooth and fluid rowing motion with your arm.

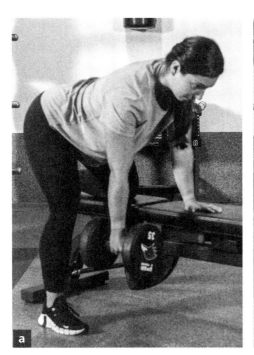 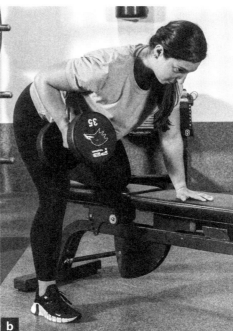

Figure 6.50 DB single-arm row: *(a)* start position and *(b)* row.

TWO DB KICKSTAND SQUAT

Improve overall strength and power in your quadriceps muscles, knee joints, patella tendons, and quadriceps tendons by performing this exercise consistently. This exercise will help you make some serious gains in the lower-body department!

HOW TO PERFORM

- Stand with your feet roughly hip-width apart.
- Hold a dumbbell in each hand on either side of your legs and keep a tall spine from start to finish (i.e., avoid arching your low back or flaring your rib cage).
- Keep the dumbbells close to the sides of your body throughout the entire range of motion within each rep.
- This is where the kickstand part comes into play. Trace your right foot back so that toes of your right foot are in line with the heel of your left foot. Prop your right heel up, press your right toes down into the floor, and keep your left foot flat.
- Bend both knees and squat down.
- In terms of how low to go, ensure that the dumbbells end up on the sides of your legs at the spot just below your knees and next to your mid-shin.
- Once you're in the bottom position, retrace the movement on the way back to the top.
- Complete all reps on one side, switch sides, and repeat.

PERFORMANCE TIPS FOR SUCCESS

- Place roughly 75% of your body weight on the foot that remains flat on the floor and roughly 25% of your body weight on the foot that remains propped up ("kickstand" foot).
- You'll need to be as stable as possible in your lower body during each rep, so don't rush. Instead, take your time and focus on the technique.

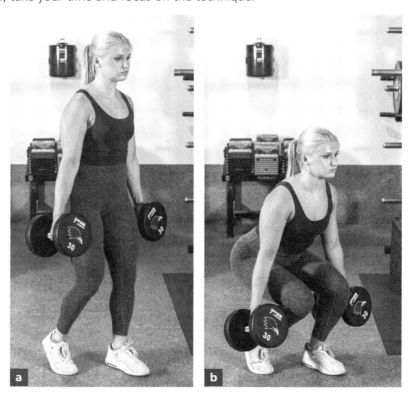

Figure 6.51 Two DB kickstand squat: (a) start position and (b) squat.

CABLE HALF-KNEELING SINGLE-ARM HIGH ROW

Most people focus only on horizontal rowing exercises, during which your arm rows from out in front of you. This exercise focuses on a vertical rowing pattern that aids in your overall shoulder health and strengthens your upper and mid-back.

HOW TO PERFORM

- Reach your right arm up high toward the handle of a cable column attached to a high anchor point and grab it with your right hand.
- Take a step back and place your right knee down on a pad on the floor with the toes of your right foot aiming directly down into the floor.
- Place your left foot flat on the floor in front of you with your left knee up.
- Row your right hand down toward the right side of your body by aiming your right elbow down toward your right pocket.
- Return your hand to the top position.
- Complete all reps in this setup, switch sides, and repeat.

PERFORMANCE TIPS FOR SUCCESS

- Perform this exercise to develop a strong upper and mid-back, in addition to benefiting from improved hip joint mobility and hip flexor flexibility.
- Allow for a subtle stretch of the rowing arm at the top of each rep when your arm is long; this will aid in both upper back muscle building and shoulder joint health.

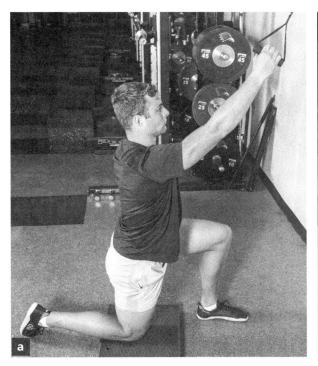
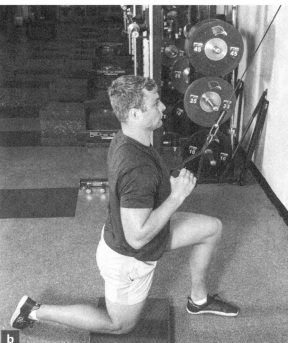

Figure 6.52 Cable half-kneeling single-arm high row: *(a)* starting position and *(b)* row.

DB FLOOR SKULL CRUSHER

Most athletes view direct triceps training as a way to build muscle in the triceps, without ever considering its benefits for developing durable elbow joints, durable wrist joints, and strong forearms. When you perform this exercise properly, you'll make gains in all of these areas.

HOW TO PERFORM

- Lie flat on your back on the floor with both knees bent and both feet flat.
- Hold a dumbbell in each hand. Keep your armpits tight to the sides of your body and avoid letting your arms sway out toward the sides. Start with both arms straight and your knuckles aiming up toward the ceiling.
- Slowly lower the dumbbells toward your ears by allowing your lower arms (forearms and wrists) to move. However, keep your upper arms straight.
- At the bottom of the rep, you'll notice that both of your elbows are aiming up toward the ceiling, which is perfect.
- Slowly raise both dumbbells back up to the starting position.

PERFORMANCE TIPS FOR SUCCESS

- Athletes need strong arms and durable wrist and elbow joints, which is why this direct arm training exercise is included in this program.
- Perform this exercise consistently to build durable elbows and wrists.

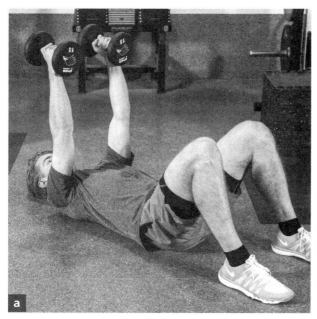 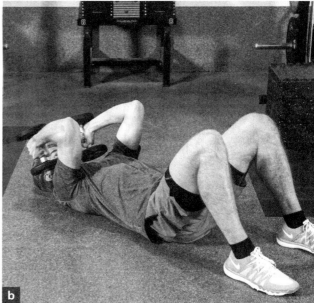

Figure 6.53 DB floor skull crusher: *(a)* starting position and *(b)* lower dumbbells.

DB FLOOR PRONE SUPERMAN ISOMETRIC

You'll benefit from not only increased lower back muscular endurance and strength, but also the anti-flexion core strength challenge provided by this exercise.

HOW TO PERFORM

- Lie flat on your front side on the floor.
- Point the toes of both feet directly down into the floor.
- Perform a subtle chin tuck and reach both arms into the overhead position in a Y shape with your thumbs up.
- In this position, grab a light dumbbell in each hand.
- Keeping your abdomen and the front of your upper hips in contact with the floor, raise your legs and arms off the floor as high as possible.
- Maintain this isometric (hold) position for the prescribed amount of time.

PERFORMANCE TIPS FOR SUCCESS

- Performing this exercise will help you improve lower back muscular strength, lower back muscular endurance, and anti-flexion core strength.
- Fight to keep both arms long and both legs long. This is much more difficult than it sounds.

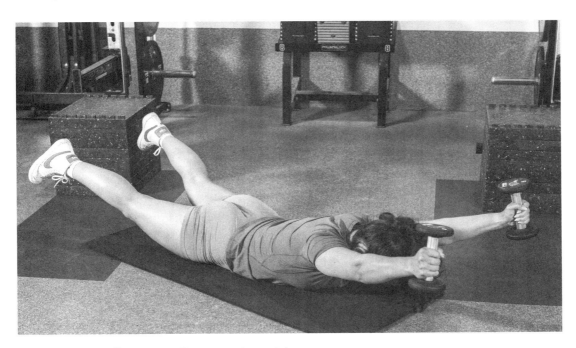

Figure 6.54 DB floor prone Superman isometric.

DB GOBLET SQUAT

The squat is a foundational movement pattern in life and athletic performance, which is why we've included it in this training program.

HOW TO PERFORM

- Stand tall with your feet roughly hip-width apart.
- Hold a dumbbell tight to your chest with both hands as if you were holding a bowl.
- Keeping both feet flat and your spine relatively straight, sink down into the bottom of a squat.
- Keep your chest proud so that I would be able to see the logo on the front of your shirt if I were standing in front of you.
- Stand back up to the top position.

PERFORMANCE TIPS FOR SUCCESS

- Perform this fundamental exercise as a way to strengthen your lower body, especially your quadriceps, knees, and hips.

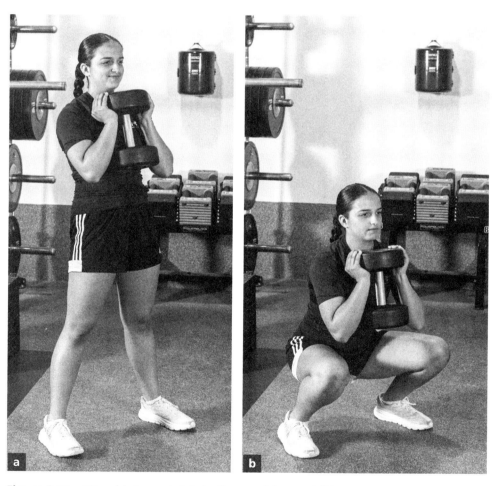

Figure 6.55 DB goblet squat: *(a)* starting position and *(b)* squat.

Strength Exercises **165**

BAND STANDING PALLOF PRESS

Use this exercise to increase overall anti-rotation core and shoulder strength from a standing position.

HOW TO PERFORM

- Anchor a band on your left-hand side to a squat rack or cable column at roughly shoulder height.
- Assume an athletic stance with a slight bend in your knees and hips and both feet flat on the floor.
- Grab the band with both hands and interlock your fingers.
- Press the band straight out in front of your shoulders until both arms are straight.
- Return your arms to the starting position.
- Complete all reps on one side, switch sides, and repeat.

PERFORMANCE TIPS FOR SUCCESS

- The most important aspect of this exercise is to press the band out and back in while using a controlled tempo as opposed to a rapid pace. The more time you spend under tension, the more challenging this exercise will be for your core and shoulder muscles.
- Make sure that you're pressing straight out in front of your shoulders during each rep; avoid any sort of upward or downward motion of your arms.

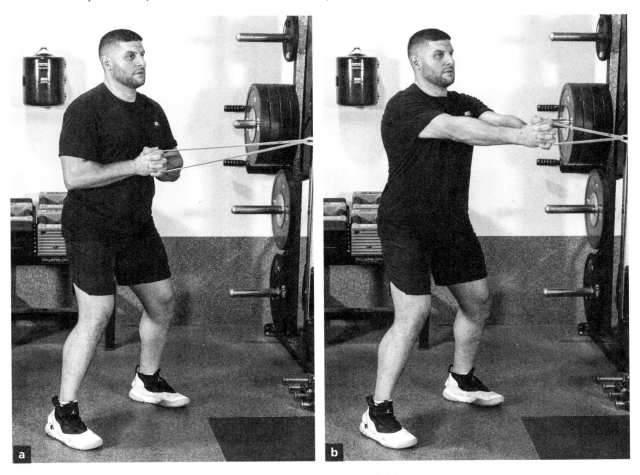

Figure 6.56 Band standing Pallof press: *(a)* starting position and *(b)* press.

BARBELL RDL

Strong and flexible hamstrings developed from performing this exercise will allow you to become more proficient in a variety of athletic skills, such as sprinting, jumping, and cutting.

HOW TO PERFORM

- Stand with your feet roughly hip-width apart.
- Hold a barbell in front of your hips with your hands roughly shoulder-width apart. Keep a tall spine from start to finish (i.e., avoid arching your low back or flaring your rib cage).
- Keep the barbell as close as possible to your body throughout the entire range of motion during each rep.
- Start by sitting your hips back behind you into the hip hinge pattern with a slight bend in your knees.
- In terms of how low to go, ensure that the barbell ends up anywhere from just below your knees to mid-shin.
- Aside from the slight knee bend, all other motion should occur at your hips.
- Once you're in the bottom position, retrace the movement back up to the top.

PERFORMANCE TIPS FOR SUCCESS

- Challenge your hamstring muscle strength and flexibility with this classic lower-body exercise, in addition to improving hip joint mobility.
- Work hard to allow only a slight knee bend while all other motion occurs at your hips.

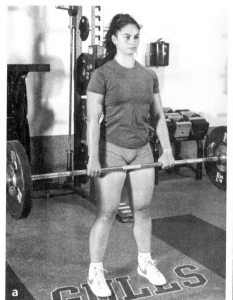 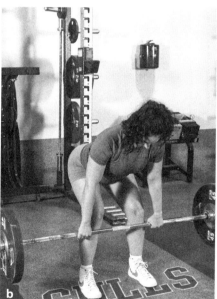 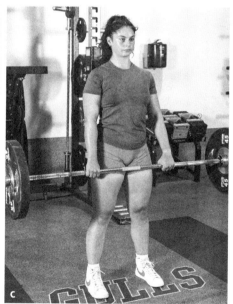

Figure 6.57 Barbell RDL: *(a)* start position, *(b)* hip hinge and lower barbell, and *(c)* return to start position.

Strength Exercises 167

KB SEATED SHOULDER PRESS (BACK SUPPORTED)

This exercise checks off a few boxes that all athletes need: shoulder strength, grip strength, and anti-extension core strength.

HOW TO PERFORM

- Sit on a sturdy bench that has a back support so your upper body remains in a relatively upright position.
- Keep both feet flat on the floor. Hold a pair of kettlebells tight to your upper chest and shoulder area in a front rack position.
- Squeeze the handles of both kettlebells hard for added stability, then press them straight up into the overhead position.
- Return the kettlebells to the starting position.
- Brace your core muscles during each rep to avoid arching at your low back or flaring your rib cage.

PERFORMANCE TIPS FOR SUCCESS

- Use this exercise to improve overhead pressing strength in your shoulders and anti-extension core strength.
- Keep your core muscles braced to avoid arching at your low back or flaring your rib cage.

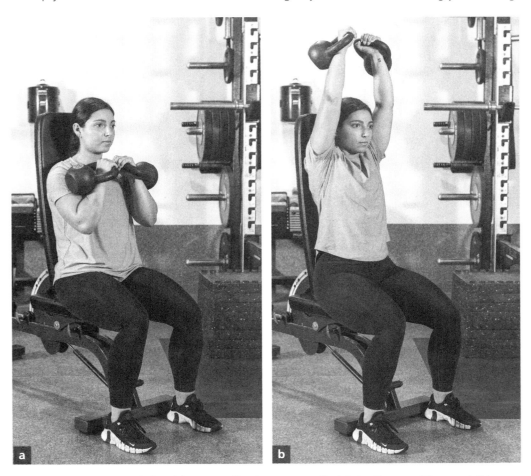

Figure 6.58 KB seated shoulder press (back supported): *(a)* starting position and *(b)* overhead press.

WALKING LUNGE

Lower body strength in the knees, quadriceps, hips, and glutes is important for success in life and sports. Walking lunges provide a great opportunity for you to develop strength in all these areas.

HOW TO PERFORM

- Stand tall with both feet roughly hip-width apart.
- Keep your feet and legs roughly hip-width apart the entire time to remain stable and balanced.
- Take a step out in front of you so that your right foot is flat on the floor, your left knee is hovering just above the floor, your left toes are in contact with the floor, and your trunk is at a slight forward lean.
- Stand up to the top and repeat this sequence on the other side.
- Each rep should feel smooth and controlled.

PERFORMANCE TIPS FOR SUCCESS

- Here you'll be able to improve lower body strength and muscular development, especially in your quadriceps and glutes.
- If you notice that you begin reaching out too far in front, simply shorten your stride.

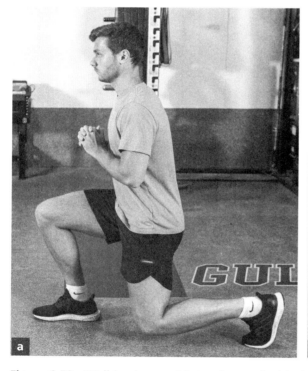 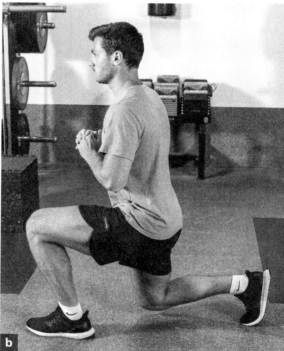

Figure 6.59 Walking lunge: *(a)* step forward with right foot and *(b)* step forward with left foot.

Strength Exercises **169**

DB STANDING BICEPS CURL

Most athletes view direct biceps training as a way to build muscle in the biceps, without considering its benefits for developing durable elbow joints, durable wrist joints, and strong forearms. When you perform this curl properly, you'll make gains in all these areas.

HOW TO PERFORM

- Stand with both feet roughly hip-width apart.
- Hold a dumbbell in each hand with your knuckles facing forward and hands down by your pockets.
- Keep the inside aspect of your arms and elbows tight to the sides of your body.
- Bend your arms so that your knuckles travel up toward your shoulders.
- Once you're there, retrace that pattern back down to the bottom.

PERFORMANCE TIPS FOR SUCCESS

- Athletes need strong arms and durable wrist and elbow joints, which is why we've included this direct arm training exercise in this program.
- Perform this exercise to keep your wrists and elbows healthy and durable.

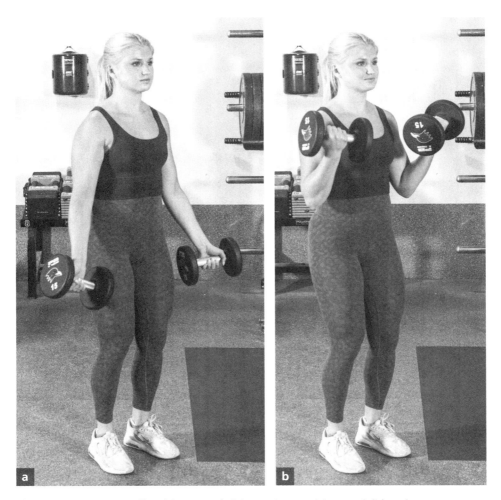

Figure 6.60 DB standing biceps curl: *(a)* starting position and *(b)* curl.

DB BENCH PRESS

Bench pressing isn't just for powerlifters and individuals seeking maximal strength. It's also a great exercise for athletes looking to develop upper-body horizontal pushing strength. The added benefit of using dumbbells in this scenario is that each arm has to work alone rather than together with one barbell, which helps you improve shoulder stability.

HOW TO PERFORM

- Lie flat on your back on a bench.
- Place your feet on either side of the bench on the floor.
- Drive both feet directly down into the floor to create leg drive, hip stability, and trunk stability to set a sturdy base to press from.
- In terms of arm position, the goal is to create a 45-degree angle with your elbows, which will allow for a stronger bench press.
- Hold a dumbbell in each hand with hands slightly outside of shoulder-width apart and press them straight up toward the ceiling. Lower both dumbbells down toward the sides of your chest, then press them back up into the top position with strength and power.
- Complete all prescribed reps.

PERFORMANCE TIPS FOR SUCCESS

- Perform this exercise consistently to improve shoulder strength, shoulder stability, muscular strength in your chest, and grip strength.
- Drive both feet down hard into the floor to increase stability in the hips and core muscles, which will make your pressing stronger.

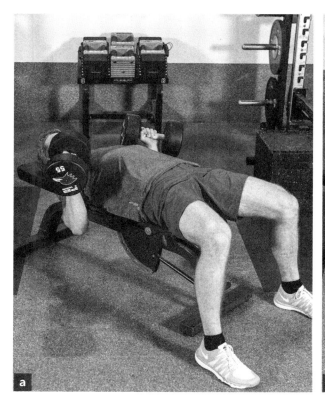
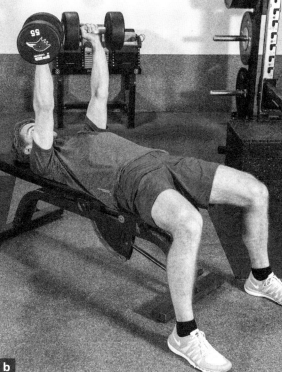

Figure 6.61 DB bench press: *(a)* starting position and *(b)* press.

SIDE PLANK

This exercise allows you to make gains in your hips, shoulders, and core muscles.

HOW TO PERFORM

- Lie on your right side on the floor and stack both legs, keeping them straight.
- Ensure that your entire body from head to heels is in a straight line.
- Place your right elbow directly under your right shoulder. From here, reach your left hand straight up toward the ceiling with a clenched fist.
- Raise your entire body up and away from the floor into the side plank position with only your right elbow, right forearm, and outside of your right foot in contact with the floor.
- Maintain this isometric (hold) position for the prescribed amount of time on one side, switch sides, and repeat.

PERFORMANCE TIPS FOR SUCCESS

- Perform this exercise to develop strength and stability in your shoulders, core, and hips, in addition to improving anti–side bend core strength.
- Work hard to keep your hips from sagging toward the floor and keep your body straight from head to feet.

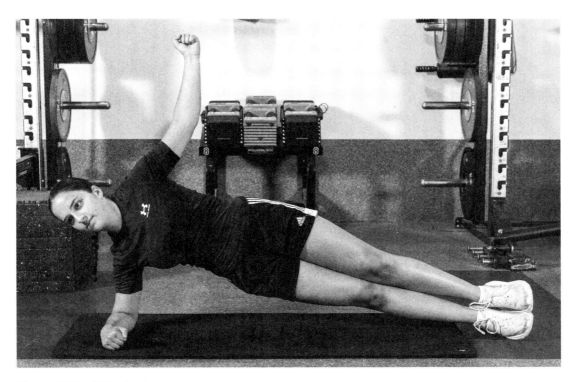

Figure 6.62 Side plank.

KB GOBLET LATERAL SQUAT

This frontal plane of motion (side-to-side) exercise is a great way to begin strengthening the inner thigh muscles (adductors) in your legs, which will help you during cutting, turning, sprinting, and other athletic movements.

HOW TO PERFORM

- Hold a kettlebell tight to your chest with both hands open as if you were holding a large bowl. In this goblet hold position, the horn of the kettlebell should be aimed down.
- Assume a wide stance with both feet flat on the floor and the toes of both feet aimed forward.
- Allow your hips to hinge back while simultaneously squatting laterally to your right side.
- In this bottom position, your left leg should remain straight, your right knee should bend, and your torso should remain straight from head to hips with a slight forward lean.
- Once you've reached the bottom position, make your way back up to the top position with both legs straight.
- Complete all reps on one side, switch sides, and repeat.

PERFORMANCE TIPS FOR SUCCESS

- The key performance tip is to maintain a straight leg on the non-working side as opposed to allowing that knee to bend.
- When performed properly, this exercise helps you develop strength in your adductor muscles, quadriceps, and glutes

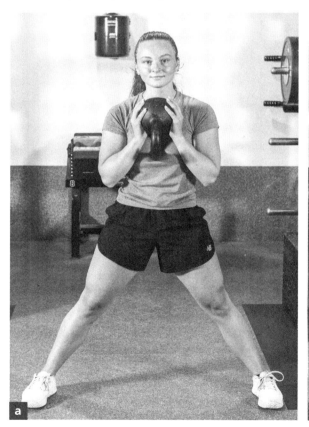
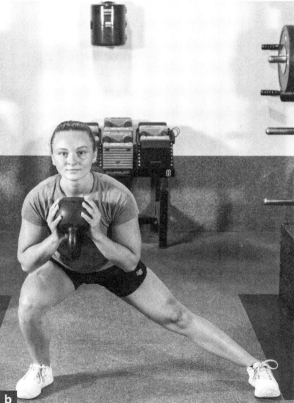

Figure 6.63 KB goblet lateral squat: *(a)* starting position and *(b)* squat to the right side..

Strength Exercises **173**

STANDING BAND PULL-APART

This is a classic upper-body exercise that strengthens your upper back and shoulders when performed consistently.

HOW TO PERFORM

- Stand tall with your feet roughly hip-width apart.
- Hold a long resistance band with both hands directly in front of your upper chest and shoulders. The band resistance should be light to medium.
- Keeping both arms long, begin to pull the band apart so that your hands travel back. Once you've reached your end point, retrace the band back to the starting position. It's important that only your arms move during this exercise and that the rest of your body remain still.

PERFORMANCE TIPS FOR SUCCESS

- When performed with proper technique, the band pull-apart is an excellent exercise for improving strength in not only the shoulders but also the postural muscles in your upper back.
- Be sure to keep your entire body still and allow motion to occur only at the arms.

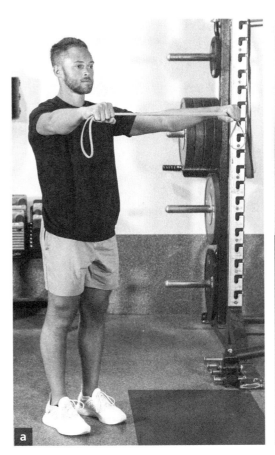 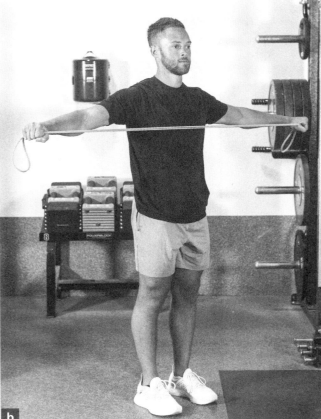

Figure 6.64 Standing band pull-apart: *(a)* starting position and *(b)* pull the band apart.

KB DEADLIFT

The deadlift is a foundational movement that helps you improve complete lower-body strength and power while also increasing your overall grip strength.

HOW TO PERFORM

- Stand directly over a kettlebell with your feet roughly hip-width apart.
- Sit your hips back into a hip hinge position as you also slightly bend your knees.
- Although the deadlift calls for a hip hinge movement pattern, this exercise requires a bit more of a knee bend than usual based on the height of the kettlebell.
- Once you're in the bottom position, grab either side of the horn of the kettlebell with both hands.
- Line up the tongues of your sneakers with your hands. This alignment with your hands and sneakers will position your hips and spine so you can be strong and powerful.
- Keeping a straight spine from head to hips with a subtle chin tuck, press both feet down into the floor as hard as possible and stand tall.
- Retrace that pattern back down the floor.

PERFORMANCE TIPS FOR SUCCESS

- Perform this exercise to develop a strong lower body and improve grip and forearm strength.
- Keep the kettlebell directly underneath you rather than allowing it to drift forward or backward.

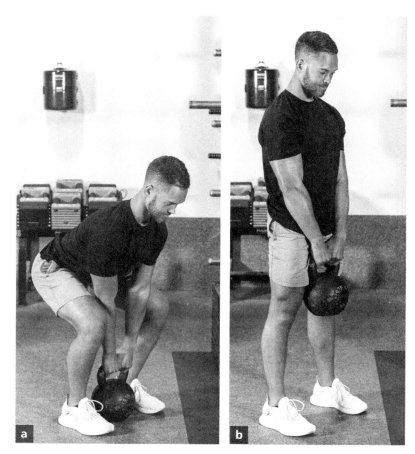

Figure 6.65 KB deadlift: *(a)* starting position and *(b)* lift.

BAND-ASSISTED PULL-UP

Upper-back strength is a major player in overall upper-body development for athletes, which is why we've included this foundational movement in the training program.

HOW TO PERFORM

- Stand on top of a sturdy bench or box.
- Hold on to a pull-up bar with your hands slightly wider than shoulder-width apart.
- Start by hanging from the pull-up bar with both arms straight.
- Straighten one leg down toward the floor directly over a long resistance band that is anchored from above on the pull-up bar. Cross this leg over the bottom leg. It's important to keep both legs straight the entire time.
- This long resistance band will support and assist your pull-ups. Use a band that provides enough assistance for you to achieve all the prescribed reps.
- Pull yourself all the way up into the top position so that your chin is just above the bar, then lower yourself back down. Move through a full range of motion each time.

PERFORMANCE TIPS FOR SUCCESS

- You'll be able to develop upper back strength, grip strength, and shoulder health when performing this exercise consistently.
- Avoid any sort of momentum or swinging during each rep. Brace your core muscles to avoid arching your low back or flaring your rib cage.

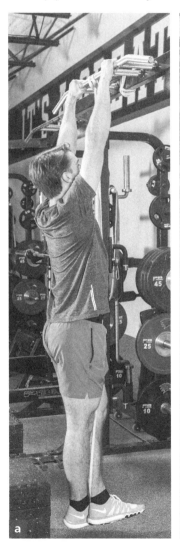
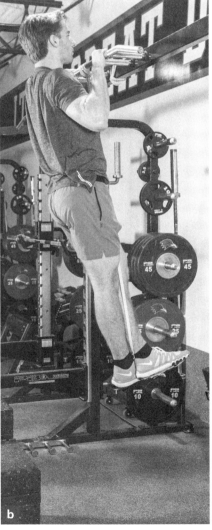

Figure 6.66 Band assisted pull-up: *(a)* starting position and *(b)* pull-up.

DB CAPTAIN STANCE SHOULDER PRESS

The benefits of the captain stance position are improving hip joint mobility, hip flexor flexibility, single-leg stability, and anti-extension core strength. You'll also improve overall shoulder strength and stability when performing this exercise.

HOW TO PERFORM

- Place your left foot flat on top of a sturdy box or bench at roughly knee height. This foot remains here the entire time.
- Keeping your right foot flat on the floor (this foot remains also remains in place the entire time) and your right leg straight, perform a slight forward lean.
- Hold a dumbbell in each hand just in front of your shoulders with your elbows bent.
- Here's where the exercise kicks in: Squeeze the dumbbells hard with both hands and press them into the overhead position until both arms are straight.
- Lower them back to the starting position.
- Complete all reps in this setup, switch sides, and repeat.

PERFORMANCE TIPS FOR SUCCESS

- This is a full-body, more-bang-for-your-buck exercise that athletes from all walks of life will benefit from.
- A major key to success is to avoid a low back arch or rib cage flare. Instead, keep your core muscles braced.

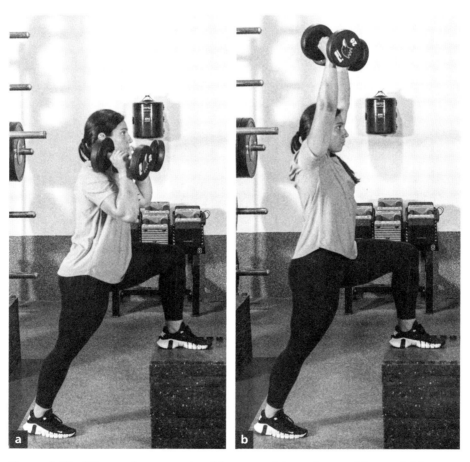

Figure 6.67 DB captain stance shoulder press: *(a)* starting position and *(b)* press.

Strength Exercises 177

DB SINGLE-LEG RDL (2 DB)

Single-leg strength and stability are hallmark traits of athleticism, and this exercise will get you on the fast track to success in this department. Make gains in single-leg strength, single-leg stability, hamstring strength, and glute strength.

HOW TO PERFORM

- Hold a dumbbell in each hand with hands down by the sides of your pockets.
- Keep your right foot flat on the floor and a subtle bend in your right knee.
- Keeping a roughly straight line from your left heel to the back of your head, hinge at the hips so that your chest lowers down to the front and your left leg raises up toward the back.
- Once you reach a point where your body is parallel to the floor, your chest is aiming down, and your heel is aiming up, slowly reverse that pattern back into the starting (top) position.
- Keep a subtle chin tuck and avoid letting the toes of your left foot rotate toward the left.

PERFORMANCE TIPS FOR SUCCESS

- Move at a slow and controlled pace to really dial in your technique.
- Grip the ground with your foot to provide more stability in the ankle. Think about scrunching the toes toward the heel as if you were grabbing the floor.

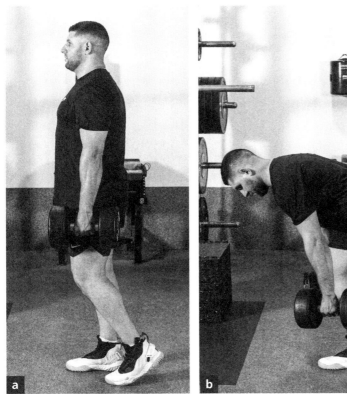 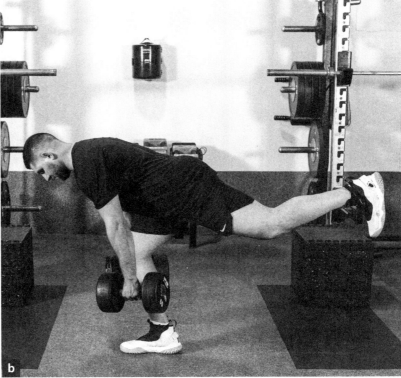

Figure 6.68 DB single-leg RDL (2 DB): *(a)* starting position and *(b)* hinge forward.

DB SINGLE-ARM BENCH PRESS

Bench pressing isn't just for powerlifters and individuals seeking maximal strength. It's also a great exercise for athletes looking to develop upper-body horizontal pushing strength. This unique exercise also incorporates an anti-rotation core challenge due to the unilateral loading setup.

HOW TO PERFORM

- Lie flat on your back on a bench and place your feet on either side of the bench on the floor.
- Drive both feet directly down into the floor when performing this exercise to create leg drive, hip stability, and trunk stability to set a sturdy base to press from.
- Hold a dumbbell in your right hand with your right arm straight just above your chest. Clench your left fist and reach your left arm just above your chest (this arm remains here the entire time).
- Lower your right arm down toward your chest and then press it back up.
- In terms of arm position, the goal is to create a 45-degree angle with your pressing elbow, which will allow for a strong bench press.
- Avoid any motion in your left (non-working) arm, and move only your right (working) arm.
- Complete all the prescribed reps in this setup, switch sides, and repeat.

PERFORMANCE TIPS FOR SUCCESS

- This exercise will help you improve shoulder strength, shoulder stability, grip strength, muscular strength in your chest, and anti-rotation core strength.
- Fight hard to avoid letting your torso rotate, and instead, drive both feet down hard into the floor to help provide lower body stability.

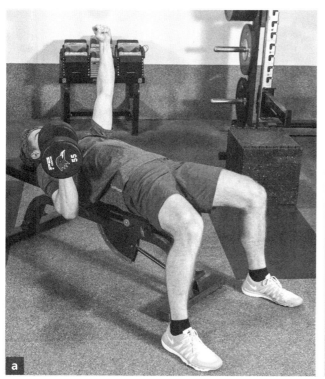 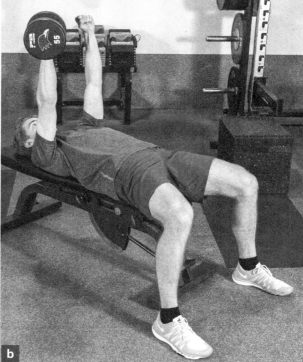

Figure 6.69 DB single-arm bench press: *(a)* lower arm down and *(b)* press.

DB FRANKENSTEIN FLOOR PRESS

Improve shoulder strength, shoulder stability, muscular strength in your chest, and grip strength. Fight through the challenge of having less leg drive in this unique variation on a traditional bench press.

HOW TO PERFORM

- Lie flat on your back on the floor with both legs long.
- Hold a dumbbell in each hand with hands slightly outside of shoulder-width apart and straight up toward the ceiling. Lower both dumbbells down to the sides of your chest, then press them back up into the top position with strength and power.
- While you press, squeeze your quadriceps muscles on both legs and drive the heels of both feet down into the floor to create hip and trunk stability and a sturdy base to press from.
- In terms of arm position, the goal is to create a 45-degree angle with your elbows, which will allow for a strong floor press.
- Complete all prescribed reps.

PERFORMANCE TIPS FOR SUCCESS

- Dumbbell pressing isn't just for powerlifters and individuals seeking maximal strength. It's also a great exercise for athletes looking to develop upper-body horizontal pushing strength.
- Drive the heels of both feet down hard into the floor to create lower-body stability.

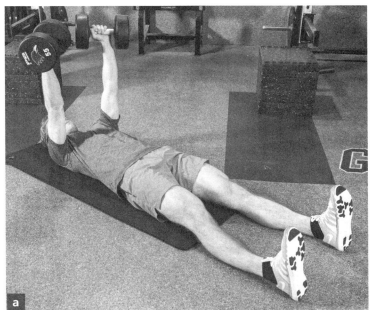

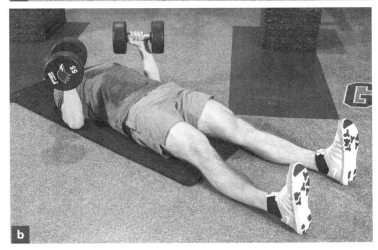

Figure 6.70 DB Frankenstein floor press: *(a)* starting position and *(b)* press.

CABLE SEATED MID ROW

There's nothing fancy here—just an age-old classic exercise that will help you develop muscle in your mid-back and shoulders.

HOW TO PERFORM

- Sit down on a sturdy box or bench with both feet flat on the floor and drive them down to create hip and trunk stability.
- With both hands, grab the handles of a cable column directly set up in front of you at mid-abdomen level.
- Make sure you are far away enough from the cable column that there is resistance on the pulley system.
- Row both hands in toward your mid-abdomen while both elbows reach back on either side of your body.
- Return your hands back to the starting position.

PERFORMANCE TIPS FOR SUCCESS

- Mid-back and shoulder strength are pivotal for upper-body posterior chain development for athletes in all walks of life.
- The key to success is to very slightly lean back for the duration of each set, which will allow for a greater range of motion at the end of each rep.

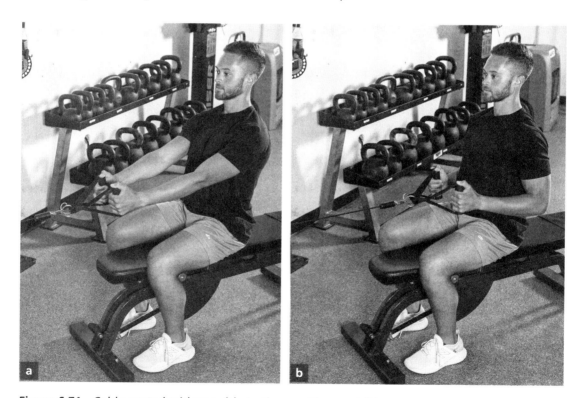

Figure 6.71 Cable seated mid row: *(a)* starting position and *(b)* row.

BAND RESISTED BENT-OVER DB LATERAL RAISE

Improve shoulder strength and health, in addition to hip joint mobility and hamstring muscle flexibility. The small muscles in and around your shoulders will also make gains when you perform this exercise.

HOW TO PERFORM

- Step on top of a long resistance band with both feet, placing the feet roughly shoulder-width apart. Loop the ends of the band around one dumbbell on each side (two total dumbbells). In this setup, the band is securely fastened around both dumbbells for safety. The band should be light to medium resistance.
- Hold a dumbbell in each hand.
- Sit your hips back into the hip hinge pattern and slightly bend both knees.
- The logo on your t-shirt should be aiming down toward the floor and slightly forward.
- Keeping a subtle chin tuck and both arms long, raise both arms up laterally until you've reached roughly shoulder level. You'll notice an increased challenge at the top of the rep where the band is stretched out.
- Slowly lower back down to the starting position.

PERFORMANCE TIPS FOR SUCCESS

- Avoid any sort of swinging motion or momentum. Instead, use a slow and controlled approach.
- A pro tip is to really sit your hips back into the hip hinge pattern to feel a stretch in the hamstrings and provide stability in your hip and core muscles.

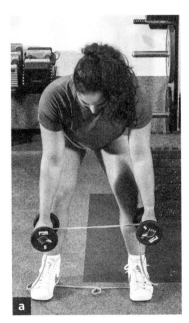
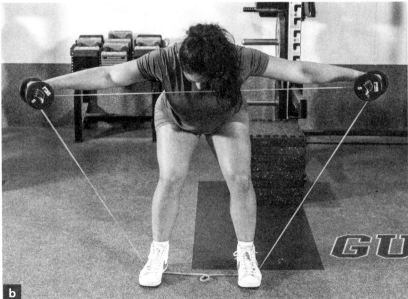

Figure 6.72 Band resisted bent-over DB lateral raise: *(a)* starting position and *(b)* lateral raise.

BAND WIDE-STANCE CROSSBODY SHORT CHOP

Benefit here by improving your overall anti-rotation core and shoulder strength, in addition to hip joint mobility and groin flexibility.

HOW TO PERFORM

- Assume a wide stance with the toes of both feet aiming forward, both feet flat, and both legs straight.
- Anchor a band to a squat rack or cable column on your left at roughly shoulder height. The band should be medium to heavy resistance.
- Grab the band with both hands, placing hands roughly shoulder-width apart. The arm furthest from the band anchor point should be bent at the elbow and close to your chest. The arm closest to the band anchor point should be straight out to the side.
- Bring the band across your body keeping both arms as close as possible to the front of your body. You'll need to straighten the outside arm, bend the inside arm, and then reverse that sequence to get back to the starting position.
- Complete all reps on one side, switch sides, and repeat.

PERFORMANCE TIPS FOR SUCCESS

- This exercise will help you increase anti-rotation core strength, shoulder strength, hip joint mobility, and groin flexibility.
- Keep the toes of both feet aimed forward and both legs straight in the wide-stance position to create a stable base.

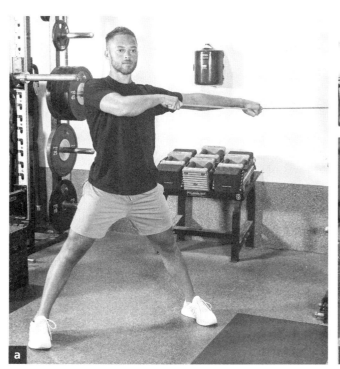 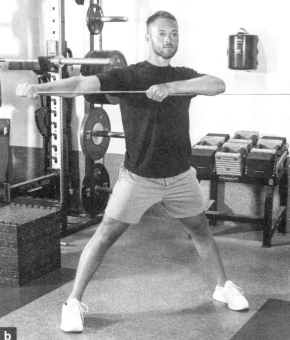

Figure 6.73 Band wide-stance crossbody short chop: *(a)* starting position and *(b)* chop.

KB HORNS-GRIP TALL-KNEELING BICEPS CURL

Most people view direct biceps training as a way to build muscle in the biceps, without ever considering its benefits for developing durable elbow joints, durable wrist joints, and strong forearms. When you perform this exercise properly, you'll make gains in all these areas.

HOW TO PERFORM

- Place both knees on top of a pad on the floor roughly hip-width apart and aim the toes of both feet directly down into the floor.
- Grab both sides (horns) of a kettlebell handle so that your thumbs are in the up position; this will look and feel like the hammer grip. Holding the kettlebell here will challenge your grip.
- Keeping your upper arms and elbows as close to the sides of your body as possible, perform the biceps curl in a slow and controlled fashion.
- Once you've reached the top position without letting anything else move, lower the kettlebell back to the bottom position.

PERFORMANCE TIPS FOR SUCCESS

- Athletes need strong arms and durable wrist and elbow joints, which is why we've included this direct arm training exercise in the program.
- Fight hard to keep your upper arm and elbows as close to the sides of your body as possible to ensure good technique.

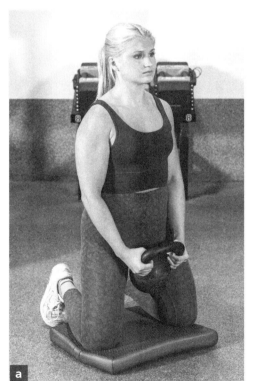 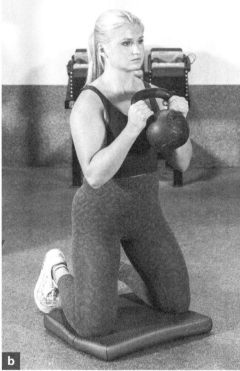

Figure 6.74 KB horns-grip tall-kneeling biceps curl: *(a)* starting position and *(b)* curl.

MINI-BAND BENT-KNEE STAR PLANK

Benefit from this exercise by developing strength and stability in your shoulders, core, and hips, in addition to improving anti-side bend core strength.

HOW TO PERFORM

- Loop a mini-band around both legs and just above both knees. The mini-band should be medium to heavy resistance.
- Lie on your right side on the floor, bend both knees, and stack your legs. Make sure your back is flush with your heels rather than your heels being behind your back.
- Place your right elbow on the floor directly underneath your right shoulder. The right elbow remains on the floor the entire time.
- From here, reach your top (left) hand straight up toward the ceiling with a clenched fist and raise up into the star plank position with both knees bent but separated, which will increase tension on the mini-band.
- Hold this position for the prescribed amount of time, switch sides, and repeat.

PERFORMANCE TIPS FOR SUCCESS

- This exercise allows you to make gains in your hips, shoulders, and core muscles.
- Raise both hips up high and away from the floor to increase the overall stability challenge.

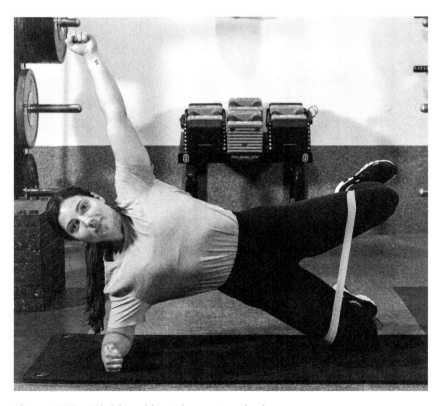

Figure 6.75 Mini-band bent-knee star plank.

DB SPLIT SQUAT

The split squat position is seen often in sports, athletic endeavors, and physical activities; perform it often in your training program to remain strong and powerful.

HOW TO PERFORM

- Place your rear foot just behind you so that only the toes of that foot are in contact with the floor.
- Position your front foot out in front of you, keeping it flat on the floor.
- Hold a dumbbell in each hand down by the sides of your pockets.
- Lower your rear knee down toward the floor, gently tap the floor with that knee, and rise back into the top position.
- Complete all reps on one side, switch sides, and repeat.

PERFORMANCE TIPS FOR SUCCESS

- Use this exercise to improve strength and power in your knees, quadriceps, hips, and glutes.
- Keep a tall torso through the duration of each rep.

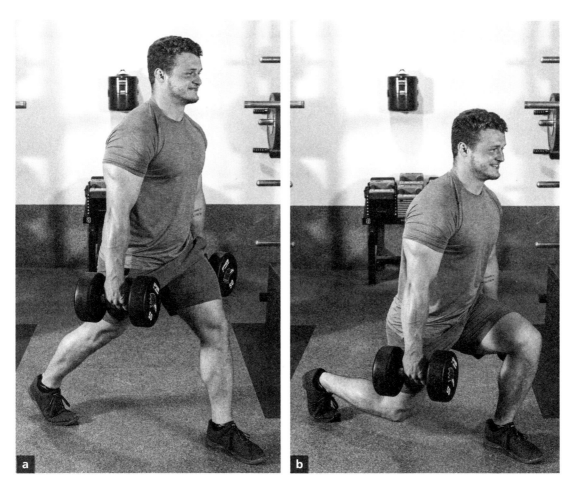

Figure 6.76 DB split squat: *(a)* starting position and *(b)* squat.

KB GOBLET KICKSTAND SQUAT

Improve overall strength and power in your quadriceps muscles, knee joints, patella tendons, and quadriceps tendons when performing this exercise consistently.

HOW TO PERFORM

- Hold a kettlebell tight to your chest with both hands as if you were holding a bowl.
- Stand with your feet roughly hip-width apart and keep a tall spine from start to finish (i.e., avoid arching your low back or flaring your rib cage).
- Keep the kettlebell tight to your chest throughout the entire range of motion within each rep.
- This is where the kickstand part comes into play. Trace your right foot back so the toes of your right foot are in line with the heel of your left foot. Prop your right heel up, press your right toes down into the floor, and keep your left foot flat.
- Bend both knees and begin squatting down.
- Once you're in the bottom position, retrace the movement back up to the top.
- Complete all reps on one side, switch sides, and repeat.

PERFORMANCE TIPS FOR SUCCESS

- When performing this exercise, place roughly 75% of your body weight on the foot that remains flat on the floor and roughly 25% on the foot that is propped up (the kickstand foot).
- Keep the entire surface of the stable foot pressing down into the floor to provide stability in your hips while using the foot of the kickstand leg for secondary support.

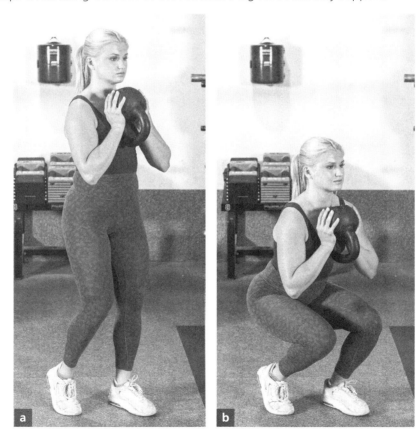

Figure 6.77 KB goblet kickstand squat: *(a)* starting position and *(b)* squat.

BARBELL FRONT SQUAT

The squat is a foundational movement pattern in life and athletic performance, which is why we've included it in this training program.

HOW TO PERFORM

- Set yourself up in the front rack position with a barbell.
- The front rack position consists of both arms roughly shoulder-width apart, both elbows bent and in front of you pointing forward, and the top edges of your fingertips sandwiched between the barbell and the upper part of your shoulders (collarbone area). This position will be easier if you have adequate mobility in your shoulder, elbow, and wrist joints, in addition to adequate flexibility in your triceps and latissimus dorsi muscles.
- If this position is too difficult to get into, use lifting straps for support or simply cross both arms into an X pattern with your fingertips resting on the upper part of your shoulders (collarbone area).
- Keeping both feet flat and your spine relatively straight, sink down into the bottom position of a squat.
- Once there, ensure that you have a proud chest so that I would be able to see the logo on the front of your shirt if I were standing in front of you.
- Stand back up to the top position.

PERFORMANCE TIPS FOR SUCCESS

- Perform this exercise to strengthen your quadriceps, knees, and hips, in addition to creating upper-back strength.
- Fight hard to keep your elbows driving up the entire time to maintain a tall and rigid spinal position.

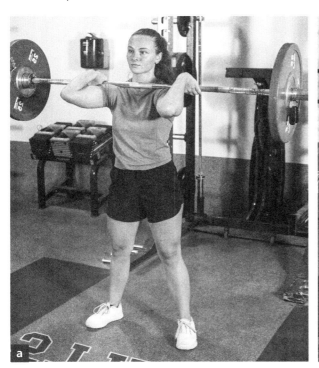 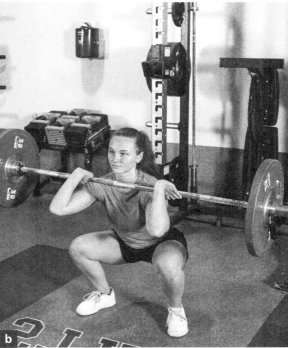

Figure 6.78 Barbell front squat: *(a)* starting position and *(b)* squat.

BAND TALL-KNEELING PALLOF PRESS

With this press you'll improve your core strength in an anti-rotation fashion by forcing the muscles in your midsection to stabilize against a rotational force, in addition to improving shoulder strength.

HOW TO PERFORM

- Kneel on the floor with knees roughly hip-width apart.
- Place a pad under both knees for comfort. Aim the toes of both feet directly down into the floor.
- Anchor a band around a squat rack or cable column at roughly chest height on your left side. Place the band inside your hands and interlock your fingers.
- Start with enough resistance from the band that it provides a challenge, but not so much that you're unable to remain stable.
- Press your arms out straight in front of your upper chest and shoulders, then return to the starting position.
- Complete all reps on one side, switch sides, and repeat.

PERFORMANCE TIPS FOR SUCCESS

- This is a classic exercise for improving your overall anti-rotation core strength and stability.
- Avoid any motion aside from the pressing motion in your arms. Fight hard to maintain stability!

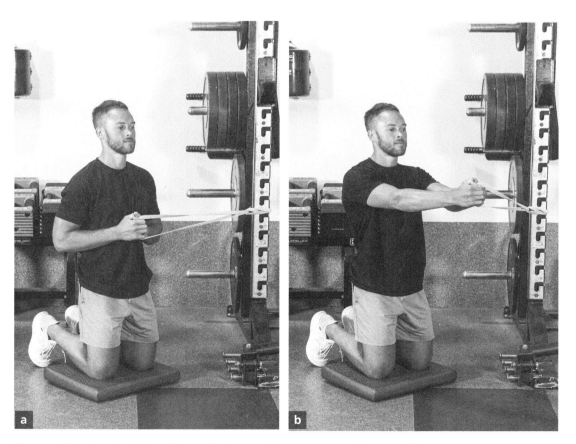

Figure 6.79 Band tall-kneeling Pallof press: *(a)* starting position and *(b)* press.

Strength Exercises 189

DB SKATER SQUAT

Knee strength and durability and strong quadriceps muscles are key components of athleticism. This exercise will build knee strength and durability.

HOW TO PERFORM

- Hold a light dumbbell in each hand down by your pockets.
- Place your left foot flat on the floor and bend your right knee so that your right heel is almost touching your left glute.
- Descend toward the floor, allowing your chest to slightly travel forward. Bend your left knee forward and past the toes of your left foot. Finally, allow your right leg to shift slightly behind you.
- At the same time you're descending with your lower body, raise both arms toward your upper chest and shoulder.
- Once you've reached the bottom, reverse the sequence to come back into the top position.
- Complete all reps on one side, switch sides, and repeat.

PERFORMANCE TIPS FOR SUCCESS

- Strong and durable knees and quadriceps are key qualities you'll develop by performing this exercise.
- Slow down, use proper technique, and keep your form in check.

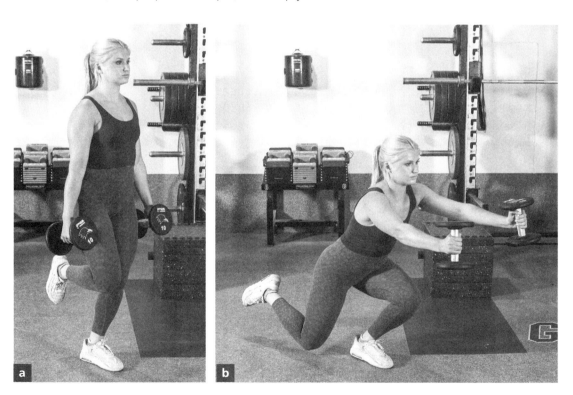

Figure 6.80 DB skater squat: *(a)* starting position and *(b)* squat.

CABLE DOUBLE-ARM SINGLE-LEG RDL WITH KNEE DRIVE AND ROW

Single-leg strength and stability are hallmark traits of athleticism, and this exercise will get you on the fast track to success in this department. The rowing pattern ties in the upper body as well.

HOW TO PERFORM

- Set up two handles at a low anchor point on a cable column.
- Grab both handles with your hands and take a few steps back.
- Keep your right foot flat on the floor with a subtle bend in your right knee.
- Keeping a roughly straight line from your left heel to the back of your head, hinge at the hips so that your chest lowers to the front and your left leg lifts toward the back.
- Keep a subtle chin tuck and avoid letting the toes of your left foot rotate toward the left. Move at a slow and controlled pace to really dial in your technique.
- Once your body is parallel to the floor, your chest is aiming down, and your heel is aiming up, slowly reverse that pattern and come back to the starting (top) position.
- As you come back to the top during each rep, simultaneously drive the knee up on the non-working leg, row both arms in toward the mid-abdomen, and straighten the working leg with your foot flat on the floor.

PERFORMANCE TIPS FOR SUCCESS

- Perform this exercise to make gains in single-leg strength, single-leg stability, hamstring strength, and glute strength.
- Be patient. Dial in technique and move at a controlled pace as opposed to rushing through your reps.

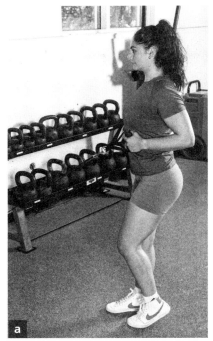
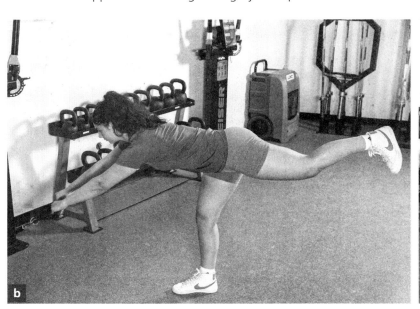
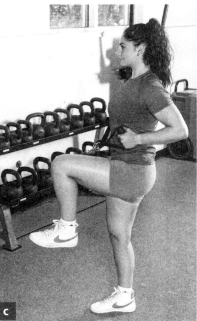

Figure 6.81 Cable double-arm single-leg RDL with knee drive and row: *(a)* starting position, *(b)* single-leg RDL, and *(c)* knee drive and row.

WEIGHTED NEUTRAL-GRIP PULL-UP

Upper-back strength is a major player in overall upper-body development, which is why we've incorporated this foundational movement in this training program. This exercise will also help you improve grip strength and shoulder health.

HOW TO PERFORM

- Stand on top of a sturdy bench or box.
- Add external load to your body (i.e., weight vest, chains, weight belt, etc.).
- The goal is to perform a full range of motion from the bottom to the top and back down again.
- Hold on to a neutral-grip pull-up bar with your hands roughly shoulder-width apart and your knuckles facing in toward each other.
- Start by hanging from the pull-up bar at the bottom with both arms straight.
- Pull yourself all the way up into the top position so that your chin is just above the bar, then lower yourself back down into the bottom position.

PERFORMANCE TIPS FOR SUCCESS

- Avoid any sort of momentum or swinging during each rep. Brace your core muscles to avoid an arch in your low back or a rib cage flare.
- Squeeze the pull-up bar hard with your hands to add stability in your wrists, elbows, and shoulders—this small detail goes a long way.

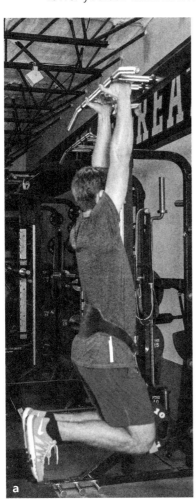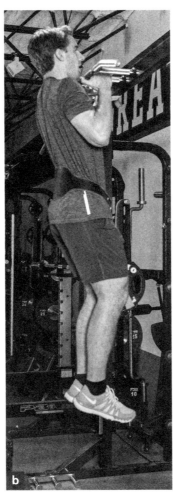

Figure 6.82 Weighted neutral-grip pull-up: *(a)* starting position and *(b)* pull-up.

DB HAND-SUPPORTED IPSILATERAL SINGLE-LEG RDL

The primary benefits of this exercise are gains in single-leg strength, single-leg stability, hamstring strength, and glute strength. You'll now be able to lift a little bit heavier than with a typical single-leg RDL based on the unique setup of this exercise.

HOW TO PERFORM

- Place your left hand on a squat rack or cable column at roughly hip height.
- Hold a dumbbell in your right hand—an ipsilateral (same-side) hold since your right foot will remain stable on the floor.
- Keep your right foot flat on the floor and a subtle bend in your right knee.
- Keeping a roughly straight line from your left heel to the back of your head, hinge at the hips so that your chest lowers to the front and your left leg lifts toward the back.
- Keep a subtle chin tuck and avoid letting the toes of your left foot rotate away toward the left. Move at a slow and controlled pace to really dial in your technique here.
- Once your body is parallel to the floor, your chest is aiming down, and your heel is aiming up, slowly reverse that pattern back into the starting (top) position.
- The additional hand support will allow you to lift a bit heavier than usual in this ipsilateral loading variation.

PERFORMANCE TIPS FOR SUCCESS

- Single-leg strength and stability are hallmark traits of athleticism, and this exercise will get you on the fast track to success in this department.
- Grip the ground with your foot to provide more stability in the ankle. Think about scrunching the toes toward the heel as if you were grabbing the floor.

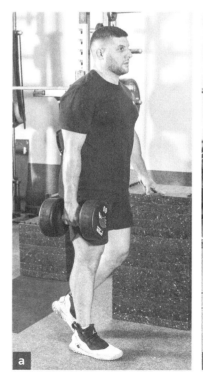 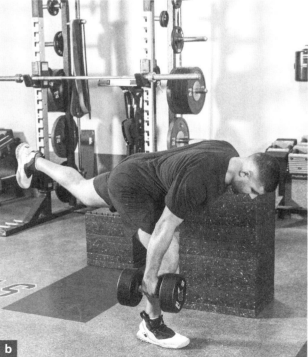

Figure 6.83 DB hand-supported ipsilateral single-leg RDL: *(a)* starting position and *(b)* single-leg RDL.

DB ALTERNATING BENCH PRESS (BOTTOM)

Here is a unique bench press variation that will help you improve shoulder strength, shoulder stability, muscular strength in your chest, and overall grip strength.

HOW TO PERFORM

- Lie flat on your back on a bench and place your feet on the floor on either side of the bench.
- Drive both feet directly down into the floor when performing this exercise to create leg drive, hip stability, and trunk stability, creating a sturdy base to press from.
- Hold a dumbbell in each hand with hands slightly wider than shoulder-width apart and down by the sides of your chest.
- In terms of arm position, the goal is to create a 45-degree angle with your elbows, which will allow for a strong bench press.
- Keeping your right arm still, press your left arm up into the top position, then return it to the bottom position. Repeat this exact sequence on the opposite side.
- Continue completing reps in this alternating fashion from the bottom until all the prescribed reps are complete.

PERFORMANCE TIPS FOR SUCCESS

- Be patient during each rep and follow through with intent during each sequence. During alternating variations of a given exercise, people often tend to rush through. Slow down and be precise.
- Work hard to root both feet down into the floor to stabilize the hips and core muscles; this will make the upper-body pressing action much stronger.

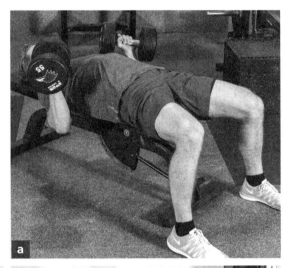

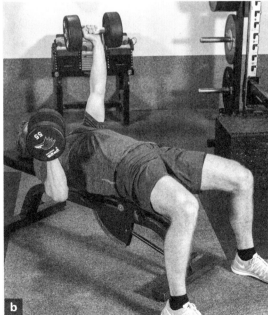

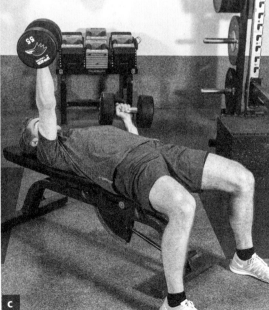

Figure 6.84 DB alternating bench press (bottom): *(a)* start position, *(b)* press left arm up, and *(c)* press right arm up.

BAND-RESISTED TALL-KNEELING AB WHEEL ROLLOUT

This is a very challenging anti-extension core strength exercise, so be sure to really dial in technique and control your pace.

HOW TO PERFORM

- Anchor a long resistance band to a sturdy object in front of you at a low anchor point and loop it around the inside of one of the ab wheel handles. The extra resistance from the long resistance band will increase the overall challenge of the exercise. The band should be light to medium resistance.
- Place both knees on top of a pad on the floor with the toes of both feet aiming directly down into the floor. Hold both sides of an ab wheel with your hands.
- Before rolling forward, hollow out your abdomen and create a slight bend (flexion) in your mid-back. Avoid any sort of shrugging at your neck.
- Keeping both arms straight, lower your body out and forward until your nose is within inches of the floor. Return to the starting position.

PERFORMANCE TIPS FOR SUCCESS

- When you perform this exercise, it is of the utmost importance to avoid any sort of arching at your low back or rib cage flare.
- Control your movement here. There's a lot going on, so keep it slow and dial in your technique within each rep.

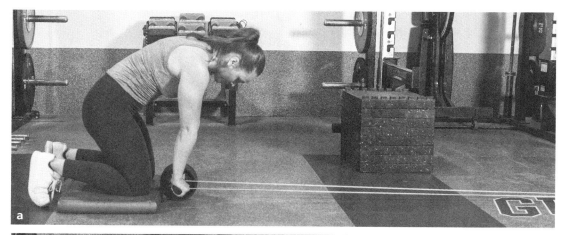

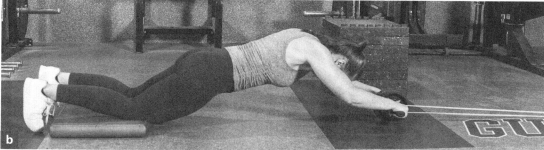

Figure 6.85 Band-resisted tall-kneeling ab wheel rollout: *(a)* starting position and *(b)* roll.

Strength Exercises 195

BARBELL POWER STEP-UP

With this exercise, develop single-leg power and explosiveness in the step-up movement pattern; this will directly transfer to activities such as sprinting and jumping.

HOW TO PERFORM

- Set up a stack of bumper plates or sturdy blocks at roughly mid-shin to kneecap height. The higher, the more challenging.
- Set a bar on your upper back so it rests just below your neck. Bend both elbows with the knuckles of both hands aiming up toward the ceiling. Pull the bar down hard into your upper back to create stability in your trunk and brace your core muscles to avoid a low back arch or rib cage flare.
- Keeping your left leg stiff and your spine tall, reach your right knee up high toward the ceiling and then aggressively stomp it down into the stack of bumper plates or sturdy blocks. This action should propel you up onto the step with your right foot while your left knee drives up toward your chest. Then step back down to the floor with your left foot and then with your right foot.
- Each rep should be powerful, fast, and explosive.
- Complete all reps on one side, switch sides, and repeat.

PERFORMANCE TIPS FOR SUCCESS

- Improve lower-body power and explosiveness with this step-up exercise.
- Explode up during each rep—this is a power-based exercise.

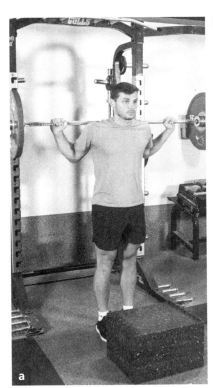 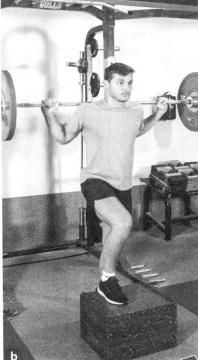 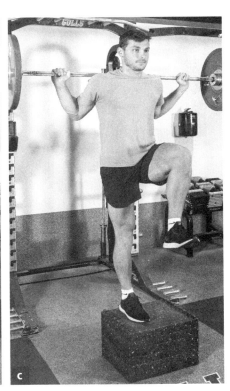

Figure 6.86 Barbell power step-up: *(a)* start position, *(b)* lift right knee and stomp on blocks, and *(c)* step up and drive knee toward chest.

BARBELL SPEED BENCH PRESS

Bench pressing isn't just for powerlifters and individuals seeking maximal strength. It's also a great exercise for anyone looking to develop upper-body horizontal pushing strength. The speed bench press is focused on moving the bar fast and explosively.

HOW TO PERFORM

- Lie flat on your back on a bench and place your feet on either side of the bench on the floor.
- Drive both feet down into the floor when performing this exercise to create leg drive, hip stability, and trunk stability, setting a sturdy base to press from.
- Hold a barbell with hands slightly more than shoulder-width apart, knuckles pointed up toward the ceiling. Remove the barbell from the rack and position it directly above your chest. Lower the bar until it gently touches your chest, then press it back up into the top position with as much speed and power as possible.
- In terms of arm position, the goal is to create a 45-degree angle with your elbows, which will allow for a strong bench press.
- Move the bar fast during each rep! However, avoid bouncing the bar off your chest.
- Complete all prescribed reps in this fashion.

PERFORMANCE TIPS FOR SUCCESS

- Perform this exercise to improve shoulder strength, shoulder stability, muscular strength in your chest, and grip strength, in addition to upper-body horizontal pressing speed.
- Complete each rep with speed but avoid bouncing the bar off your chest.

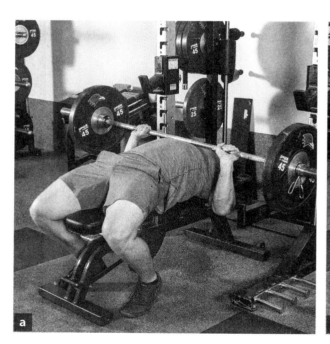 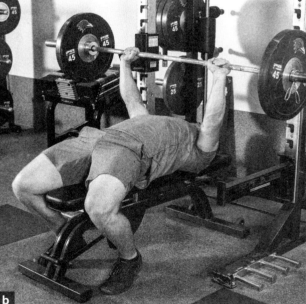

Figure 6.87 Barbell speed bench press: *(a)* starting position and *(b)* press.

Plyometrics and Power Exercises

Plyometrics and power training allow you to unleash your inner athlete through jumps, hops, bounds, and skips. The exercises in this chapter also include equipment such as medicine balls to challenge your ability to move in a fast and powerful manner. If your goal is to improve your overall athleticism, plyometrics and power training will put you on the fast track to success!

Exercises that fall under the category of *plyometrics* use what is known as the stretch-shortening cycle to create maximum force in the shortest amount of time possible. We typically see these exercises performed with assistance (e.g., resistance bands) using body weight or light forms of resistance (e.g., medicine balls). In terms of power training, these types of exercise will have a maximum speed and power component and use light to moderate external loads (e.g., dumbbells).

BAND-ASSISTED CONTINUOUS SQUAT JUMP

Repeating a series of squat jumps with continuous effort directly translates to being able to perform similar movements in competition. Using the band for assistance helps you develop the ability to jump higher as you progress.

HOW TO PERFORM

- Anchor two large resistance bands to a pull-up bar above you roughly shoulder-width apart.
- Stand under the bar and grasp a band in each hand.
- Sit your hips back in a quarter-depth squat and jump straight up toward the bar.
- Land softly back in the quarter-depth squat and immediately continue into the next squat jump for the number of reps prescribed.

PERFORMANCE TIPS FOR SUCCESS

- A band with stronger resistance will provide you with more assistance, and one with weaker resistance will provide less. A good rule of thumb is to start out using a band of medium resistance and adjust if needed after performing the first set.
- The goal is to spend as little time as possible on the floor between jumps, which is why you go only a quarter of the way down in the squat during each rep. Think of your continuous squat jump effort as rebounding off the floor as rapidly as possible during each rep.
- Using your lower body to repeat a series of squat jumps through a continuous effort directly translates to your ability to perform acts like this in sports and other physical activities.

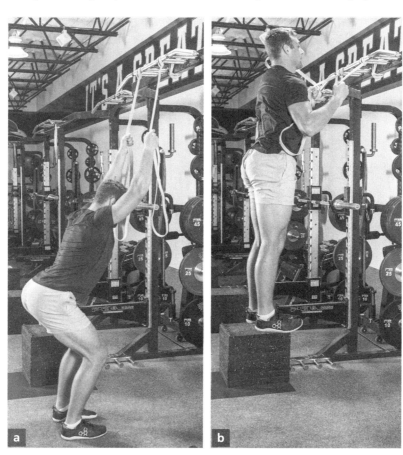

Figure 7.1 Band-assisted continuous squat jump: *(a)* start position and *(b)* squat jump.

MB TALL-KNEELING SLAM WITH HIP HINGE

Slamming the medicine ball without assistance from your lower body helps develop upper-body power.

HOW TO PERFORM

- Kneel with knees hip-width apart on a pad on the floor with the laces of both feet kissing the floor.
- Holding a medicine ball in both bands, raise the ball overhead.
- Slam the ball down into the floor while explosively shooting your hips back.
- Keep your arms long the entire time; don't bend your elbows. As the ball slams down into the floor, continue the swinging motion of your arms behind you.

PERFORMANCE TIPS FOR SUCCESS

- Slamming the medicine ball down into the floor while standing lets you use your entire body to develop power. When you kneel, your upper body must take over completely to produce power.
- It may take some time to truly master the sequencing and coordination of the upper and lower body. Start by performing a few practice reps slowly to master the movement and, most importantly, coordinate the simultaneous movement of the upper and lower body.
- Once your coordination and sequencing are ready, go at full speed and work your way through the prescribed sets and reps.

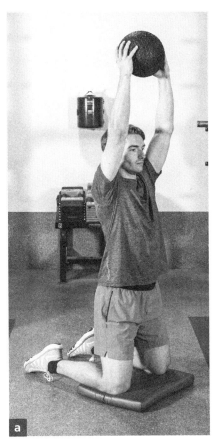
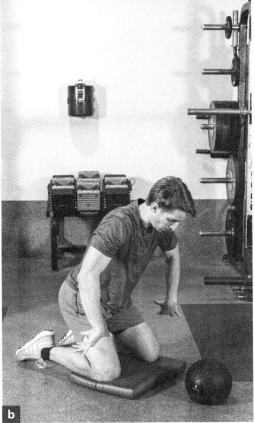

Figure 7.2 MB tall-kneeling slam with hip hinge: *(a)* start position and *(b)* slam ball.

MB SKATER HOP WITH CHOP AND STICK

This exercise will help you develop the ability to hop from side-to-side in the frontal plane, a common movement in a variety of sporting activities. The medicine ball in your hands acts as a form of resistance to increase the overall intensity.

HOW TO PERFORM

- Stand holding a 4- to 12-pound medicine ball in both hands.
- Begin by placing your body weight onto your right foot. Hold the medicine ball out toward the right side of your body. Both knees and hips should have a slight bend while your left foot hovers above the floor.
- Explosively hop to your left while chopping the medicine ball to the left and sticking your landing on your left foot. Pause for a moment.
- Repeat, hopping the right side with another brief pause when you stick the landing. Continue until all reps are complete.

PERFORMANCE TIPS FOR SUCCESS

- Start with a light medicine ball and master the movement with perfect technique. Once you've done that, increase the weight slightly over time.
- The goal of this exercise is not necessarily to increase weight as much as to move with power and precision. In other words, produce and absorb force in an athletic and controlled manner.

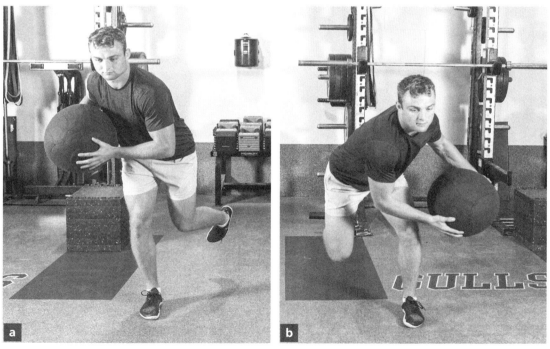

Figure 7.3 MB skater hop with chop and stick: *(a)* medicine ball to right, weight on right foot, and *(b)* hop to left and chop medicine ball to left side.

Plyometrics and Power Exercises **201**

MB HALF-KNEELING LATERAL WALL TOSS

This exercise will help you improve your upper body rotational power and stability in your hips and core muscles. Think of the medicine ball in your hands as a form of resistance to increase the overall intensity.

HOW TO PERFORM

- Set up in a half-kneeling position roughly one to two feet from the wall with the knee closest to the wall remaining up while the knee furthest from the wall rests on a pad on the floor.
- Hold the medicine ball in both hands and bring it across your body and away from the wall. Quickly toss the medicine ball across your body with both hands directly into the wall and catch it when it bounces back to you.
- Keep your lower body strong and stable in the half-kneeling position. To do this, drive the entire surface of your front foot down into the floor. Keep the toes of your back foot bent and pointing down into the floor to provide some additional grip and stability.
- This stable base of support in your hips is what will allow your upper body to rotate powerfully with the medicine ball as you toss it laterally into the wall.

PERFORMANCE TIPS FOR SUCCESS

- Start with a light medicine ball weighing about 4 to 6 pounds. You can increase the medicine ball weight over time as long as it does not slow the speed of your movement. Remember: Your goal is to be powerful!
- The half-kneeling position will create lower-body stability in your hips, knees, and ankles.

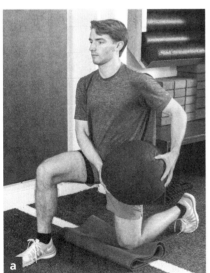 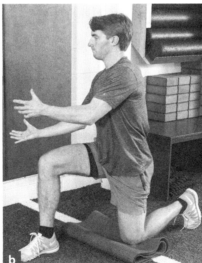 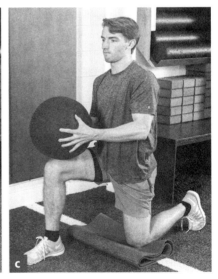

Figure 7.4 MB half-kneeling lateral wall toss: *(a)* start position, *(b)* toss medicine ball to wall, and *(c)* catch medicine ball on rebound.

90-DEGREE ROTATIONAL SINGLE-LEG HOP WITH STICK

Here's an exercise that you can use to build lower-body power and landing ability while rotating in the transverse plane. Couple that with the strength and stability benefits of using only one leg, and you'll find that this exercise packs a punch.

HOW TO PERFORM

- Start with your right foot on the floor and your left foot off the floor. Keep a subtle bend in the knee of the down leg (i.e., your right knee). Bend the up (i.e., left) leg a bit more to create space.
- Use the right leg to hop rotationally 90 degrees toward the left side and land on the left leg. Essentially, your legs will switch positions.
- You will hop in a 90-degree arc; hence the name of the exercise.
- Be sure to stick your landing on each rep.

PERFORMANCE TIPS FOR SUCCESS

- Use your arms for momentum as you hop to create power during the initial hop and maintain balance during the landing.
- Control your landing during each rep. Think about sinking down slightly by bending the hips and knees during each landing to absorb force.

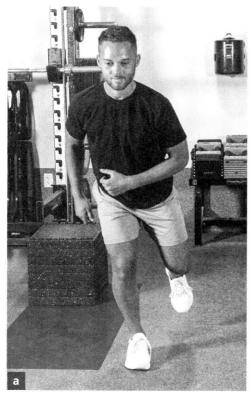 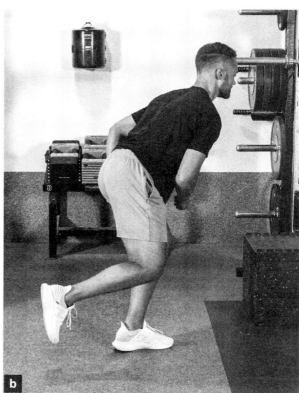

Figure 7.5 90-degree rotational single-leg hop with stick: *(a)* hop on one leg and *(b)* rotate 90 degrees and land on the other foot.

MB HALF-KNEELING AROUND-THE-WORLD SLAM

In this exercise, you'll develop the ability to maintain a stable trunk and hip position while performing an upper-body rotational power movement. This will translate to a variety of athletic movements and skills, in addition to improving balance and stability in your day-to-day life.

HOW TO PERFORM

- Place your right knee down on a pad on the floor and leave your left knee up.
- Keep your left foot flat on the floor and the toes of your right foot in contact with the floor.
- Keep a stable core and hip position during the upper body movement.
- Hold a medicine ball in both hands. Perform a circular ("around-the-world") motion above and around your head, then slam the ball down on the floor toward the outside of your left knee.

PERFORMANCE TIPS FOR SUCCESS

- Start with a light medicine ball in the ballpark of 4 to 6 pounds. You can increase the medicine ball weight over time as long as it does not slow down the speed of your movement. Remember: Your goal is to be powerful!
- The coordination this requires is a hallmark trait of some of the best athletes in the world—and some of the best everyday gymgoers! Competitive sports, recreational pickup sports, and day-to-day life all require you to be powerful rotationally, which is why this type of exercise is crucial for success.
- As a bonus, the half-kneeling position will help you improve stability in your hips, knees, and ankles.

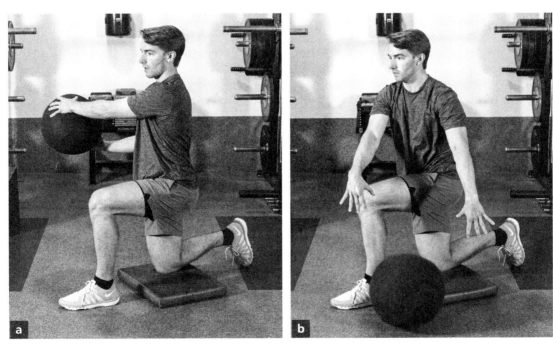

Figure 7.6 MB half-kneeling around-the-world slam: *(a)* around the world and *(b)* slam medicine ball.

BAND-RESISTED ACCELERATION POWER STEP

Your first steps in any sprinting activity are crucial if your goal is to be fast and powerful. First-step speed is a game-changer in sports, athletics, and physical activities; use this exercise to develop it.

HOW TO PERFORM

- Anchor a large resistance band around your waist from behind at roughly mid-abdomen level to something sturdy like a squat rack.
- Set up a sturdy bench or box in front of you.
- Set up your feet on the floor in a staggered stance similar to how you would start a race if someone challenged you in a sprint. I've always been right-foot dominant, so I tend to begin with my right foot forward.
- From here, power out from the starting position on the floor with lightning speed and land with your opposite foot (in my case, it would be my left foot) flat on the sturdy bench or box in a controlled manner.

PERFORMANCE TIPS FOR SUCCESS

- When some folks sprint, run, or perform any other type of locomotion, they completely forget about their arms. If you start out with your right foot in front, make sure that your left arm is out in front, and vice versa. This will be key!
- Use a bench or box roughly 18 to 24 inches high and anchor the band roughly 6 to 8 feet from it. These are general guidelines and may need to be adjusted based on your height.

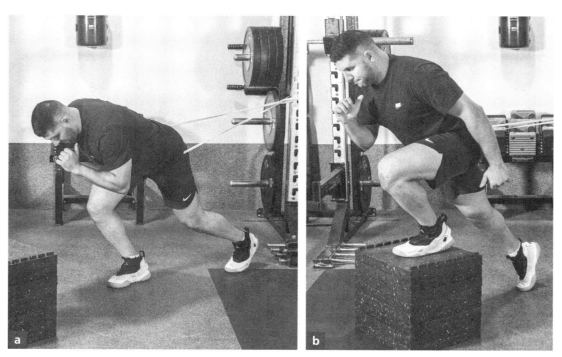

Figure 7.7 Band-resisted acceleration power step: *(a)* start position and *(b)* land on box.

Plyometrics and Power Exercises **205**

BARBELL EXPLOSIVE INVERTED ROW WITH HIP THRUST ISOMETRIC

Use this exercise to start building upper-body power, specifically in the horizontal pulling pattern. When it comes to athletic development and training for power, this pattern isn't trained nearly enough! This exercise is beneficial for competitive athletes and everyday gymgoers since it helps you unlock upper-body power and explosiveness—vastly undertrained in most programs.

HOW TO PERFORM

- Position your body directly underneath a barbell on a squat rack at roughly hip height. Be sure to place your upper chest directly underneath the bar.
- Bend both knees while keeping both feet flat on the floor. Reach out with both hands in an overhand position and grab the barbell, hands roughly shoulder-width apart.
- Raise your hips to create a straight line that begins at your knees and ends at your shoulders. Keep this hip position the entire time to ensure that your hips and core remain stable.
- Use your arms to explosively pull your body up toward the barbell with as much power as you can. This is much more challenging than it looks. Your finishing position is with your chest roughly an inch from the barbell. Then reset back to the bottom.

PERFORMANCE TIPS FOR SUCCESS

- Power is a quality in athletic development that tends to fade when we don't train it. Athletes often think of power as lower body jumping, hopping, and sprinting, but the upper body is just as important—that's why we added this exercise into the rotation.
- Since upper-body power is neglected, people tend to be unaware of how to really dial in and be powerful with their arms. Be very powerful when you pull your body up to the bar. This movement should occur with lightning speed!
- Plant both feet down into the floor to create a sturdy foundation with your feet and hips.

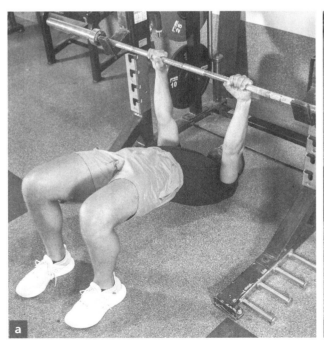
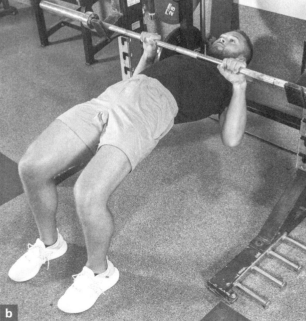

Figure 7.8 Barbell explosive inverted row with hip thrust isometric: *(a)* start position and *(b)* row.

MB STANDING DOUBLE CLUTCH SLAM

In the double clutch slam, you'll use additional momentum to create more force than a traditional slam with a medicine ball. Consider this exercise a level up from the traditional version that will aid in your overall athletic development!

HOW TO PERFORM

- Stand tall with both feet roughly hip-width apart on the floor.
- Hold a medicine ball with both hands just out in front of you with your elbows slightly bent.
- Quickly raise the ball up into the overhead position while standing tall, pull it back down hard to the starting position while bending both knees roughly halfway down, quickly raise it back up into the overhead position while standing tall again, and lastly, slam it down into the floor with everything you have.
- Welcome to the double clutch slam, which is packed with power!

PERFORMANCE TIPS FOR SUCCESS

- Start with a light medicine ball in the ballpark of 4 to 6 pounds. You can increase the medicine ball weight over time as long as it does not slow down the speed of your movement. Remember: Your goal is to be powerful!
- This sequencing and coordination take time to develop, so be patient with the process and dial in on how powerful you can be with each rep.

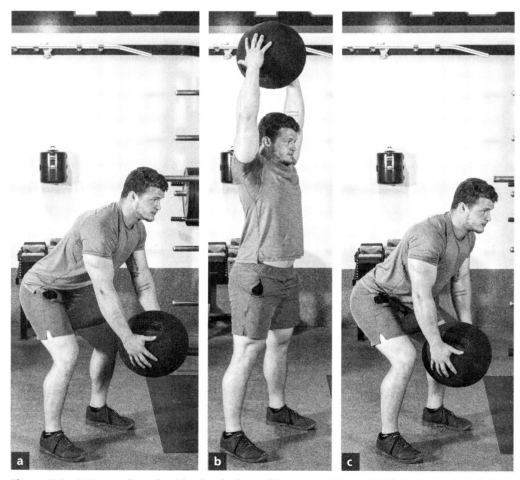

Figure 7.9 MB standing double clutch slam: *(a)* start position, *(b)* lift ball overhead, *(c)* swing ball down, *(continued)*

Plyometrics and Power Exercises 207

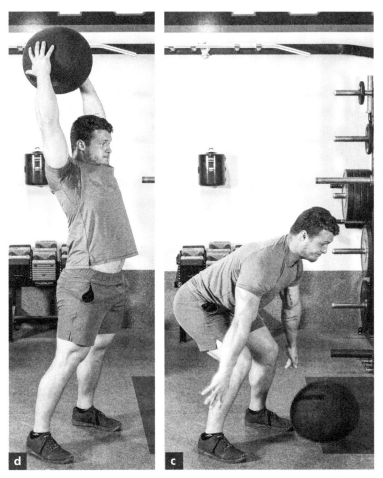

Figure 7.9 *(continued)* *(d)* lift ball overhead again, and *(e)* slam ball to ground.

BAND-RESISTED SKATER HOP WITH STICK (LATERAL ORIENTATION)

Sports require lower-body power in all three planes of motion: sagittal, frontal, and transverse. Life also requires you to remain powerful in your lower body (i.e., jumping, sprinting, etc.), but this physical quality diminishes quickly if not trained frequently. This lower-body power exercise focuses on the frontal plane, in which your body moves from side to side.

HOW TO PERFORM

- Anchor a resistance band around your waist and out toward the right side of your body around a sturdy squat rack or cable column.
- Walk away from the anchor point toward your left so that the anchor point is still on your right side. You'll want to get far enough away that the band is under near-full tension without much slack remaining.
- Place all your weight onto your right leg. Keep your right foot flat on the floor and a bend in your right knee and right hip.
- Bend your left knee and left hip much more and pick your left foot up off the floor.
- From here, hop out laterally from your right foot to your left foot, and stick the landing. This hop should be as explosive as possible, with a controlled and stable landing.
- Once all reps are complete on that side, turn around to the other side so that you're facing in the opposite direction, switch legs, and repeat.

PERFORMANCE TIPS FOR SUCCESS

- People tend to perform lower-body power movements with their legs only and forget to use their arms. We know how important leg motion is when performing lower body power movements, but keeping the arms active as well can be a true game-changer.
- Use your arms for momentum as you perform the skater hop. This will not only allow you to create more power during the initial hop, but provide more balance when you land.

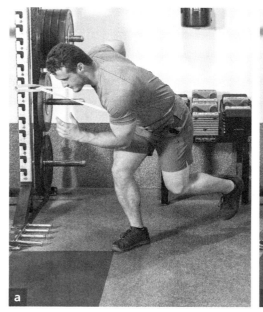 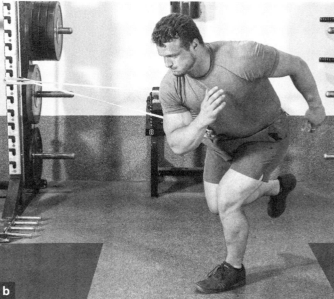

Figure 7.10 Band-resisted skater hop with stick (lateral orientation): *(a)* start position and *(b)* hop to other foot.

SINGLE-LEG BROAD JUMP TO DOUBLE-LEG STICK

This exercise takes the traditional broad jump exercise and ramps it up a notch! Here you'll develop the ability to hop out in front horizontally with one leg and then land on both feet, which is a precursor to single-leg lower-body power.

HOW TO PERFORM

- Start out standing on your left foot with a slight bend in your left knee and hip. Keep your right foot off the floor and your right knee bent.
- Swing both arms and your right leg to create momentum as you broad jump out in front with your left leg.
- Be sure to stick the landing with both feet.
- Complete the prescribed number of reps starting on your left foot, then complete the prescribed reps starting on your right foot. Your landing in each rep will be on both feet.

PERFORMANCE TIPS FOR SUCCESS

- Really commit to only using one foot at the beginning and then sticking your landing with both feet at the end. It feels a bit more awkward than it sounds, but it's worth it for building lower-body power!
- Jumping out in front and exploding forward with your lower body is an athletic skill we often see in activities such as running, sprinting, and playing recreational sports. This athletic skill is rarely performed on both feet, which is why performing this 1 to 2-foot lower-body power exercise will benefit your overall athletic performance.

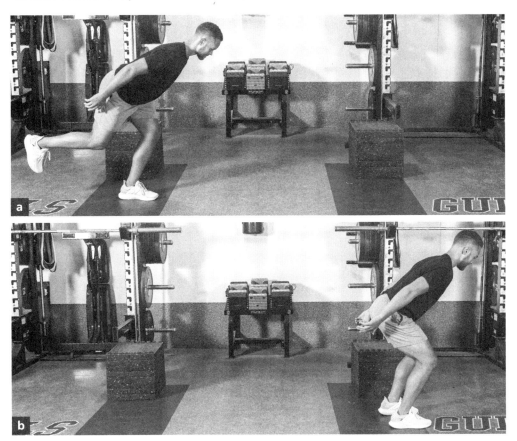

Figure 7.11 Single-leg broad jump to double-leg stick: *(a)* start position and *(b)* landing.

DB RELEASE SQUAT JUMP TO BROAD JUMP WITH STICK

Lower-body power and explosiveness are important for athletes regardless of what sport or physical activity they participate in. Performing this combo lower-body power exercise is a surefire way to improve your overall athleticism.

HOW TO PERFORM

- Stand tall with your feet roughly hip-width apart.
- Hold a dumbbell in each hand down by the sides of your pockets. Aim to keep the total weight of both dumbbells between 10-20% of your total body weight to ensure that you're able to move rapidly when performing this exercise. For example, if your body weight is 200 pounds, start with 10 pounds in each hand, totaling out to 20 pounds, which represents 10%.
- In a rapid motion, perform a squat jump up and away from the floor.
- When you land back down on the floor, quickly release the dumbbells behind you, and simultaneously swing both arms forward to perform a broad (horizontal) jump out in front.
- Stick your landing with body control.

PERFORMANCE TIPS FOR SUCCESS

- There's a lot going on here; break down each of the movements, and attempt the first few reps with only your body weight. Perform the squat jump and stick the landing. Then perform the broad jump and stick the landing. Now perform a squat jump, immediately transition into a broad jump, and stick the landing. Sometimes putting the pieces together like that helps you to improve your coordination. Add in both dumbbells once you feel ready to roll.
- Don't think of the broad jump as the only important motion here: The squat jump is important as well. Focus on lower body power during both motions of this combo exercise.

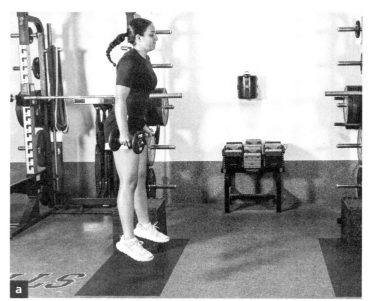
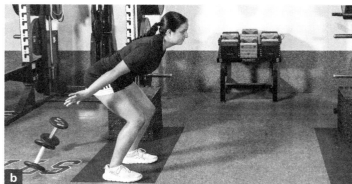
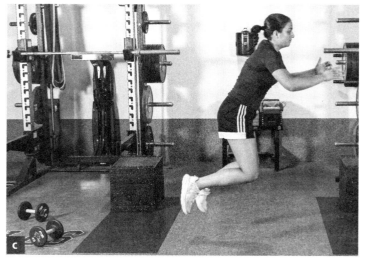

Figure 7.12 DB release squat jump to broad jump with stick: *(a)* jump up, *(b)* land and drop weights, and *(c)* broad jump.

MB STEP-THROUGH WALL CHEST PASS (STAGGERED-STANCE START)

Using your entire body to generate power while moving forward is the primary benefit of performing this exercise, and one that will contribute to your overall athleticism.

HOW TO PERFORM

- Hold a medicine ball on the sides with both hands.
- Set up your feet in a staggered stance (one foot in front and one behind) and crouch down as if you were about to shoot out in a track-and-field sprinting event .
- First, power forward with as much force as possible through an explosive first step.
- Next, perform a chest pass with a medicine ball into the sturdy wall in front of you.
- Leave enough space (roughly 10 to 15 feet) between your starting point and the eventual chest pass so that you're able to catch the medicine ball in a controlled manner after it bounces off the wall.

PERFORMANCE TIPS FOR SUCCESS

- To make this combined movement less complex, break it down into each of its parts. First, master powering out in front from the staggered stance position. Second, master the medicine ball wall chest pass motion. Then perform the entire sequence with your body weight only. Once you're ready, use the medicine ball to perform the entire exercise in one fluid motion.
- Start out with a light medicine ball in the ballpark of 4 to 6 pounds. You can increase the medicine ball weight over time as long as it does not slow down the speed of your movement. Remember: Your goal is to be powerful!

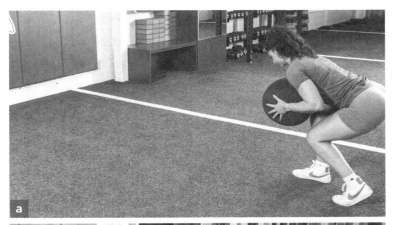

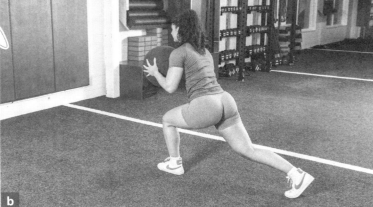

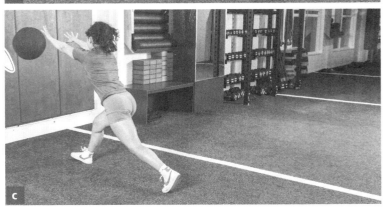

Figure 7.13 MB step-through wall chest pass (staggered-stance start): *(a)* start position, *(b)* step forward, and *(c)* chest pass to wall.

CONTINUOUS BROAD JUMP

The ability to repeat a lower body movement with power is highly coveted in athleticism, and you'll develop it with this exercise.

HOW TO PERFORM

- Stand tall with your feet roughly hip-width apart.
- In a rapid motion, swing your arms to create momentum and launch your body out in front of you, using as much lower body power as possible.
- Rather than sticking your landing, complete as many consecutive reps as the training program calls for (typically between 3 and 5). Stick the landing on the final rep.

PERFORMANCE TIPS FOR SUCCESS

- Many people make the mistake of being powerful only on the first rep, then coasting during the remaining reps. Don't let that be you! Be powerful during all reps.
- The goal is to use a continuous effort, which means that your job is to perform all reps consecutively, one after the other. However, if you need to break it down and simplify at first, perform a few reps as singles. Once you're ready, perform reps in a continuous manner. It's never a bad idea to focus on technique until you've mastered it!

Plyometrics and Power Exercises **213**

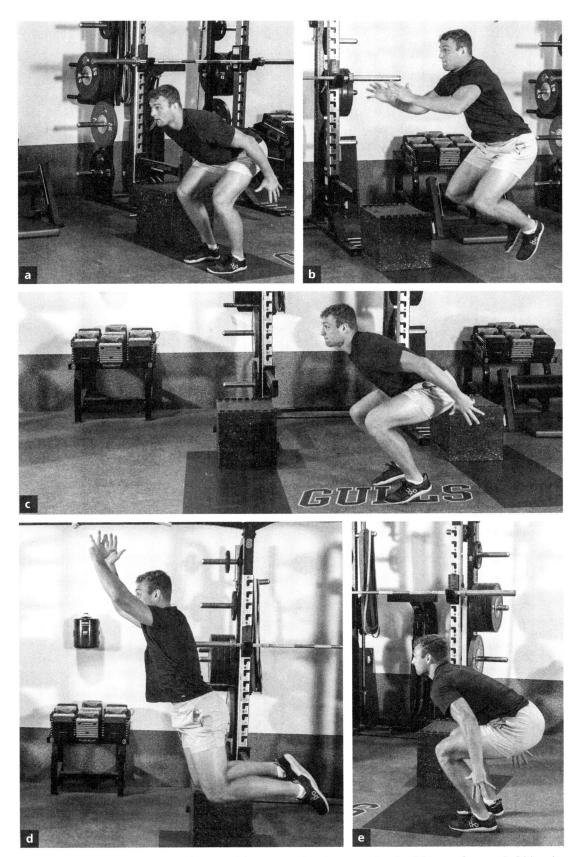

Figure 7.14 Continuous broad jump: *(a)* squat and swing arms back, *(b)* jump forward, *(c)* land and prepare for next jump, *(d)* jump forward, and *(e)* land and prepare for next jump.

MB STEP-BACK ROTATIONAL SINGLE-ARM WALL CHEST PASS

Transferring weight from the lower body through the core and finishing through the upper body is a skill possessed by some of the world's best athletes. You can build it, too! Use this exercise to help you get there.

HOW TO PERFORM

- Hold a medicine ball on the sides with both hands slightly in front of your body and both elbows bent.
- Keep your feet on the floor, slightly wider than hip-width apart.
- With the wall on your left, quickly step away from the wall toward the right.
- Rotate your entire body toward the wall (left side).
- Perform a single-arm wall pass with the medicine ball, throwing it at the wall.
- Perform this sequence as explosively as possible.

PERFORMANCE TIPS FOR SUCCESS

- Go through a few practice reps at a slow pace to make sure your technique is dialed in before performing the exercise at full speed. Remember, practice makes perfect.
- Start with a light medicine ball in the ballpark of 4 to 6 pounds. You can increase the weight over time as long as it does not slow down the speed of your movement. Remember, your goal is to be powerful!

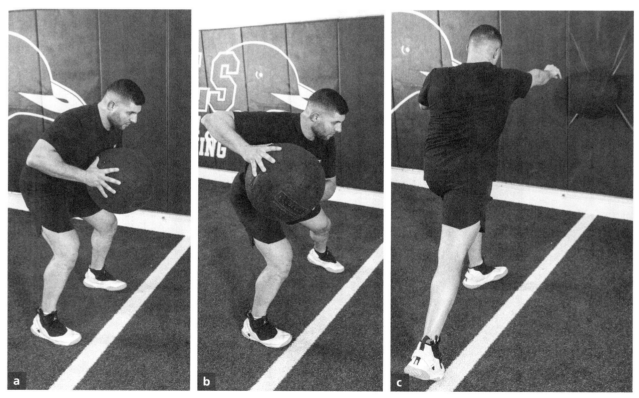

Figure 7.15 MB step-back rotational single-arm wall chest pass: *(a)* start position, *(b)* step away from wall, and *(c)* rotate toward the wall and throw the medicine ball to the wall.

BAND STANDING CONTINUOUS POWER PUNCH

Repeat power is a skill that some of the most talented athletes in the world possess. You can develop this same skill with consistent practice. This exercise will benefit you greatly in this area!

HOW TO PERFORM

- Anchor a resistance band directly behind you at mid-chest height around a sturdy squat rack or cable column.
- Step into the band and slightly bend both knees and hips to assume an athletic position.
- Set up both hands on the band at roughly shoulder-width apart with an overhand grip.
- Rapidly perform the power punch motion with your arms in a continuous effort while avoiding movement in the rest of your body.
- Keep both arms roughly shoulder-width apart throughout the duration of each set.

PERFORMANCE TIPS FOR SUCCESS

- Start with a band that feels moderately challenging. Try a few reps and see if it feels like the right amount of tension. If it's too easy, use a band with more resistance, and if it's too hard, use a band with less resistance.
- It's important to move at a rapid and continuous pace.
- Begin each set with enough tension on the band to be able to punch against. That's the key!

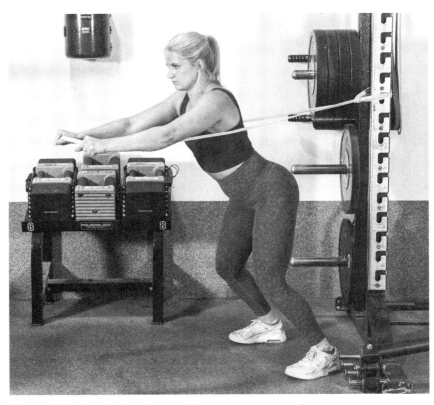

Figure 7.16 Band standing continuous power punch.

PLATE SKATER HOP WITH QUICK, STICK, AND PUNCH

Being able to quickly hop out laterally to one side, immediately hop back to the other side, and then stick your landing is a challenge—even more so when you add in a punch while holding a weight plate. You'll develop both power and force absorption with this exercise.

HOW TO PERFORM

- Hold a weight plate with both hands out by your right pocket.
- Stand on your right foot with a slight bend in your right knee and hip. Keep your left foot off the floor with a slight bend in your left knee and hip as well.
- Lean into your right hip, then hop out laterally toward your left foot.
- As you bring the weight plate across your body toward your left side, land on your left foot, then immediately hop back toward your right side.
- Finally, stick the landing on your right foot while also punching the weight plate down toward the right side of your body, which will make the landing that much more challenging.

PERFORMANCE TIPS FOR SUCCESS

- When learning a complex movement, it's easier to break it down into individual parts. If this exercise is a challenge, simply perform one motion at a time at a slow speed to get the hang of things. When you're ready, bump it up to full speed and go through the entire exercise.
- Hopping laterally can feel awkward for some people, especially if you don't do it often. This movement might seem silly, but think of the motion as a dance you perform from side to side with your hips. This is an important concept you can use to truly feel the lower body produce and absorb force during each hop and stick.

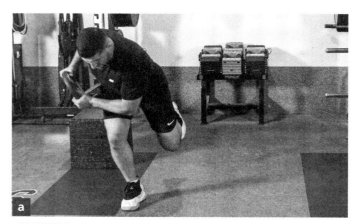

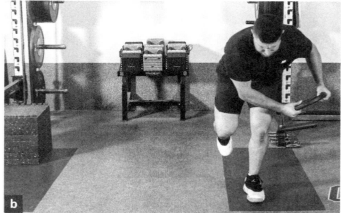

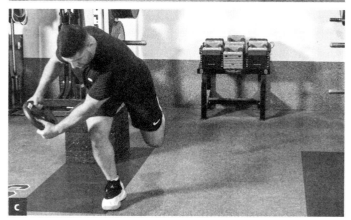

Figure 7.17 Plate skater hop with quick, stick, and punch: *(a)* starting position on right foot, *(b)* hop laterally to left side and land on left foot, and *(c)* hop back to right side and punch the weight plate down to the right.

DB REACTIVE SPLIT SQUAT JUMP

Reactive lower-body power is a key skill that can tell you a lot about an athlete's overall power and explosiveness. Use this exercise to improve your ability in this area.

HOW TO PERFORM

- Hold a dumbbell in each hand down by your pockets.
- Position your lower body in a split squat stance. The front foot should be flat, and the rear toes should be in contact with the floor.
- Rather than simply jumping up and landing back down on the floor as you would in a traditional split squat jump, rapidly jab down hard into the floor with your feet.
- This will allow you to produce a greater amount of force going down into the floor, and in turn, help you power up toward the sky a bit higher.
- Make sure to stick your landing and reset during each rep.

PERFORMANCE TIPS FOR SUCCESS

- It's best to hit a few practice reps with body weight only, because the motion takes a little time to get accustomed to. When you're ready, use the dumbbells to increase the overall intensity.
- Think of the "jab" as a quick stomp: It should be performed rapidly and take up only a little space between your feet and the floor.

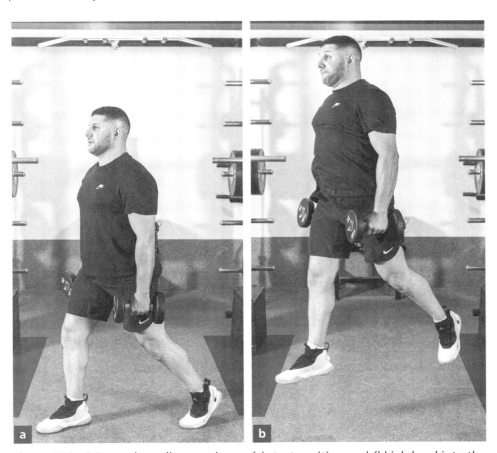

Figure 7.18 DB reactive split squat jump: *(a)* start position and *(b)* jab hard into the floor with your feet and jump up.

CABLE SPLIT-STANCE SINGLE-ARM LOW ROW WITH BOX STOMP

Coordinating powerful movements with your entire body isn't easy, but pays off tremendously in sports and athletics. You'll develop this ability when performing this exercise. You'll also improve in balance, stability, and coordination, all of which fitness enthusiasts need!

HOW TO PERFORM

- Set up a handle on a cable column machine from a low anchor point.
- Set up a sturdy box or stack of bumper plates (roughly mid-shin height) a few feet away from the cable column machine.
- Grab the handle with your left hand and walk back so that you're positioned just behind the box or stack of bumper plates.
- Place your right foot flat on the floor a few inches from the box or bumper plates. Place your left foot a couple of feet behind you with just your toes in contact with the floor.
- Perform a rapid row with your left hand while your left foot rises up toward the box or bumper plates and stomps down.
- This movement must occur rapidly.
- Perform all reps one side, switch sides, and repeat.

PERFORMANCE TIPS FOR SUCCESS

- Break down this movement using body weight only when you first try it. Get a feel for it. Start slow and then build up speed during each rep. Once you've got the hang of it, grab the handle from the cable column machine and let it rip!
- Focus on being smooth and powerful as opposed to loading the machine heavily. Remember, this is a power-based movement—power is key in developing your overall athleticism.

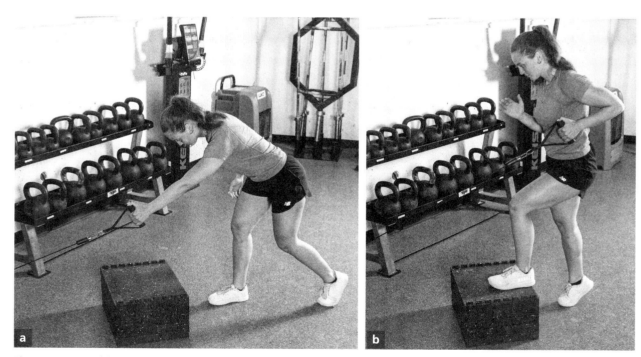

Figure 7.19 Cable split-stance single-arm low row with box stomp: *(a)* start position and *(b)* row with left hand and stomp with left foot.

CHAPTER 8

Change of Direction, Agility, and Speed Exercises

Changing directions rapidly, moving with agility in tight spaces, and doing all of this with speed and precision: These skills aren't exclusive to competitive athletes in sports. They're valuable for everyone. That's why this book was created—to help you train like a pro and boost your skills in change-of-direction ability, reactive agility, and speed. More often than not, these are the skills and exercises that most people skip, since going to the gym to lift weights seems like enough. However, when you combine these skills with lifting weights, your overall athleticism will skyrocket!

In this chapter, you'll be exposed to a variety of exercises that challenge your ability to change directions quickly. This is the starting point. As you improve and advance, you'll progress to more difficult exercises that challenge your ability to quickly react with agility, speed, and precision. Whether you're stepping onto the playing field in a professional sport or the court in a pickup basketball game, or just playing around in the backyard with your kids, developing your change-of-direction ability and reactive agility will be a game-changer for you.

10-YARD SPRINT AND REHEARSED STOP

This is an excellent way to develop the ability to accelerate and decelerate in a fast and athletic manner. Sprinting for 10 yards trains acceleration with regard to first-step speed. The addition of the rehearsed stop at the end develops your ability to decelerate and control eccentric forces in an abrupt athletic motion, which frequently occurs in a variety of sports.

HOW TO PERFORM

- Start in a two-point or three-point stance so that you're prepared to shoot out like a cannon when it comes time to sprint.
- Once your coach or training partner instructs you to sprint, explode out in front as fast as humanly possible.
- Since you have only 10 yards to work with, it's important to plan for your rehearsed stop ahead of time rather than at the last second. Begin preparing to stop within 2 or 3 yards from the 10-yard finish line. In doing so, you'll be able to control your body and stop on a dime.

PERFORMANCE TIPS FOR SUCCESS

- It's important to situate yourself in the two-point or three-point stance as a way to shrink the amount of space your body is taking up. Think of this as like winding up a toy car. Once that toy car is completely wound up, it has stored energy that will help launch it straight out as soon as you let go of it.
- Really drive your front knee out explosively during the initial sprint—this will improve your sprinting ability.

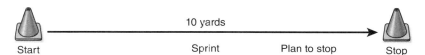

Figure 8.1 10-yard sprint and rehearsed stop.

MULTIDIRECTIONAL PLYO STEP FROM HALF-KNEELING START TO 5-YARD SPRINT

The purpose of the plyo step is to redirect your lower-body force and power to take off in a different direction. This redirection, or plyo step, occurs frequently in sports where the athlete has to quickly change directions. This is the perfect exercise to perform if your goal is mastering this skill.

HOW TO PERFORM

- Start in a half-kneeling position with your left knee down on the ground and your right foot flat on the floor. In this setup, your right leg will be the working leg.
- You have the option of selecting which direction to sprint: forward (north), backward (south), right (east), or left (west).
- Quickly lift the foot that's on the floor, jab the floor, and sprint for a total of 5 yards in a direction other than the way you are facing in the initial kneeling position.
- The entire sequence should take place rapidly and explosively.
- Complete all reps with the right leg acting as the working leg, switch sides, and repeat.

PERFORMANCE TIPS FOR SUCCESS

- Rather than thinking about all of the steps it takes to complete this exercise, think about "getting out of there" as quickly as possible. You can liken this concept to playing a game of tag or being between the bases in a game of baseball.
- Be as explosive as possible with your lower body. Think about using an explosive first step to launch your body out of the starting position and in a different direction as if a car was speeding toward you.

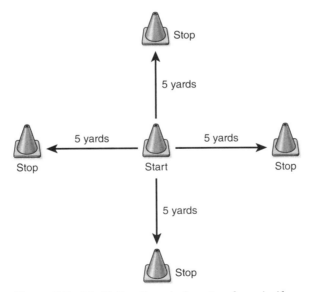

Figure 8.2 Multidirectional plyo step from half-kneeling start to 5-yard sprint.

100-YARD TEMPO RUN

Performing this type of exercise will help you develop efficient running mechanics at a specific tempo or intensity that is typically a bit lower than maximal effort. Incorporating this into your training is useful for building up running volume as you eventually work your way into lower volumes at higher intensities (i.e., sprinting at shorter distances).

HOW TO PERFORM

- Start in a two-point or three-point stance so that you're prepared to shoot out like a cannon when it's time to run.
- Take off, running at a specific tempo or intensity level (e.g., 75% effort or intensity) for 100 yards.
- The goal of a tempo run is to maintain a specific intensity level as prescribed by your coach or training program.

PERFORMANCE TIPS FOR SUCCESS

- This exercise is as simple as it looks. Don't overthink it. Simply run for the prescribed amount of distance at the prescribed tempo or intensity level.
- Stay true to the percentage of effort that is prescribed—this is easier said than done, especially if you're new to tempo runs.

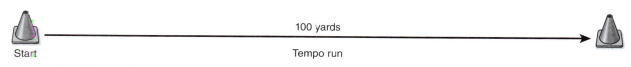

Figure 8.3 100-yard tempo run.

10-YARD SPRINT AND REHEARSED Y-TURN

This drill develops the ability to accelerate fast, in addition to rapidly changing direction into a Y-turn, a movement that occurs in a variety of sports. Sprinting for 10 yards develops acceleration with regard to first-step speed. The addition of the Y-turn at the end develops your ability to quickly change direction and continue sprinting.

HOW TO PERFORM

- Start in a two-point or three-point stance so that you're prepared to shoot out like a cannon when it's time to sprint.
- Once your coach or training partner instructs you to sprint, explode out in front as fast as possible.
- Since you have 10 yards to work with prior to the Y-turn, it's important to plan for your rehearsed turn ahead of time. Begin preparing for your rehearsed Y-turn within 2 or 3 yards from the 10-yard line. By doing so, you'll be able to control your body and efficiently take your Y-turn at the 10-yard line.
- At the Y-turn, quickly turn right or left at a 45-degree angle and sprint for 5 to 10 yards.
- Complete all reps on one side, switch sides, and repeat.

PERFORMANCE TIPS FOR SUCCESS

- Situate yourself in the two-point or three-point stance to shrink the amount of space your body is taking up. Think of this in the same way as similar to winding up a remote-control toy car. Once that toy car is completely wound up, it has stored energy that will help launch it straight out once you let go of it.
- Drive your front knee forward during the initial sprint to improve your sprinting ability.

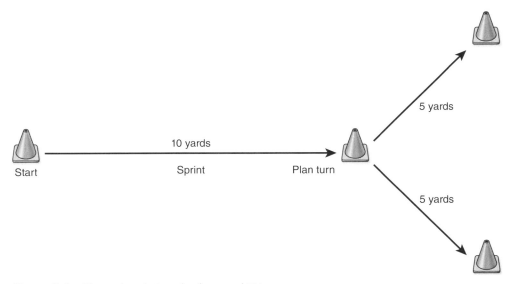

Figure 8.4 10-yard sprint and rehearsed Y-turn.

10-YARD SPRINT FROM LATERAL HALF-KNEELING START

Develop the ability to rapidly plant your outside foot in the ground to push hard, turn laterally, and then sprint in the other direction for 10 yards. Enhancing this skill will directly benefit your ability to change directions in competitive sports and various activities of life that require lower-body power and explosiveness.

HOW TO PERFORM

- Start in a half-kneeling position on the ground with your left knee down and right knee up.
- Set up your body so that you can eventually turn left and sprint in that direction.
- Consider your left knee as your inside knee and your right knee as your outside knee. This position will allow for a quick and efficient turn and sprint. Drive your right foot into the ground and away toward the right as you explosively turn left and sprint for a distance of 10 yards.

PERFORMANCE TIPS FOR SUCCESS

- It's much more common and natural to sprint from a linear starting position, like in track-and-field races. However, sports occur in all planes of movement, so it's important to be able to sprint from any position.
- Slightly lean into the direction that you plan to sprint toward.

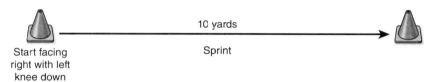

Figure 8.5 10-yard sprint from lateral half-kneeling start.

20-YARD DASH

This drill will improve your ability to sprint short distances and increase your overall speed with more reps.

HOW TO PERFORM

- Start in a two-point or three-point stance so that you're prepared to shoot out like a cannon when it's time to sprint.
- Once your coach or training partner instructs you to sprint, explode out in front as fast as possible and sprint for a total of 20 yards.
- Keep sprinting as explosively as possible from start to finish.

PERFORMANCE TIPS FOR SUCCESS

- Situate yourself in a two-point or three-point stance to shrink the amount of space your body is taking up. Think of this as like winding up a remote-control toy car. Once that toy car is completely wound up, it has stored energy that will help launch it straight out once you let go of it.
- Many professional sports leagues, such as the NFL, use the 40-yard dash, which allows the athlete to build up speed over a greater distance. However, since the 20-yard dash covers less distance, you have to get up to speed more quickly.

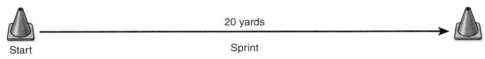

Figure 8.6 20-yard dash.

10-YARD SPRINT AND REHEARSED T-TURN

This drill develops the ability to accelerate fast and rapidly change direction in a 90-degree T-turn, a movement that occurs in a variety of sports. Sprinting for 10 yards develops acceleration with regard to first-step speed. The T-turn at the end develops your ability to quickly change directions and continue sprinting.

HOW TO PERFORM

- Start in a two-point or three-point stance so that you're prepared to shoot out like a cannon when it's time to sprint.
- Once your coach or training partner instructs you to sprint, explode out in front as fast as possible.
- Since you have 10 yards to work with prior to your T-turn, it's important to plan for your rehearsed turn ahead of time. Begin preparing for your rehearsed T-turn within 2 or 3 yards from the 10-yard line. By doing so, you'll be able to control your body and efficiently turn 90 degrees at the 10-yard line.
- Quickly turn at a 90-degree angle, then sprint for 5 to 10 more yards.
- Complete all reps on one side, switch sides, and repeat.

PERFORMANCE TIPS FOR SUCCESS

- Situate yourself in the two-point or three-point stance to shrink the amount of space your body takes up. Think of this as like winding up a remote-control toy car. Once that toy car is completely wound up, it has stored energy that will help launch it straight out once you let go of it.
- Drive your front knee forward during the initial sprint to improve your sprinting ability.

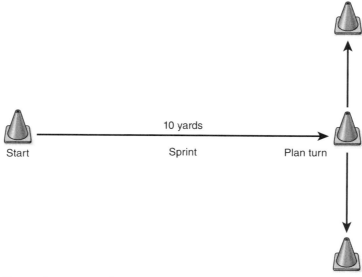

Figure 8.7 10-yard sprint and rehearsed T-turn.

5-10-5 PRO AGILITY SHUTTLE

The pro agility shuttle is a classic exercise used in professional, collegiate, and high school sports to gauge an athlete's ability to rapidly change directions in tight spaces. Performing this exercise routinely will enhance your ability to change directions through a pre-planned path.

HOW TO PERFORM

- Start in an athletic stance with both knees and hips bent, leaning slightly to one side (right or left).
- When the coach instructs you to do so, rapidly turn and sprint in the direction that you were slightly leaning toward for 5 yards.
- Immediately drop down low toward the ground, turn in the opposite direction, and sprint for 10 yards.
- Again, drop down low toward the ground once you reach that point, turn in the opposite direction, and sprint 5 more yards to the finish line.
- You will cover a total distance of 20 yards during 1 rep.

PERFORMANCE TIPS FOR SUCCESS

- Stay low to the ground. This can be a challenge due to the rapid direction changes, but if you can do it, you'll increase your ability to make rapid and efficient turns.
- Angle your torso in the direction that you want your body to move in. In other words, if you're moving toward the right side and you're planning a rapid turn to the left, transition your torso to the left just before this turn. This will make a big difference in your change of direction and agility skills.

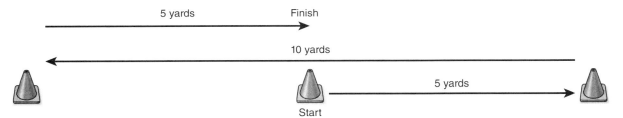

Figure 8.8 5-10-5 pro agility shuttle.

20-YARD CURVILINEAR SPRINT

Performing this drill consistently will improve your speed when sprinting in a curved fashion. Although linear sprinting occurs in sports and life, it's more common that you'll need to move in a curve or angle based on sudden changes or reactions. That's why performing the curvilinear sprint can be a game-changer!

HOW TO PERFORM

- Start in a two-point or three-point stance so that you're prepared to shoot out like a cannon when it's time to sprint.
- Once your coach or training partner instructs you to sprint, explode out in front as fast as possible and sprint over a curved line for 20 yards.

PERFORMANCE TIPS FOR SUCCESS

- Not all sprints happen in a straight line—using a curvilinear pattern allows you to angle your sprints similar to the penalty arc at the top of a soccer field.
- Situate yourself in a two-point or three-point stance to shrink the amount of space your body takes up. Think of this as like winding up a remote-control toy car. Once that toy car is completely wound up, it has stored energy that will help launch it out once you let go of it.
- When sprinting in a curvilinear fashion, slightly lean into the side that you're moving toward in order to make your sprinting feel smoother. If you're sprinting toward the left, lean and angle your body toward the left.

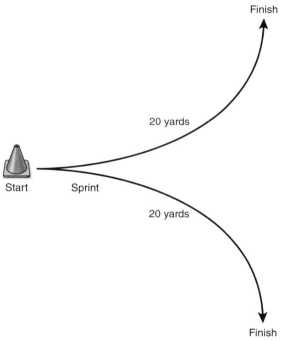

Figure 8.9 20-yard curvilinear sprint.

CHAPTER 9

Conditioning Exercises and Protocols

Let's face it: Conditioning is never fun. It's not uncommon to avoid it—even coaches sometimes talk about needing to put conditioning back into strength and conditioning. Fun or not, it's definitely an important part of your overall health and performance. The conditioning protocols and exercises in this book will help you elevate your health, performance, and overall athleticism. The cardiorespiratory endurance and stamina you'll gain from these protocols and exercises will make a huge impact on how well you move in your training, physical activities, or sports.

When we think about conditioning, we often think of someone stepping onto the treadmill and trudging along until they're sweaty enough to step off and call it quits. That's exactly the opposite of the conditioning exercises and protocols that you'll be exposed to in this book. Each one has been programmed with a specific purpose and intent so that you can make the athletic gains you desire. Conditioning exercises and protocols will be broken down based on focus—aerobic (i.e., lower intensity and longer duration) or anaerobic (i.e., higher intensity and shorter duration)—to help you turn over every stone in the process of becoming a healthier, more athletic version of yourself.

First, an overview of this chapter. The one conditioning day per week in phase 1 is identical for all four of the 12-week training programs (Train Like a Pro, GPP/hypertrophy, strength, and power) within each of their individual phase 1 blocks. The one conditioning day per week in phase 2 is identical for all four of the 12-week training programs within each of their individual phase 2 blocks. Lastly, the one conditioning day per week in phase 3 is identical for all four of the 12-week training programs within each of their individual phase 3 blocks. The programs were designed this way to help keep you consistent on your path toward achieving your health and athletic performance goals!

PHASE 1 CONDITIONING: Thursday

Focus: aerobic and anaerobic development

Warm-up: same for Tuesday (multidirectional athletic development: change of direction and agility) and Thursday (general conditioning: aerobic and anaerobic development)

Workout:
- Objective: steady-state aerobic conditioning
- Pick one: erg rower, air bike, ski erg, or treadmill
- Total duration: 30 to 40 minutes
- Target heart rate: 130 to 150 bpm
- Target RPE: 6 or 7 (60%-70% of max HR)

PHASE 2 CONDITIONING: Thursday

Focus: aerobic and anaerobic development

Warm-up: same for Tuesday (multidirectional athletic development: change of direction and agility) and Thursday (general conditioning: aerobic and anaerobic development)

Workout:
- Objective: aerobic conditioning intervals
- Pick one: erg rower, air bike, ski erg, or treadmill
- Total duration: 15 to 20 minutes
- Interval protocol: 15 seconds of hard work (RPE 8-9; 80%-90% of max HR) followed by 45 seconds of easy work (RPE 5; 50% of max HR)

PHASE 3 CONDITIONING: Thursday

Focus: aerobic and anaerobic development

Warm-up: same for Tuesday (multidirectional athletic development: change of direction and agility) and Thursday (general conditioning: aerobic and anaerobic development)

Workout:
- Objective: high-intensity sprint intervals
- Pick one: incline treadmill (20%-30% incline), outdoor hill (20%-30% incline), or sled (empty—no weight added)
- Total duration: 8 to 12 sets
- Interval protocol: 6 to 8 seconds of all-out sprint (RPE 10; 100% of max HR) followed by 45 to 60 seconds of complete rest (goal is to bring HR back down during this time)

LISS and HIIT: What Is the Difference, and When and How Should I Implement Each Type of Conditioning?

Low-intensity steady state (LISS) refers to a sustained pace of conditioning that's typically moderately challenging. *High-intensity interval training (HIIT)* refers to a form of training that combines short bouts of high-intensity effort with periods of complete rest or very low intensity. A weekly combination of LISS and HIIT, provides many benefits for your overall stamina and endurance and expands your capacity in the aerobic and anaerobic departments by making your heart more efficient. A good guideline is to include LISS one or two days per week and HIIT one or two days per week. Since these values can vary dependent on your training goals, injury history, and level of fitness, it's best to include them within an overall strength and conditioning program that provides the right volume and intensity for you. For more specific recommendations, see the training programs in chapters 10 to 13.

STEADY-STATE AEROBIC CONDITIONING

Steady-state aerobic conditioning is crucial in athletic development for building the engine. Build your base of aerobic capacity, and enjoy the fruits of your labor down the line by lasting longer in your workouts, recreational sports, and other activities!

HOW TO PERFORM

Choose one of the following conditioning tools: erg rower, air bike, ski erg, or treadmill.

- When using the erg rower, be sure to clip both feet to the straps. To begin, pull the handle back toward your mid-abdomen with both hands while pushing your torso back and straightening your legs. Finish with your torso leaning back slightly, but not so much that you become parallel to the floor. Aim for a roughly 45-degree angle.
- When using the air bike, set the seat to a height in line with the bone on the side of your hip. This will ensure that you don't have to reach your foot down too far during each pedal motion. Be sure to work just as hard with your arms as you do with your legs.
- When using the ski erg, take a small step back to leave room for your arms to move and set your feet roughly hip-width apart. Reach up to grab the handles with both hands. Pull both handles down and back toward your pockets while dropping your torso down and sitting your hips back.
- When running on the treadmill, use the same technique as you would if you were running outside on a track or a field. It should feel smooth and controlled.

The goal is to stay within the target HR zone of 130 to 150 beats per minute (bpm). On the scale of perceived exertion, this will feel like an RPE of 6 or 7 (60%-70% of max HR). Perform the activity for 30 to 40 minutes.

PERFORMANCE TIPS FOR SUCCESS

- This type of conditioning helps to improve your steady-state aerobic capacity, which improves stamina and endurance and aids in your overall recovery in between bouts of power, speed, and strength training.
- Exercises that produce power, speed, and strength get all the hype, but make no mistake—steady-state aerobic conditioning is the foundation on which to build.

AEROBIC CONDITIONING INTERVALS

This type of conditioning improves your ability to efficiently change intensity levels from high to moderate. This may not sound like a big deal, but packs a punch in terms of your ability to recover from and within your strength and power training sessions. It also boosts your stamina and endurance.

HOW TO PERFORM

You can use any of the following conditioning tools: erg rower, air bike, ski erg, or treadmill.

- When using the erg rower, be sure to clip both feet into the straps. To begin, pull the handle back toward your mid-abdomen with both hands while pushing your torso back and straightening your legs. Finish with your torso leaning back slightly, but not so much that you become parallel to the floor. Aim for a roughly 45-degree angle.
- When using the air bike, set the seat to a height in line with the bone on the side of your hip. This will ensure that you don't have to reach your foot down too far during each pedal motion. Be sure to work just as hard with your arms as you do with your legs.
- When using the ski erg, take a small step back to leave room for your arms to move and set your feet roughly hip-width apart. Reach up to grab the handles with both hands. Pull both handles down and back toward your pockets while dropping your torso down and sitting your hips back.
- When running on the treadmill, use the same technique as you would if you were running outside on a track or a field. It should feel smooth and controlled.

The goal is to work hard for 15 seconds at 80% to 90% of your max HR (RPE 8-9) and then perform easy work for 45 seconds at 50% of your max HR (RPE 5). Complete these intervals for a total of 15 to 20 minutes.

PERFORMANCE TIPS FOR SUCCESS

- Athleticism requires the ability to change speeds and intensities quickly. Sports are naturally intermittent and call for constant changes in movement. Aerobic conditioning intervals prepare you for these challenges and boost your overall athleticism.
- Think of this type of conditioning protocol as a major boost in your overall health and performance, even though it may not always be exciting or fun. It's like brushing your teeth. You know it's important and you have to do it often, even though it can be annoying and redundant.

HIGH-INTENSITY SPRINT INTERVALS

Exerting all-out effort at max HR is customary in sports and athletics. Your heart's ability to navigate between high-intensity and low-intensity intervals is a hallmark trait of athleticism that is often overlooked and underappreciated.

HOW TO PERFORM

Use any of the following conditioning tools: incline treadmill (20%-30% incline), outdoor hill (20%-30% incline), or an empty sled (no weight added).

- When running on the incline treadmill, use the same technique as you would if you were running outside on a track or a field. It should feel smooth and controlled. However, keep in mind that the 20% to 30% incline will increase the overall intensity.
- When running on the outdoor hill, use the same technique as you would if you were running on a treadmill or outside on a flat track. It should feel smooth and controlled. However, keep in mind that the 20% to 30% incline will increase the overall intensity.
- When conditioning with the sled, do not add any weights. The weight of the sled and the friction caused by pushing it on the turf will provide enough resistance. Grab the sled handles near the top with both hands and angle your body down at roughly 45 degrees. Think about pushing the ground away from you during each step forward.

Perform an all-out sprint at 100% of your max HR (RPE 10) for 6 to 8 seconds and then take a complete rest for 45 to 60 seconds. Complete 8 to 12 sets.

PERFORMANCE TIPS FOR SUCCESS

- High-intensity sprint intervals will not only help you become faster and more powerful, but improve how quickly you can react in sports, athletics, and life. Sprinting is one of those things that become even more important after our high school and college days.
- Really dial in to the specific percentage of effort prescribed—this will become easier with frequent practice.

CHAPTER 10

The Train Like a Pro Training Program

This 12-week training program has three consecutive phases (four-week training blocks) that build off each other. In phase 1, the primary emphasis is on general physical preparedness and hypertrophy, with a splash of isometric exercises to help you master key positions and movements. Essentially, we want you to get a solid number of reps in while building some muscle (i.e., body armor) as an athlete. In phase 2, we will be emphasizing strength with a primary goal of helping you become a stronger overall athlete, and we'll include eccentric-based exercises to master body control. Lastly, in phase 3, you'll notice an emphasis on overall power and explosive capabilities, in addition to full-range-of-motion exercises. This is the final phase, where you put everything together for elite athleticism!

The following training program is the flagship 12-week program that this book is centered around. If your goal is to tap into your inner athlete and become the strongest, fastest, most powerful version of yourself while staying healthy, this is the program for you. If you're an athlete, this is the perfect training program to use as you head into your upcoming season of competition.

When it comes to overall intensity and how heavy your weights should be in each exercise, it's important to use a standard to make it easy to learn and apply. This is why we'll be using the rating of perceived exertion (RPE) 10-point scale to help you each step of the way. When using RPE, you can think of the number on the 1-10 scale as being multiplied by 10 to represent a percentage of intensity. In other words, if RPE 7 is recommended, the exercise should feel like you're working at 70% of your maximum intensity. If RPE 5 is recommended, it should feel like 50%. The bonus with our RPE 1-10 scale is the addition of *reps in reserve*, a concept that helps provide even more clarity about your intensity and weight selection. Table 10.1 outlines the RPE scale based on reps in reserve.

Table 10.1 Rating of Perceived Exertion Based on Reps in Reserve

Rating	Reps in reserve
10	Could not do more reps or load.
9.5	Could not do more reps, but could do slightly more load.
9	Could do 1 more rep.
8.5	Could definitely do 1 more rep, and a chance at 2 reps.
8	Could do 2 more reps.
7.5	Could definitely do 2 more reps, and a chance at 3 reps.
7	Could do 3 more reps.
5-6	Could do 4-6 more reps.
1-4	Very light to light effort.

Table 10.2   Train Like a Pro Training Program: Phase 1 (Weeks 1-4)

DAY 1: MONDAY			
Warm-up			
Exercise	**Reps/time/distance**	**Notes**	**Page #**
Band cat-cow	8		42
Heels-up single-leg bridge isometric with knee drive isometric	15 sec per side		43
Catcher rockback isometric with reach and rotate	5 per side		44
Floor bent-knee Copenhagen plank	15 sec per side		45
Alternating Spiderman	3 per side		46
Split squat isometric	15 sec per side		47
Squat rack Kang squat	5		48
Extensive pogo hop	15		49
Drop squat to stick	8		50
Linear skip	20 yd		51
Workout			
Exercise	**Sets × reps at RPE**	**Notes**	**Page #**
Power block • A1: Band-assisted continuous squat jump • A2: MB tall-kneeling slam with hip hinge	3 × 5 at RPE 6-7 3 × 5 at RPE 6-7	Complete A block (A1 and A2) with no rest between exercises, then rest for 45-60 sec. That equals 1 set. Complete all sets in this way, then move on to B block.	198 199
Strength block • B1: KB goblet squat with 3-second isometric • B2: Band tall-kneeling Pallof press isometric	3 × 8 at RPE 8 3 × 20 sec per side at RPE 7-8	Complete B block (B1 and B2) with no rest between exercises, then rest for 45-60 sec. That equals 1 set. Complete all sets in this way, then move on to C block.	110 111
Hypertrophy block • C1: DB RDL • C2: KB half-kneeling shoulder press with 3-second isometric	3 × 10, 12, 15 at RPE 8, 7, 7 3 × 8 per side at RPE 8	Complete C block (C1 and C2) with no rest between exercises, then rest for 45-60 sec. That equals 1 set. Complete all sets in this way, then move on to D block.	112 113
Accessory block • D1: Suspension skater squat with 3-second isometric • D2: DB standing hammer curl	3 × 8 per side at RPE 7-8 3 × 15 at RPE 7-8	Complete D block (D1 and D2) with no rest between exercises, then rest for 45-60 sec. That equals 1 set. Complete all sets in this way, then move on to recovery.	114 115
Recovery			
Exercise	**Reps/time**	**Notes**	**Page #**
Hamstring floss	12 per side		N/A
Book opener isometric	20 sec per side		N/A
Rear foot elevated half-kneeling hip flexor stretch	20 sec per side		N/A

(continued)

Table 10.2 Train Like a Pro Training Program: Phase 1 (Weeks 1-4) *(continued)*

DAY 2: TUESDAY			
Warm-up			
Exercise	Reps/time/distance	Notes	Page #
Long bridge isometric	15 sec		52
Wall press with alternating dead bug	8 per side		53
Wall stork	15 sec per side		54
Wall single-leg heel raise isometric	15 sec per side		55
Alternating yoga plex	3 per side		56
Stationary inchworm	3		57
Hinge to squat	5		58
Wall linear single exchange	5 per side		59
Stationary hamstring scoop	5 per side		60
Walking alternating Spiderman	2 × 10 yd		61
Lateral shuffle with arm swing	2 × 10 yd per side		62
Backpedal	2 × 10 yd		63
Workout			
Exercise	Reps at RPE	Notes	Page #
A: 10-yard sprint and rehearsed stop	3 at RPE 8-9	Complete 1 rep, then rest for 30-45 sec. That equals 1 set. Complete all sets in this way, then move on to the next exercise.	220
B: Multidirectional plyo step from half-kneeling start to 5-yard sprint	2 per direction (4 total directions) at RPE 8-9	Complete 1 rep per direction then rest for 45-60 sec. That equals 1 set. Complete all sets in this way, then move on to the next exercise.	221
C: 100-yard tempo run	6 at 80% effort	30-45 sec rest between reps	222
Recovery			
Exercise	Reps/time	Notes	Page #
Hamstring floss	12 per side		N/A
Book opener isometric	20 sec per side		N/A
Rear foot elevated half-kneeling hip flexor stretch	20 sec per side		N/A

DAY 3: WEDNESDAY

Warm-up

Exercise	Reps/time/distance	Notes	Page #
Band cat-cow	8		42
Heels-up single-leg bridge isometric with knee drive isometric	15 sec per side		43
Catcher rockback isometric with reach and rotate	5 per side		44
Floor bent-knee Copenhagen plank	15 sec per side		45
Alternating Spiderman	3 per side		46
Split squat isometric	15 sec per side		47
Squat rack Kang squat	5		48
Extensive pogo hop	15		49
Drop squat to stick	8		50
Linear skip	20 yd		51

Workout

Exercise	Sets × reps at RPE	Notes	Page #
Power block • A1: MB skater hop with chop and stick • A2: MB half-kneeling lateral wall toss	3 × 5 per side at RPE 6-7 3 × 5 per side at RPE 6-7	Complete A block (A1 and A2) with no rest between exercises, then rest for 45-60 sec. That equals 1 set. Complete all sets in this way, then move on to B block.	200 201
Strength block • B1: DB bench press with 3-second isometric (top) • B2: Bent-knee star plank with top leg long	3 × 8 at RPE 8 3 × 15 sec per side at RPE 7-8	Complete B block (B1 and B2) with no rest between exercises, then rest for 45-60 sec. That equals 1 set. Complete all sets in this way, then move on to C block.	116 117
Hypertrophy block • C1: DB chest-supported row • C2: KB single-arm offset lateral squat with 1-second isometric	3 × 10, 12, 15 at RPE 8, 7, 7 3 × 8 per side at RPE 8	Complete C block (C1 and C2) with no rest between exercises, then rest for 45-60 sec. That equals 1 set. Complete all sets in this way, then move on to D block.	118 119
Accessory block • D1: KB goblet carry • D2: Band tall-kneeling pull-apart	3 × 40 yd at RPE 7-8 3 × 15 at RPE 7-8	Complete D block (D1 and D2) with no rest between exercises, then rest for 45-60 sec. That equals 1 set. Complete all sets in this way, then move on to recovery.	120 121

Recovery

Exercise	Reps/time	Notes	Page #
Hamstring floss	12 per side		N/A
Book opener isometric	20 sec per side		N/A
Rear foot elevated half-kneeling hip flexor stretch	20 sec per side		N/A

(continued)

Table 10.2 Train Like a Pro Training Program: Phase 1 (Weeks 1-4) *(continued)*

DAY 4: THURSDAY			
Warm-up			
Exercise	Reps/time/distance	Notes	Page #
Long bridge isometric	15 sec		52
Wall press with alternating dead bug	8 per side		53
Wall stork	15 sec per side		54
Wall single-leg heel raise isometric	15 sec per side		55
Alternating yoga plex	3 per side		56
Stationary inchworm	3		57
Hinge to squat	5		58
Wall linear single exchange	5 per side		59
Stationary hamstring scoop	5 per side		60
Walking alternating Spiderman	2 × 10 yd		61
Lateral shuffle with arm swing	2 × 10 yd per side		62
Backpedal	2 × 10 yd		63
Workout			
Exercise	Parameters	Notes	Page #
Objective: Steady-state aerobic conditioning Pick one: erg rower, air bike, ski erg, or treadmill	Total duration: 30-40 min Target heart rate: 130-150 bpm Target RPE: 6-7 (60%-70% of max HR)		232
Recovery			
Exercise	Reps/time	Notes	Page #
Hamstring floss	12 per side		N/A
Book opener isometric	20 sec per side		N/A
Rear foot elevated half-kneeling hip flexor stretch	20 sec per side		N/A

DAY 5: FRIDAY				
Warm-up				
Exercise	**Reps/time/distance**	**Notes**		**Page #**
Band cat-cow	8			42
Heels-up single-leg bridge isometric with knee drive isometric	15 sec per side			43
Catcher rockback isometric with reach and rotate	5 per side			44
Floor bent-knee Copenhagen plank	15 sec per side			45
Alternating Spiderman	3 per side			46
Split squat isometric	15 sec per side			47
Squat rack Kang squat	5			48
Extensive pogo hop	15			49
Drop squat to stick	8			50
Linear skip	20 yd			51
Workout				
Exercise	**Sets × reps at RPE**	**Notes**		**Page #**
Power block • A1: 90-degree rotational single-leg hop with stick • A2: MB half-kneeling around-the-world slam	3 × 5 per side at RPE 6-7 3 × 5 per side at RPE 6-7	Complete A block (A1 and A2) with no rest between exercises, then rest for 45-60 sec. That equals 1 set. Complete all sets in this way, then move on to B block.		202 203
Strength block • B1: Trap bar deadlift • B2: PB push–pull	3 × 6 at RPE 8 3 × 12 at RPE 7-8	Complete B block (B1 and B2) with no rest between exercises, then rest for 45-60 sec. That equals 1 set. Complete all sets in this way, then move on to C block.		122 123
Hypertrophy block • C1: Two DB foam roller hack squat against a wall • C2: Cable half-kneeling high row with 1-second isometric	3 × 10, 12, 15 at RPE 8, 7, 7 3 × 8 per side at RPE 8	Complete C block (C1 and C2) with no rest between exercises, then rest for 45-60 sec. That equals 1 set. Complete all sets in this way, then move on to D block.		124 125
Accessory block • D1: Cable double-arm single-leg RDL with knee drive and row • D2: Band standing triceps extension	3 × 8 per side at RPE 7-8 3 × 15 at RPE 7-8	Complete D block (D1 and D2) with no rest between exercises, then rest for 45-60 sec. That equals 1 set. Complete all sets in this way, then move on to recovery.		190 127
Recovery				
Exercise	**Reps/time**	**Notes**		**Page #**
Hamstring floss	12 per side			N/A
Book opener isometric	20 sec per side			N/A
Rear foot elevated half-kneeling hip flexor stretch	20 sec per side			N/A

Table 10.3 Train Like a Pro Training Program: Phase 2 (Weeks 5-8)

DAY 1: MONDAY				
Warm-up				
Exercise	Reps/time/distance	Notes		Page #
Cat-cow	8			64
Single-leg bridge isometric with bent-knee leg whip	5 per side			65
Catcher rockback	5 per side			66
Elevated bent-knee Copenhagen plank	15 sec per side			67
Alternating Spiderman to yoga pike	3			68
Heels-up split squat isometric	15 sec per side			69
MB hug Kang squat	5			70
Extensive single-leg pogo hop	10 per side			71
Drop reverse lunge to stick	3 per side			72
Lateral skip	10 yd per side			73
Workout				
Exercise	Sets x reps at RPE	Notes		Page #
Strength and power block • A1: DB step-up • A2: Band-resisted acceleration power step	3 x 6 per side at RPE 7-8 3 x 3 per side at RPE 6-7	Complete A block (A1 and A2) with no rest between exercises, then rest for 45-60 sec. That equals 1 set. Complete all sets in this way, then move on to B block.		128 204
Strength and power block • B1: DB heels-up three-point row with 3-second eccentric • B2: Barbell explosive inverted row with hip thrust isometric	3 x 8 per side at RPE 7-8 3 x 5 at RPE 6-7	Complete B block (B1 and B2) with no rest between exercises, then rest for 45-60 sec. That equals 1 set. Complete all sets in this way, then move on to C block.		129 205
Hypertrophy block • C1: DB cyclist squat (2 DB) • C2: Cable seated lat pull-down with 3-second eccentric	3 x 8, 10, 12 at RPE 8, 7, 7 3 x 8, 10, 12 at RPE 8, 7, 7	Complete C block (C1 and C2) with no rest between exercises, then rest for 45-60 sec. That equals 1 set. Complete all sets in this way, then move on to D block.		130 131
Accessory block • D1: KB front rack carry • D2: Cable tall-kneeling rope triceps extension	3 x 40 yd at RPE 7-8 3 x 12 at RPE 7-8	Complete D block (D1 and D2) with no rest between exercises, then rest for 45-60 sec. That equals 1 set. Complete all sets in this way, then move on to recovery.		132 133
Recovery				
Exercise	Reps/time	Notes		Page #
Band single-leg lower	8 per side			N/A
Band Brettzel stretch	20 sec per side			N/A
Rear foot elevated half-kneeling hip flexor stretch with single-arm overhead reach	20 sec per side			N/A

DAY 2: TUESDAY				
Warm-up				
Exercise	Reps/time/distance	Notes		Page #
Single-leg long bridge isometric with knee drive isometric	15 sec per side			74
Cross-connect dead bug (opposite side)	8 sec per side			75
Mini-band stork	15 sec per side			76
Wall bent-knee single-leg heel raise isometric	15 sec per side			77
Alternating yoga plex to yoga pike	3 per side			78
Walking inchworm	3			79
Hinge to squat with alternating rotation	3			80
Wall linear double exchange	5 per side			81
Walking alternating hamstring scoop	2 x 10 yd			82
Walking alternating Spiderman to reach and rotate	2 x 10 yd			83
Double lateral shuffle with alternating lateral squat	2 x 10 yd per side			84
Backward reach run	2 x 10 yd			85
Workout				
Exercise	Reps at RPE	Notes		Page #
A: 10-yard sprint and rehearsed Y-turn	3 per side at RPE 8-9	Complete 1 rep per side, then rest for 30-45 sec. That equals 1 set. Complete all sets in this way, then move on to the next exercise.		223
B: 10-yard sprint from lateral half-kneeling start	3 per side at RPE 8-9	Complete 1 rep per side, then rest for 30-45 sec. That equals 1 set. Complete all sets in this way, then move on to the next exercise.		224
C: 20-yard dash	4 at 100% effort	Rest 60-75 sec between reps.		225
Recovery				
Exercise	Reps/time	Notes		Page #
Band single-leg lower	8 per side			N/A
Band Brettzel stretch	20 sec per side			N/A
Rear foot elevated half-kneeling hip flexor stretch with single-arm overhead reach	20 sec per side			N/A

(continued)

Table 10.3 Train Like a Pro Training Program: Phase 2 (Weeks 5-8) *(continued)*

DAY 3: WEDNESDAY			
Warm-up			
Exercise	Reps/time/distance	Notes	Page #
Cat-cow	8		64
Single-leg bridge isometric with bent-knee leg whip	5 per side		65
Catcher rockback	5 per side		66
Elevated bent-knee Copenhagen plank	15 sec per side		67
Alternating Spiderman to yoga pike	3		68
Heels-up split squat isometric	15 sec per side		69
MB hug Kang squat	5		70
Extensive single-leg pogo hop	10 per side		71
Drop reverse lunge to stick	3 per side		72
Lateral skip	10 yd per side		73
Workout			
Exercise	Sets x reps at RPE	Notes	Page #
Strength and power block • A1: Weighted eccentric-only neutral grip pull-up with 5-second eccentric • A2: MB standing double clutch slam	3 x 5 at RPE 7-8 3 x 5 at RPE 6-7	Complete A block (A1 and A2) with no rest between exercises, then rest for 45-60 sec. That equals 1 set. Complete all sets in this way, then move on to B block.	134 206
Strength and power block • B1: Landmine goblet lateral squat • B2: Band-resisted skater hop with stick (lateral orientation)	3 x 6 per side at RPE 7-8 3 x 5 per side at RPE 6-7	Complete B block (B1 and B2) with no rest between exercises, then rest for 45-60 sec. That equals 1 set. Complete all sets in this way, then move on to C block.	135 208
Hypertrophy block • C1: DB captain stance single-arm shoulder press • C2: Cable plank single-arm row to triceps extension	3 x 8, 10, 12 each side at RPE 8, 7, 7 3 x 8 per side at RPE 8	Complete C block (C1 and C2) with no rest between exercises, then rest for 45-60 sec. That equals 1 set. Complete all sets in this way, then move on to D block.	136 137
Accessory block • D1: KB suitcase carry • D2: DB incline bench trap raise (Y) with 3-second eccentric	3 x 40 yd per side at RPE 7-8 3 x 12 at RPE 7-8	Complete D block (D1 and D2) with no rest between exercises, then rest for 45-60 sec. That equals 1 set. Complete all sets in this way, then move on to recovery.	138 139
Recovery			
Exercise	Reps/time	Notes	Page #
Band single-leg lower	8 per side		N/A
Band Brettzel stretch	20 sec per side		N/A
Rear foot elevated half-kneeling hip flexor stretch with single-arm overhead reach	20 sec per side		N/A

DAY 4: THURSDAY				
Warm-up				
Exercise	**Reps/time/distance**	**Notes**		**Page #**
Single-leg long bridge isometric with knee drive isometric	15 sec per side			74
Cross-connect dead bug (opposite side)	8 sec per side			75
Mini-band stork	15 sec per side			76
Wall bent-knee single-leg heel raise isometric	15 sec per side			77
Alternating yoga plex to yoga pike	3 per side			78
Walking inchworm	3			79
Hinge to squat with alternating rotation	3			80
Wall linear double exchange	5 per side			81
Walking alternating hamstring scoop	2 x 10 yd			82
Walking alternating Spiderman to reach and rotate	2 x 10 yd			83
Double lateral shuffle with alternating lateral squat	2 x 10 yd per side			84
Backward reach run	2 x 10 yd			85
Workout				
Exercise	**Parameters**	**Notes**		**Page #**
Objective: Aerobic conditioning intervals Pick one: erg rower, air bike, ski erg, or treadmill	Total duration: 15-20 min Interval protocol: 15 sec of hard work (RPE 8-9; 80%-90% of max HR) followed by 45 sec of easy work (RPE 5; 50% of max HR)			233
Recovery				
Exercise	**Reps/time**	**Notes**		**Page #**
Band single-leg lower	8 per side			N/A
Band Brettzel stretch	20 sec per side			N/A
Rear foot elevated half-kneeling hip flexor stretch with single-arm overhead reach	20 sec per side			N/A

(continued)

Table 10.3 Train Like a Pro Training Program: Phase 2 (Weeks 5-8) *(continued)*

DAY 5: FRIDAY				
Warm-up				
Exercise	Reps/time/distance	Notes		Page #
Cat-cow	8			64
Single-leg bridge isometric with bent-knee leg whip	5 per side			65
Catcher rockback	5 per side			66
Elevated bent-knee Copenhagen plank	15 sec per side			67
Alternating Spiderman to yoga pike	3			68
Heels-up split squat isometric	15 sec per side			69
MB hug Kang squat	5			70
Extensive single-leg pogo hop	10 per side			71
Drop reverse lunge to stick	3 per side			72
Lateral skip	10 yd per side			73
Workout				
Exercise	Sets x reps at RPE	Notes		Page #
Strength and power block • A1: DB single-leg RDL • A2: Single-leg broad jump to double-leg stick	3 x 6 per side at RPE 7-8 3 x 3 per side at RPE 6-7	Complete A block (A1 and A2) with no rest between exercises, then rest for 45-60 sec. That equals 1 set. Complete all sets in this way, then move on to B block.		140 209
Strength and power block • B1: DB single-arm bench press with single-leg hip thrust isometric • B2: MB step-through wall chest pass (staggered-stance start)	3 x 8 per side at RPE 7-8 3 x 3 per side at RPE 6-7	Complete B block (B1 and B2) with no rest between exercises, then rest for 45-60 sec. That equals 1 set. Complete all sets in this way, then move on to C block.		141 211
Hypertrophy block • C1: Cable pull-through • C2: DB seal row	3 x 12, 15, 20 at RPE 8, 7, 6 3 x 8, 10, 12 at RPE 8, 7, 7	Complete C block (C1 and C2) with no rest between exercises, then rest for 45-60 sec. That equals 1 set. Complete all sets in this way, then move on to D block.		142 143
Accessory block • D1: Band wide-stance vertical Pallof press • D2: Cable tall-kneeling straight bar biceps curl	3 x 8 per side at RPE 7-8 3 x 12 at RPE 7-8	Complete D block (D1 and D2) with no rest between exercises, then rest for 45-60 sec. That equals 1 set. Complete all sets in this way, then move on to recovery.		144 145
Recovery				
Exercise	Reps/time	Notes		Page #
Band single-leg lower	8 per side			N/A
Band Brettzel stretch	20 sec per side			N/A
Rear foot elevated half-kneeling hip flexor stretch with single-arm overhead reach	20 sec per side			N/A

Table 10.4 Train Like a Pro Training Program: Phase 3 (Weeks 9-12)

DAY 1: MONDAY				
Warm-up				
Exercise	Reps/time/distance	Notes		Page #
Segmental cat-cow	5			86
Bridge isometric with alternating reach	5 per side			87
Catcher rockback with toe turn	6 per side			88
Floor bent-knee Copenhagen plank with liftoff	5 per side			89
Alternating Spiderman to stationary inchworm	3 per side			90
Rear foot elevated split squat isometric	15 sec per side			91
KB goblet Kang squat	5			92
Intensive pogo hop	10			93
Drop skater squat to stick	5 per side			94
Lateral crossover skip	20 yd per side			95
Workout				
Exercise	Sets × reps at RPE	Notes		Page #
Strength and power block • A1: Landmine single-leg RDL (lateral orientation) • A2: Continuous broad jump	3 × 6 per side at RPE 8 3 × 4 at RPE 7	Complete A block (A1 and A2) with no rest between exercises, then rest for 45-60 sec. That equals 1 set. Complete all sets in this way, then move on to B block.		146 212
Strength and power block • B1: DB single-arm bench press with single-arm fixed (top) • B2. MB step-back rotational single-arm wall chest pass	3 × 8 per side at RPE 8 3 × 4 per side at RPE 7	Complete B block (B1 and B2) with no rest between exercises, then rest for 45-60 sec. That equals 1 set. Complete all sets in this way, then move on to C block.		147 214
Strength block • C1: DB neutral grip kickstand RDL • C2: Cable split-stance single-arm mid row with opposite hand reach	3 × 8 per side at RPE 7-8 3 × 8 per side at RPE 7-8	Complete C block (C1 and C2) with no rest between exercises, then rest for 45-60 sec. That equals 1 set. Complete all sets in this way, then move on to D block.		148 149
Accessory block • D1: DB bent-over lateral raise • D2: Ab wheel tall-kneeling rollout	3 × 12 at RPE 7-8 3 × 10 at RPE 7-8	Complete D block (D1 and D2) with no rest between exercises, then rest for 45-60 sec. That equals 1 set. Complete all sets in this way, then move on to recovery.		150 151
Recovery				
Exercise	Reps/time	Notes		Page #
Three-way hamstring floss	5 each direction per side			N/A
Brettzel stretch with breathing	8 breaths per side			N/A
Rear foot elevated half-kneeling hip flexor stretch with single-arm overhead reach and rotate	20 sec per side			N/A

(continued)

Table 10.4 Train Like a Pro Training Program: Phase 3 (Weeks 9-12) *(continued)*

DAY 2: TUESDAY			
Warm-up			
Exercise	Reps/time/distance	Notes	Page #
Single-leg long bridge isometric with power switch	3 per side		96
Wall press with single-leg lower	8 per side		97
Mini-band stork with clam lift	8 per side		98
Tempo wall heel raise (3 seconds up/3 seconds iso/3 seconds down)	6		99
Hand-supported alternating reverse lunge with single-arm overhead reach	3 per side		100
Walking inchworm to push-up	3		101
Hinge to squat isometric with alternating rotation	3 per side		102
Wall press single-leg RDL with power drive	3 per side		103
Reverse walking single-leg RDL	2 × 10 yd		104
Walking alternating Spiderman to yoga push-up	2 × 10 yd		105
5-yard lateral shuffle to turn and 10-yard sprint	2 × 15 yd per side		106
5-yard backpedal to turn and 10-yard sprint	2 × 15 yd per side		107
Workout			
Exercise	Reps at RPE	Notes	Page #
A: 10-yard sprint and rehearsed T-turn	3 per side at RPE 8-9	Complete 1 rep per side, then rest for 30-45 sec. That equals 1 set. Complete all sets in this way, then move on to the next exercise.	226
B: 5-10-5 pro agility shuttle	3 per side at RPE 8-9	Complete 1 rep per side, then rest for 45-60 sec. That equals 1 set. Complete all sets in this way, then move on to the next exercise.	227
C: 20-yard curvilinear sprint	3 per side at 100% effort	Rest 60-75 sec between reps.	228
Recovery			
Exercise	Reps/time	Notes	Page #
Three-way hamstring floss	5 each direction per side		N/A
Brettzel stretch with breathing	8 breaths per side		N/A
Rear foot elevated half-kneeling hip flexor stretch with single-arm overhead reach and rotate	20 sec per side		N/A

DAY 3: WEDNESDAY

Warm-up

Exercise	Reps/time/distance	Notes	Page #
Segmental cat-cow	5		86
Bridge isometric with alternating reach	5 per side		87
Catcher rockback with toe turn	6 per side		88
Floor bent-knee Copenhagen plank with liftoff	5 per side		89
Alternating Spiderman to stationary inchworm	3 per side		90
Rear foot elevated split squat isometric	15 sec per side		91
KB goblet Kang squat	5		92
Intensive pogo hop	10		93
Drop skater squat to stick	5 per side		94
Lateral crossover skip	20 yd per side		95

Workout

Exercise	Sets × reps at RPE	Notes	Page #
Strength and power block • A1: Barbell bench press • A2: Band standing continuous power punch	3 × 6 at RPE 8 3 × 5 at RPE 7	Complete A block (A1 and A2) with no rest between exercises, then rest for 45-60 sec. That equals 1 set. Complete all sets in this way, then move on to B block.	152 215
Strength and power block • B1: DB single-arm offset band slider lateral lunge • B2: Plate skater hop with quick, stick, and punch	3 × 8 per side at RPE 8 3 × 3 per side at RPE 7	Complete B block (B1 and B2) with no rest between exercises, then rest for 45-60 sec. That equals 1 set. Complete all sets in this way, then move on to C block.	153 216
Strength block • C1: Landmine standing Viking shoulder press • C2: Band wide-stance crossbody long chop	3 × 8 at RPE 7-8 3 × 10 per side at RPE 7-8	Complete C block (C1 and C2) with no rest between exercises, then rest for 45-60 sec. That equals 1 set. Complete all sets in this way, then move on to D block.	154 155
Accessory block • D1: KB towel standing hammer curl • D2: Bent-knee star plank with clamshell	3 × 12 at RPE 7-8 3 × 8 per side at RPE 7-8	Complete D block (D1 and D2) with no rest between exercises, then rest for 45-60 sec. That equals 1 set. Complete all sets in this way, then move on to recovery.	156 157

Recovery

Exercise	Reps/time	Notes	Page #
Three-way hamstring floss	5 each direction per side		N/A
Brettzel stretch with breathing	8 breaths per side		N/A
Rear foot elevated half-kneeling hip flexor stretch with single-arm overhead reach and rotate	20 sec per side		N/A

(continued)

Table 10.4 Train Like a Pro Training Program: Phase 3 (Weeks 9-12) *(continued)*

DAY 4: THURSDAY			
Warm-up			
Exercise	Reps/time/distance	Notes	Page #
Single-leg long bridge isometric with power switch	3 per side		96
Wall press with single-leg lower	8 per side		97
Mini-band stork with clam lift	8 per side		98
Tempo wall heel raise (3 seconds up/3 seconds iso/3 seconds down)	6		99
Hand-supported alternating reverse lunge with single-arm overhead reach	3 per side		100
Walking inchworm to push-up	3		101
Hinge to squat isometric with alternating rotation	3 per side		102
Wall press single-leg RDL with power drive	3 per side		103
Reverse walking single-leg RDL	2 × 10 yd		104
Walking alternating Spiderman to yoga push-up	2 × 10 yd		105
5-yard lateral shuffle to turn and 10-yard sprint	2 × 15 yd per side		106
5-yard backpedal to turn and 10-yard sprint	2 × 15 yd per side		107
Workout			
Exercise	Parameters	Notes	Page #
Objective: High-intensity sprint interval Pick one: Incline treadmill (20%-30% incline), outdoor hill (20%-30% incline), or empty sled (no weight added)	Total duration: 8-12 sets Interval protocol: 6-8 sec of all-out sprint (RPE 10; 100% of max HR) followed by 45-60 sec of complete rest (goal is to bring HR back down during this time)		234
Recovery			
Exercise	Reps/time	Notes	Page #
Three-way hamstring floss	5 each direction per side		N/A
Brettzel stretch with breathing	8 breaths per side		N/A
Rear foot elevated half-kneeling hip flexor stretch with single-arm overhead reach and rotation	20 sec per side		N/A

DAY 5: FRIDAY

Warm-up

Exercise	Reps/time/distance	Notes	Page #
Segmental cat-cow	5		86
Bridge isometric with alternating reach	5 per side		87
Catcher rockback with toe turn	6 per side		88
Floor bent-knee Copenhagen plank with liftoff	5 per side		89
Alternating Spiderman to stationary inchworm	3 per side		90
Rear foot elevated split squat isometric	15 sec per side		91
KB goblet Kang squat	5		92
Intensive pogo hop	10		93
Drop skater squat to stick	5 per side		94
Lateral crossover skip	20 yd per side		95

Workout

Exercise	Sets × reps at RPE	Notes	Page #
Strength and power block • A1: DB rear foot elevated split squat • A2: DB reactive split squat jump	3 × 6 per side at RPE 8 3 × 5 per side at RPE 7	Complete A block (A1 and A2) with no rest between exercises, then rest for 45-60 sec. That equals 1 set. Complete all sets in this way, then move on to B block.	158 217
Strength and power block • B1: DB single-arm row • B2: Cable split-stance single-arm low row with box stomp	3 × 8 per side at RPE 8 3 × 4 per side at RPE 7	Complete B block (B1 and B2) with no rest between exercises, then rest for 45-60 sec. That equals 1 set. Complete all sets in this way, then move on to C block.	159 218
Strength block • C1: KB goblet kickstand squat (2 DB) • C2: Cable half-kneeling single-arm high row	3 × 8 per side at RPE 7-8 3 × 8 per side at RPE 7-8	Complete C block (C1 and C2) with no rest between exercises, then rest for 45-60 sec. That equals 1 set. Complete all sets in this way, then move on to D block.	186 161
Accessory block • D1: DB floor skull crusher • D2: DB floor prone Superman isometric	3 × 12 at RPE 7-8 3 × 15 sec at RPE 7-8	Complete D block (D1 and D2) with no rest between exercises, then rest for 45-60 sec. That equals 1 set. Complete all sets in this way, then move on to recovery.	162 163

Recovery

Exercise	Reps/time	Notes	Page #
Three-way hamstring floss	5 each direction per side		N/A
Brettzel stretch with breathing	8 breaths per side		N/A
Rear foot elevated half-kneeling hip flexor stretch with single-arm overhead reach and rotation	20 sec per side		N/A

The GPP/Hypertrophy Training Program

This 12-week training program has three consecutive phases (four-week training blocks) that build off each other. In all three phases, the primary emphasis is on general physical preparedness (GPP) and hypertrophy. The goal is to increase your overall volume of training while building muscle and body armor to show off in sports and competition!

The GPP/hypertrophy training program was designed to complement the initial flagship program described in chapter 10 and help you tap into your inner athlete while packing on muscle. This training program can be used at various times and seasons throughout the year since the primary goal is muscular development, which supports athletic performance. Because of the uptick in volume it requires, this program is best used outside of in-season competition.

Table 11.1 GPP/Hypertrophy Training Program: Phase 1 (Weeks 1-4)

DAY 1: MONDAY				
Warm-up				
Exercise	Reps/time/distance	Notes		Page #
Band cat-cow	8			42
Heels-up single-leg bridge isometric with knee drive isometric	15 sec per side			43
Catcher rockback isometric with reach and rotate	5 per side			44
Floor bent-knee Copenhagen plank	15 sec per side			45
Alternating Spiderman	3 per side			46
Split squat isometric	15 sec per side			47
Squat rack Kang squat	5			48
Extensive pogo hop	15			49
Drop squat to stick	8			50
Linear skip	20 yd			51
Workout				
Exercise	Sets × reps at RPE	Notes		Page #
Power block • A1: Band-assisted continuous squat jump • A2: MB tall-kneeling slam with hip hinge	3 × 5 at RPE 6-7 3 × 5 at RPE 6-7	Complete A block (A1 and A2) with no rest between exercises, then rest for 45-60 sec. That equals 1 set. Complete all sets in this way, then move on to B block.		198 199
Strength block • B1: DB goblet squat • B2: Band standing Pallof press	3 × 12 at RPE 8 3 × 12 per side at RPE 7-8	Complete B block (B1 and B2) with no rest between exercises, then rest for 45-60 sec. That equals 1 set. Complete all sets in this way, then move on to C block.		164 165
Hypertrophy block • C1: Barbell RDL • C2: KB seated shoulder press (back-supported)	3 × 12 at RPE 8 3 × 12 at RPE 8	Complete C block (C1 and C2) with no rest between exercises, then rest for 45-60 sec. That equals 1 set. Complete all sets in this way, then move on to D block.		166 167
Accessory block • D1: Walking lunge • D2: DB standing biceps curl	3 × 15 per side at RPE 7-8 3 × 15 per side at RPE 7-8	Complete D block (D1 and D2) with no rest between exercises, then rest for 45-60 sec. That equals 1 set. Complete all sets in this way, then move on to recovery.		168 169
Recovery				
Exercise	Reps/time	Notes		Page #
Hamstring floss	12 per side			N/A
Book opener isometric	20 sec per side			N/A
Rear foot elevated half-kneeling hip flexor stretch	20 sec per side			N/A

DAY 2: TUESDAY				
Warm-up			
Exercise	Reps/time/distance	Notes	Page #
Long bridge isometric	15 sec		52
Wall press with alternating dead bug	8 per side		53
Wall stork	15 sec per side		54
Wall single-leg heel raise isometric	15 sec per side		55
Alternating yoga plex	3 per side		56
Stationary inchworm	3		57
Hinge to squat	5		58
Wall linear single exchange	5 per side		59
Stationary hamstring scoop	5 per side		60
Walking alternating Spiderman	2 × 10 yd		61
Lateral shuffle with arm swing	2 × 10 yd per side		62
Backpedal	2 × 10 yd		63
Workout			
Exercise	Reps at RPE	Notes	Page #
A: 10-yard sprint and rehearsed stop	3 at RPE 8-9	Complete 1 rep, then rest for 30-45 sec. That equals 1 set. Complete all sets in this way, then move on to the next exercise.	220
B: Multidirectional plyo step from half-kneeling start to 5-yard sprint	2 per direction (4 total directions) at RPE 8-9	Complete 1 rep per direction, then rest for 45-60 sec. That equals 1 set. Complete all sets in this way, then move on to the next exercise.	221
C: 100-yard tempo run	6 at 80% effort	30-45 sec rest between reps	222
Recovery			
Exercise	Reps/time	Notes	Page #
Hamstring floss	12 per side		N/A
Book opener isometric	20 sec per side		N/A
Rear foot elevated half-kneeling hip flexor stretch	20 sec per side		N/A

(continued)

Table 11.1 GPP/Hypertrophy Training Program: Phase 1 (Weeks 1-4) *(continued)*

DAY 3: WEDNESDAY				
Warm-up				
Exercise	Reps/time/distance	Notes		Page #
Band cat-cow	8			42
Heels-up single-leg bridge isometric with knee drive isometric	15 sec per side			43
Catcher rockback isometric with reach and rotate	5 per side			44
Floor bent-knee Copenhagen plank	15 sec per side			45
Alternating Spiderman	3 per side			46
Split squat isometric	15 sec per side			47
Squat rack Kang squat	5			48
Extensive pogo hop	15			49
Drop squat to stick	8			50
Linear skip	20 yd			51
Workout				
Exercise	Sets × reps at RPE	Notes		Page #
Power block • A1: MB skater hop with chop and stick • A2: MB half-kneeling lateral wall toss	3 × 5 per side at RPE 6-7 3 × 5 per side at RPE 6-7	Complete A block (A1 and A2) with no rest between exercises, then rest for 45-60 sec. That equals 1 set. Complete all sets in this way, then move on to B block.		200 201
Strength block • B1: DB bench press • B2: Side plank	3 × 12 at RPE 8 3 × 20 sec per side at RPE 7-8	Complete B block (B1 and B2) with no rest between exercises, then rest for 45-60 sec. That equals 1 set. Complete all sets in this way, then move on to C block.		170 171
Hypertrophy block • C1: DB chest-supported row • C2: KB goblet lateral squat	3 × 12 at RPE 8 3 × 10 per side at RPE 8	Complete C block (C1 and C2) with no rest between exercises, then rest for 45-60 sec. That equals 1 set. Complete all sets in this way, then move on to D block.		118 172
Accessory block • D1: KB goblet carry • D2: Standing band pull-apart	3 × 40 yd at RPE 7-8 3 × 20 at RPE 7-8	Complete D block (D1 and D2) with no rest between exercises, then rest for 45-60 sec. That equals 1 set. Complete all sets in this way, then move on to recovery.		120 173
Recovery				
Exercise	Reps/time	Notes		Page #
Hamstring floss	12 per side			N/A
Book opener isometric	20 sec per side			N/A
Rear foot elevated half-kneeling hip flexor stretch	20 sec per side			N/A

DAY 4: THURSDAY			
Warm-up			
Exercise	**Reps/time/distance**	**Notes**	**Page #**
Long bridge isometric	15 sec		52
Wall press with alternating dead bug	8 per side		53
Wall stork	15 sec per side		54
Wall single-leg heel raise isometric	15 sec per side		55
Alternating yoga plex	3 per side		56
Stationary inchworm	3		57
Hinge to squat	5		58
Wall linear single exchange	5 per side		59
Stationary hamstring scoop	5 per side		60
Walking alternating Spiderman	2 × 10 yd		61
Lateral shuffle with arm swing	2 × 10 yd per side		62
Backpedal	2 × 10 yd		63
Workout			
Workout	**Parameters**	**Notes**	**Page #**
Objective: Steady-state aerobic conditioning Pick one: erg rower, air bike, ski erg, or treadmill	Total duration: 30-40 min Target heart rate: 130-150 bpm Target RPE: 6-7 (60%-70% of max HR)		232
Recovery			
Exercise	**Reps/time**	**Notes**	**Page #**
Hamstring floss	12 per side		N/A
Book opener isometric	20 sec per side		N/A
Rear foot elevated half-kneeling hip flexor stretch	20 sec per side		N/A

(continued)

Table 11.1 GPP/Hypertrophy Training Program: Phase 1 (Weeks 1-4) *(continued)*

DAY 5: FRIDAY			
Warm-up			
Exercise	Reps/time/distance	Notes	Page #
Band cat-cow	8		42
Heels-up single-leg bridge isometric with knee drive isometric	15 sec per side		43
Catcher rockback isometric with reach and rotate	5 per side		44
Floor bent-knee Copenhagen plank	15 sec per side		45
Alternating Spiderman	3 per side		46
Split squat isometric	15 sec per side		47
Squat rack Kang squat	5		48
Extensive pogo hop	15		49
Drop squat to stick	8		50
Linear skip	20 yd		51
Workout			
Exercise	Sets × reps at RPE	Notes	Page #
Power block • A1: 90-degree rotational single-leg hop with stick • A2: MB half-kneeling around-the-world slam	3 × 5 per side at RPE 6-7 3 × 5 per side at RPE 6-7	Complete A block (A1 and A2) with no rest between exercises, then rest for 45-60 sec. That equals 1 set. Complete all sets in this way, then move on to B block.	202 203
Strength block • B1: KB deadlift • B2: PB push–pull	3 × 12 at RPE 8 3 × 12 at RPE 7-8	Complete B block (B1 and B2) with no rest between exercises, then rest for 45-60 sec. That equals 1 set. Complete all sets in this way, then move on to C block.	174 123
Hypertrophy block • C1: Two DB foam roller hack squat against a wall • C2: Cable half-kneeling high row with 1-second isometric	3 × 12 at RPE 8 3 × 10 per side at RPE 8	Complete C block (C1 and C2) with no rest between exercises, then rest for 45-60 sec. That equals 1 set. Complete all sets in this way, then move on to D block.	124 125
Accessory block • D1: Cable double-arm single-leg RDL with knee drive and row • D2: Band standing triceps extension	3 × 10 per side at RPE 7-8 3 × 20 at RPE 7-8	Complete D block (D1 and D2) with no rest between exercises, then rest for 45-60 sec. That equals 1 set. Complete all sets in this way, then move on to recovery.	190 127
Recovery			
Exercise	Reps/time	Notes	Page #
Hamstring floss	12 per side		N/A
Book opener isometric	20 sec per side		N/A
Rear foot elevated half-kneeling hip flexor stretch	20 sec per side		N/A

Table 11.2 GPP/Hypertrophy Training Program: Phase 2 (Weeks 5-8)

DAY 1: MONDAY

Warm-up

Exercise	Reps/time/distance	Notes	Page #
Cat-cow	8		64
Single-leg bridge isometric with bent-knee leg whip	5 per side		65
Catcher rockback	5 per side		66
Elevated bent-knee Copenhagen plank	15 sec per side		67
Alternating Spiderman to yoga pike	3 per side		68
Heels-up split squat isometric	15 sec per side		69
MB hug Kang squat	5		70
Extensive single-leg pogo hop	10 per side		71
Drop reverse lunge to stick	3 per side		72
Lateral skip	20 yd per side		73

Workout

Exercise	Sets × reps at RPE	Notes	Page #
Strength and power block • A1: DB step-up • A2: Band-resisted acceleration power step	3 × 8 per side at RPE 7-8 3 × 3 per side at RPE 6-7	Complete A block (A1 and A2) with no rest between exercises, then rest for 45-60 sec. That equals 1 set. Complete all sets in this way, then move on to B block.	128 204
Strength and power block • B1: DB heels-up three-point row with 3-second eccentric • B2: Barbell explosive inverted row with hip thrust isometric	3 × 12 per side at RPE 7-8 3 × 5 at RPE 6-7	Complete B block (B1 and B2) with no rest between exercises, then rest for 45-60 sec. That equals 1 set. Complete all sets in this way, then move on to C block.	129 205
Hypertrophy block • C1: DB cyclist squat (2 DB) • C2: Cable seated lat pull-down with 3-second eccentric	3 × 12 at RPE 8 3 × 15 RPE 8	Complete C block (C1 and C2) with no rest between exercises, then rest for 45-60 sec. That equals 1 set. Complete all sets in this way, then move on to D block.	130 131
Accessory block • D1: KB front rack carry • D2: Cable tall-kneeling rope triceps extension	3 × 40 yd at RPE 7-8 3 ×15 at RPE 7-8	Complete D block (D1 and D2) with no rest between exercises, then rest for 45-60 sec. That equals 1 set. Complete all sets in this way, then move on to recovery.	132 133

Recovery

Exercise	Reps/time	Notes	Page #
Band single-leg lower	8 per side		N/A
Band Brettzel stretch	20 sec per side		N/A
Rear foot elevated half-kneeling hip flexor stretch with single-arm overhead reach	20 sec per side		N/A

(continued)

Table 11.2 GPP/Hypertrophy Training Program: Phase 2 (Weeks 5-8) *(continued)*

DAY 2: TUESDAY			
Warm-up			
Exercise	Reps/time/distance	Notes	Page #
Single-leg long bridge isometric with knee drive isometric	15 sec per side		74
Cross-connect dead bug (opposite side)	8 sec per side		75
Mini-band stork	15 sec per side		76
Wall bent-knee single-leg heel raise isometric	15 sec per side		77
Alternating yoga plex to yoga pike	3 per side		78
Walking inchworm	3		79
Hinge to squat with alternating rotation	3		80
Wall linear double exchange	5 per side		81
Walking alternating hamstring scoop	2 × 10 yd		82
Walking alternating Spiderman to reach and rotate	2 × 10 yd		83
Double lateral shuffle with alternating lateral squat	2 × 10 yd per side		84
Backward reach run	2 × 10 yd		85
Workout			
Exercise	Reps at RPE	Notes	Page #
A. 10-yard sprint and rehearsed Y-turn	3 per side at RPE 8-9	Complete 1 rep per side then rest for 30-45 sec. That equals 1 set. Complete all sets in this way, then move on to the next exercise.	223
B. 10-yard sprint from lateral half-kneeling start	3 per side at RPE 8-9	Complete 1 rep per side, then rest for 30-45 sec. That equals 1 set. Complete all sets in this way, then move on to the next exercise.	224
C. 20-yard dash	4 at 100% effort	Rest 60-75 sec between reps.	225
Recovery			
Exercise	Reps/time	Notes	Page #
Band single-leg lower	8 per side		N/A
Band Brettzel stretch	20 sec per side		N/A
Rear foot elevated half-kneeling hip flexor stretch with single-arm overhead reach	20 sec per side		N/A

The GPP/Hypertrophy Training Program

DAY 3: WEDNESDAY

Warm-up

Exercise	Reps/time/distance	Notes	Page #
Cat-cow	8		64
Single-leg bridge isometric with bent-knee leg whip	5 per side		65
Catcher rockback	5 per side		66
Elevated bent-knee Copenhagen plank	15 sec per side		67
Alternating Spiderman to yoga pike	3		68
Heels-up split squat isometric	15 sec per side		69
MB hug Kang squat	5		70
Extensive single-leg pogo hop	10 per side		71
Drop reverse lunge to stick	3 per side		72
Lateral skip	20 yd per side		73

Workout

Exercise	Sets × reps at RPE	Notes	Page #
Strength and power block • A1: Band-assisted pull-up • A2: MB standing double clutch slam	3 × 12 at RPE 7-8 3 × 5 at RPE 6-7	Complete A block (A1 and A2) with no rest between exercises, then rest for 45-60 sec. That equals 1 set. Complete all sets in this way, then move on to B block.	175 206
Strength and power block • B1: Landmine goblet lateral squat • B2: Band-resisted skater hop with stick (lateral orientation)	3 × 10 per side at RPE 7-8 3 × 5 per side at RPE 6-7	Complete B block (B1 and B2) with no rest between exercises, then rest for 45-60 sec. That equals 1 set. Complete all sets in this way, then move on to C block.	135 208
Hypertrophy • C1: DB captain stance shoulder press • C2: Cable plank single-arm row to triceps extension	3 × 10 per side at RPE 8 3 × 10 per side at RPE 8	Complete C block (C1 and C2) with no rest between exercises, then rest for 45-60 sec. That equals 1 set. Complete all sets in this way, then move on to D block.	176 137
Accessory block • D1: KB suitcase carry • D2: DB incline bench trap raise (Y) with 3-second eccentric	3 × 40 yd per side at RPE 7-8 3 × 15 at RPE 7-8	Complete D block (D1 and D2) with no rest between exercises, then rest for 45-60 sec. That equals 1 set. Complete all sets in this way, then move on to recovery.	138 139

Recovery

Exercise	Reps/time	Notes	Page #
Band single-leg lower	8 per side		N/A
Band Brettzel stretch	20 sec per side		N/A
Rear foot elevated half-kneeling hip flexor stretch with single-arm overhead reach	20 sec per side		N/A

(continued)

Table 11.2 GPP/Hypertrophy Training Program: Phase 2 (Weeks 5-8) *(continued)*

DAY 4: THURSDAY			
Warm-up			
Exercise	Reps/time/distance	Notes	Page #
Single-leg long bridge isometric with knee drive isometric	15 sec per side		74
Cross-connect dead bug (opposite side)	8 sec per side		75
Mini-band stork	15 sec per side		76
Wall bent-knee single-leg heel raise isometric	15 sec per side		77
Alternating yoga plex to yoga pike	3 per side		78
Walking inchworm	3		79
Hinge to squat with alternating rotation	3		80
Wall linear double exchange	5 per side		81
Walking alternating hamstring scoop	2 × 10 yd		82
Walking alternating Spiderman to reach and rotate	2 × 10 yd		83
Double lateral shuffle with alternating lateral squat	2 × 10 yd per side		84
Backward reach run	2 × 10 yd		85
Workout			
Exercise	Parameters	Notes	Page #
Objective: Aerobic conditioning intervals Pick one: erg rower, air bike, ski erg, or treadmill	Total duration: 15-20 minutes Interval protocol: 15 sec of hard work (RPE 8-9; 80%-90% of max HR) followed by 45 sec of easy work (RPE 5; 50% of max HR)		233
Recovery			
Exercise	Reps/time	Notes	Page #
Band single-leg lower	8 per side		N/A
Band Brettzel stretch	20 sec per side		N/A
Rear foot elevated half-kneeling hip flexor stretch with single-arm overhead reach	20 sec per side		N/A

DAY 5: FRIDAY				
Warm-up			
Exercise	Reps/time/distance	Notes	Page #
Cat-cow	8		64
Single-leg bridge isometric with bent-knee leg whip	5 per side		65
Catcher rockback	5 per side		66
Elevated bent-knee Copenhagen plank	15 sec per side		67
Alternating Spiderman to yoga pike	3		68
Heels-up split squat isometric	15 sec per side		69
MB hug Kang squat	5		70
Extensive single-leg pogo hop	10 per side		71
Drop reverse lunge to stick	3 per side		72
Lateral skip	20 yd per side		73
Workout			
Exercise	Sets × reps at RPE	Notes	Page #
Strength and power block • A1: DB single-leg RDL (2 DB) • A2: Single-leg broad jump to double-leg stick	3 × 8 per side at RPE 7-8 3 × 3 per side at RPE 6-7	Complete A block (A1 and A2) with no rest between exercises, then rest for 45-60 sec. That equals 1 set. Complete all sets in this way, then move on to B block.	177 209
Strength and power block • B1: DB single-arm bench press • B2: MB step-through wall chest pass (staggered-stance start)	3 × 12 per side at RPE 7-8 3 × 3 per side at RPE 6-7	Complete B block (B1 and B2) with no rest between exercises, then rest for 45-60 sec. That equals 1 set. Complete all sets in this way, then move on to C block.	178 211
Hypertrophy block • C1: Cable pull-through • C2: DB seal row	3 × 20 at RPE 8 3 × 12 at RPE 8	Complete C block (C1 and C2) with no rest between exercises, then rest for 45-60 sec. That equals 1 set. Complete all sets in this way, then move on to D block.	142 143
Accessory block • D1: Band wide-stance vertical Pallof press • D2: Cable tall-kneeling straight bar biceps curl	3 × 10 per side at RPE 7-8 3 × 15 at RPE 7-8	Complete D block (D1 and D2) with no rest between exercises, then rest for 45-60 sec. That equals 1 set. Complete all sets in this way, then move on to recovery.	144 145
Recovery			
Exercise	Reps/time	Notes	Page #
Band single-leg lower	8 per side		N/A
Band Brettzel stretch	20 sec per side		N/A
Rear foot elevated half-kneeling hip flexor stretch with single-arm overhead reach	20 sec per side		N/A

Table 11.3 GPP/Hypertrophy Training Program: Phase 3 (Weeks 9-12)

DAY 1: MONDAY				
Warm-up				
Exercise	Reps/time/distance	Notes		Page #
Segmental cat-cow	5			86
Bridge isometric with alternating reach	5 per side			87
Catcher rockback with toe turn	6 per side			88
Floor bent-knee Copenhagen plank with liftoff	5 per side			89
Alternating Spiderman to stationary inchworm	3 per side			90
Rear foot elevated split squat isometric	15 sec per side			91
KB goblet Kang squat	5			92
Intensive pogo hop	10			93
Drop skater squat to stick	5 per side			94
Lateral crossover skip	20 yd per side			95
Workout				
Exercise	Sets × reps at RPE	Notes		Page #
Strength and power block • A1: Landmine single-leg RDL (lateral orientation) • A2: Continuous broad jump	3 × 8 per side at RPE 8 3 × 4 at RPE 7	Complete A block (A1 and A2) with no rest between exercises, then rest for 45-60 sec. That equals 1 set. Complete all sets in this way, then move on to B block.		146 212
Strength and power block • B1: DB Frankenstein floor press • B2: MB step-back rotational single-arm wall chest pass	3 × 12 at RPE 8 3 × 4 per side at RPE 7	Complete B block (B1 and B2) with no rest between exercises, then rest for 45-60 sec. That equals 1 set. Complete all sets in this way, then move on to C block.		179 214
Strength block • C1: DB neutral grip kickstand RDL • C2: Cable seated mid row	3 × 10 per side at RPE 7-8 3 × 15 at RPE 7-8	Complete C block (C1 and C2) with no rest between exercises, then rest for 45-60 sec. That equals 1 set. Complete all sets in this way, then move on to D block.		148 180
Accessory block • D1: Band resisted bent-over DB lateral raise • D2: Ab wheel tall-kneeling rollout	3 × 12 at RPE 7-8 3 × 12 at RPE 7-8	Complete D block (D1 and D2) with no rest between exercises, then rest for 45-60 sec. That equals 1 set. Complete all sets in this way, then move on to recovery.		181 151
Recovery				
Exercise	Reps/time	Notes		Page #
Three-way hamstring floss	5 each direction per side			N/A
Brettzel stretch with breathing	8 breaths per side			N/A
Rear foot elevated half-kneeling hip flexor stretch with single-arm overhead reach and rotate	20 sec per side			N/A

DAY 2: TUESDAY

Warm-up

Exercise	Reps/time/distance	Notes	Page #
Single-leg long bridge isometric with power switch	3 per side		96
Wall press with single-leg lower	8 per side		97
Mini-band stork with clam lift	8 per side		98
Tempo wall heel raise (3 seconds up/3 seconds iso/3 seconds down)	6		99
Hand-supported alternating reverse lunge with single-arm overhead reach	3 per side		100
Walking inchworm to push-up	3		101
Hinge to squat isometric with alternating rotation	3 per side		102
Wall press single-leg RDL with power drive	3 per side		103
Reverse walking single-leg RDL	2 × 10 yd		104
Walking alternating Spiderman to yoga push-up	2 × 10 yd		105
5-yard lateral shuffle to turn and 10-yard sprint	2 × 15 yd per side		106
5-yard backpedal to turn and 10-yard sprint	2 × 15 yd per side		107

Workout

Exercise	Reps at RPE	Notes	Page #
A: 10-yard sprint and rehearsed T-turn	3 per side at RPE 8-9	Complete 1 rep per side then rest for 30-45 sec. That equals 1 set. Complete all sets in this way, then move on to the next exercise.	226
B: 5-10-5 pro agility shuttle	3 per side at RPE 8-9	Complete 1 rep per side then rest for 45-60 sec. That equals 1 set. Complete all sets in this way, then move on to the next exercise.	227
C: 20-yard curvilinear sprint	3 per side at 100% effort	Rest 60-75 sec between reps.	228

Recovery

Exercise	Reps/time	Notes	Page #
Three-way hamstring floss	5 each direction per side		N/A
Brettzel stretch with breathing	8 breaths per side		N/A
Rear foot elevated half-kneeling hip flexor stretch with single-arm overhead reach and rotate	20 sec per side		N/A

(continued)

Table 11.3 GPP/Hypertrophy Training Program: Phase 3 (Weeks 9-12) *(continued)*

DAY 3: WEDNESDAY				
Warm-up				
Exercise	Reps/time/distance	Notes		Page #
Segmental cat-cow	5			86
Bridge isometric with alternating reach	5 per side			87
Catcher rockback with toe turn	6 per side			88
Floor bent-knee Copenhagen plank with liftoff	5 per side			89
Alternating Spiderman to stationary inchworm	3 per side			90
Rear foot elevated split squat isometric	15 sec per side			91
KB goblet Kang squat	5			92
Intensive pogo hop	10			93
Drop skater squat to stick	5 per side			94
Lateral crossover skip	20 yd per side			95
Workout				
Exercise	Sets × reps at RPE	Notes		Page #
Strength and power block • A1: Barbell bench press • A2: Band standing continuous power punch	3 × 8 at RPE 8 3 × 5 at RPE 7	Complete A block (A1 and A2) with no rest between exercises, then rest for 45-60 sec. That equals 1 set. Complete all sets in this way, then move on to B block.		152 215
Strength and power block • B1: DB single-arm offset band slider lateral lunge • B2: Plate skater hop with quick, stick, and punch	3 × 10 per side at RPE 8 3 × 3 per side at RPE 7	Complete B block (B1 and B2) with no rest between exercises, then rest for 45-60 sec. That equals 1 set. Complete all sets in this way, then move on to C block.		153 216
Strength block • C1: Landmine standing Viking shoulder press • C2: Band wide-stance crossbody short chop	3 × 12 at RPE 7-8 3 × 12 per side at RFE 7-8	Complete C block (C1 and C2) with no rest between exercises, then rest for 45-60 sec. That equals 1 set. Complete all sets in this way, then move on to D block.		154 182
Accessory block • D1: KB horns-grip tall-kneeling biceps curl • D2: Mini-band bent-knee star plank	3 × 15 at RPE 7-8 3 × 20 sec per side at RPE 7-8	Complete D block (D1 and D2) with no rest between exercises, then rest for 45-60 sec. That equals 1 set. Complete all sets in this way, then move on to recovery.		183 184
Recovery				
Exercise	Reps/time	Notes		Page #
Three-way hamstring floss	5 each direction per side			N/A
Brettzel stretch with breathing	8 breaths per side			N/A
Rear foot elevated half-kneeling hip flexor stretch with single-arm overhead reach and rotate	20 sec per side			N/A

The GPP/Hypertrophy Training Program **267**

DAY 4: THURSDAY				
Warm-up			
Exercise	Reps/time/distance	Notes	Page #
Single-leg long bridge isometric with power switch	3 per side		96
Wall press with single-leg lower	8 per side		97
Mini-band stork with clam lift	8 per side		98
Tempo wall heel raise (3 seconds up/3 seconds iso/3 seconds down)	6		99
Hand-supported alternating reverse lunge with single-arm overhead reach	3 per side		100
Walking inchworm to push-up	3		101
Hinge to squat isometric with alternating rotation	3 per side		102
Wall press single-leg RDL with power drive	3 per side		103
Reverse walking single-leg RDL	2 × 10 yd		104
Walking alternating Spiderman to yoga push-up	2 × 10 yd		105
5-yard lateral shuffle to turn and 10-yard sprint	2 × 15 yd per side		106
5-yard backpedal to turn and 10-yard sprint	2 × 15 yd per side		107
Workout			
Exercise	Parameters	Notes	Page #
Objective: High-intensity sprint intervals Pick one: Incline treadmill (20%-30% incline), outdoor hill (20%-30% incline), or empty sled (no weight added)	Total duration: 8-12 sets Interval protocol: 6-8 sec of all-out sprint (RPE 10; 100% of max HR) followed by 45-60 sec of complete rest (goal is to bring HR back down at this time)		234
Recovery			
Exercise	Reps/time	Notes	Page #
Three-way hamstring floss	5 each direction per side		N/A
Brettzel stretch with breathing	8 breaths per side		N/A
Rear foot elevated half-kneeling hip flexor stretch with single-arm overhead reach and rotate	20 sec per side		N/A

(continued)

Table 11.3 GPP/Hypertrophy Training Program: Phase 3 (Weeks 9-12) *(continued)*

DAY 5: FRIDAY			
Warm-up			
Exercise	Reps/time/distance	Notes	Page #
Segmental cat-cow	5		86
Bridge isometric with alternating reach	5 per side		87
Catcher rockback with toe turn	6 per side		88
Floor bent-knee Copenhagen plank with liftoff	5 per side		89
Alternating Spiderman to stationary inchworm	3 per side		90
Rear foot elevated split squat isometric	15 sec per side		91
KB goblet Kang squat	5		92
Intensive pogo hop	10		93
Drop skater squat to stick	5 per side		94
Lateral crossover skip	20 yd per side		95
Workout			
Exercise	Sets × reps at RPE	Notes	Page #
Strength and power block • A1: DB split squat • A2: DB reactive split squat jump	3 × 10 per side at RPE 8 3 × 5 per side at RPE 7	Complete A block (A1 and A2) with no rest between exercises, then rest for 45-60 sec. That equals 1 set. Complete all sets in this way, then move on to B block.	185 217
Strength and power block • B1: DB single-arm row • B2: Cable split-stance single-arm low row with box stomp	3 × 12 per side at RPE 8 3 × 4 per side at RPE 7	Complete B block (B1 and B2) with no rest between exercises, then rest for 45-60 sec. That equals 1 set. Complete all sets in this way, then move on to C block.	159 218
Strength block • C1: KB goblet kickstand squat • C2: Cable half-kneeling single-arm high row	3 × 10 per side at RPE 7-8 3 × 12 per side at RPE 7-8	Complete C block (C1 and C2) with no rest between exercises, then rest for 45-60 sec. That equals 1 set. Complete all sets in this way, then move on to D block.	186 161
Accessory block • D1: DB floor skull crusher • D2: DB floor prone Superman isometric	3 × 15 at RPE 7-8 3 × 20 sec at RPE 7-8	Complete D block (D1 and D2) with no rest between exercises, then rest for 45-60 sec. That equals 1 set. Complete all sets in this way, then move on to recovery.	162 163
Recovery			
Exercise	Reps/time	Notes	Page #
Three-way hamstring floss	5 each direction per side		N/A
Brettzel stretch with breathing	8 breaths per side		N/A
Rear foot elevated half-kneeling hip flexor stretch with single-arm overhead reach and rotate	20 sec per side		N/A

CHAPTER 12

The Strength Training Program

This 12-week training program has three consecutive phases (four-week training blocks) that build off each other. In all three phases, the primary emphasis is on strength development. The goal is to help you increase your overall strength in order to produce force faster and more efficiently in your competition!

The strength training program was designed to complement the initial flagship program, Train Like a Pro. If your goal is to tap into your inner athlete while improving full-body strength and force production, this is the program for you. This training program can be used at a variety of times and seasons throughout the year since the primary goal is strength development, which supports athletic performance. Because it's focused on strength, it would be best to use this program in the middle of the pre-season as you're gearing for the season to begin.

Table 12.1 Strength Training Program: Phase 1 (Weeks 1-4)

DAY 1: MONDAY				
Warm-up				
Exercise	Reps/time/distance	Notes		Page #
Band cat-cow	8			42
Heels-up single-leg bridge isometric with knee drive isometric	15 sec per side			43
Catcher rockback isometric with reach and rotate	5 per side			44
Floor bent-knee Copenhagen plank	15 sec per side			45
Alternating Spiderman	3 per side			46
Split squat isometric	15 sec per side			47
Squat rack Kang squat	5			48
Extensive pogo hop	15			49
Drop squat to stick	8			50
Linear skip	20 yd			51
Workout				
Exercise	Sets × reps at RPE	Notes		Page #
Power block • A1: Band-assisted continuous squat jump • A2: MB tall-kneeling slam with hip hinge	3 × 5 at RPE 6-7 3 × 5 at RPE 6-7	Complete A block (A1 and A2) with no rest between exercises, then rest for 45-60 sec. That equals 1 set. Complete all sets in this way, then move on to B block.		198 199
Strength block • B1: Barbell front squat • B2: Band tall-kneeling Pallof press isometric	3 × 6 at RPE 8 3 × 10 sec per side at RPE 7-8	Complete B block (B1 and B2) with no rest between exercises, then rest for 45-60 sec. That equals 1 set. Complete all sets in this way, then move on to C block.		187 188
Hypertrophy block • C1: DB RDL • C2: KB half-kneeling shoulder press with 3-second isometric	3 × 10 at RPE 8 3 × 10 per side at RPE 8	Complete C block (C1 and C2) with no rest between exercises, then rest for 45-60 sec. That equals 1 set. Complete all sets in this way, then move on to D block.		112 113
Accessory block • D1: DB skater squat • D2: DB standing hammer curl	3 × 8 per side at RPE 8 3 × 15 at RPE 7-8	Complete D block (D1 and D2) with no rest between exercises, then rest for 45-60 sec. That equals 1 set. Complete all sets in this way, then move on to recovery.		189 115
Recovery				
Exercise	Reps/time	Notes		Page #
Hamstring floss	12 per side			N/A
Book opener isometric	20 sec per side			N/A
Rear foot elevated half-kneeling hip flexor stretch	20 sec per side			N/A

DAY 2: TUESDAY

Warm-up

Exercise	Reps/time/distance	Notes	Page #
Long bridge isometric	15 sec		52
Wall press with alternating dead bug	8 per side		53
Wall stork	15 sec per side		54
Wall single-leg heel raise isometric	15 sec per side		55
Alternating yoga plex	3 per side		56
Stationary inchworm	3		57
Hinge to squat	5		58
Wall linear single exchange	5 per side		59
Stationary hamstring scoop	5 per side		60
Walking alternating Spiderman	2 × 10 yd		61
Lateral shuffle with arm swing	2 × 10 yd per side		62
Backpedal	2 × 10 yd		63

Workout

Exercise	Reps at RPE	Notes	Page #
A. 10-yard sprint and rehearsed stop	3	Complete 1 rep, then rest for 30-45 sec. That equals 1 set. Complete all sets in this way, then move on to the next exercise.	220
B. Multidirectional plyo step from half-kneeling start to 5-yard sprint	2 each direction (4 directions total)	Complete 1 rep per side, then rest for 30-45 sec. That equals 1 set. Complete all sets in this way, then move on to the next exercise.	221
C. 100-yard tempo run	6 at 80% effort	Rest 60-75 sec between reps.	222

Recovery

Exercise	Reps/time	Notes	Page #
Hamstring floss	12 per side		N/A
Book opener isometric	20 sec per side		N/A
Rear foot elevated half-kneeling hip flexor stretch	20 sec per side		N/A

(continued)

Table 12.1 Strength Training Program: Phase 1 (Weeks 1-4) *(continued)*

DAY 3: WEDNESDAY			
Warm-up			
Exercise	Reps/time/distance	Notes	Page #
Band cat-cow	8		42
Heels-up single-leg bridge isometric with knee drive isometric	15 sec per side		43
Catcher rockback isometric with reach and rotate	5 per side		44
Floor bent-knee Copenhagen plank	15 sec per side		45
Alternating Spiderman	3 per side		46
Split squat isometric	15 sec per side		47
Squat rack Kang squat	5		48
Extensive pogo hop	15		49
Drop squat to stick	8		50
Linear skip	20 yd		51
Workout			
Exercise	Sets × reps at RPE	Notes	Page #
Power block • A1: MB skater hop with chop and stick • A2: MB half-kneeling lateral wall toss	3 × 5 per side at RPE 6-7 3 × 5 per side at RPE 6-7	Complete A block (A1 and A2) with no rest between exercises, then rest for 45-60 sec. That equals 1 set. Complete all sets in this way, then move on to B block.	200 201
Strength block • B1: Barbell bench press • B2: Bent-knee star plank with top leg long	3 × 6 at RPE 8 3 × 15 sec per side at RPE 7-8	Complete B block (B1 and B2) with no rest between exercises, then rest for 45-60 sec. That equals 1 set. Complete all sets in this way, then move on to C block.	152 117
Hypertrophy block • C1: DB chest-supported row • C2: KB single-arm offset lateral squat with 1-second isometric	3 × 10 at RPE 8 3 × 8 per side at RPE 8	Complete C block (C1 and C2) with no rest between exercises, then rest for 45-60 sec. That equals 1 set. Complete all sets in this way, then move on to D block.	118 119
Accessory block • D1: KB goblet carry • D2: Band tall-kneeling pull-apart	3 × 40 yd at RPE 7-8 3 × 15 at RPE 7-8	Complete D block (D1 and D2) with no rest between exercises, then rest for 45-60 sec. That equals 1 set. Complete all sets in this way, then move on to recovery.	120 121
Recovery			
Exercise	Reps/time	Notes	Page #
Hamstring floss	12 per side		N/A
Book opener isometric	20 sec per side		N/A
Rear foot elevated half-kneeling hip flexor stretch	20 sec per side		N/A

DAY 4: THURSDAY				
Warm-up				
Exercise	**Reps/time/distance**	**Notes**		**Page #**
Long bridge isometric	15 sec			52
Wall press with alternating dead bug	8 per side			53
Wall stork	15 sec per side			54
Wall single-leg heel raise isometric	15 sec per side			55
Alternating yoga plex	3 per side			56
Stationary inchworm	3			57
Hinge to squat	5			58
Wall linear single exchange	5 per side			59
Stationary hamstring scoop	5 per side			60
Walking alternating Spiderman	2 × 10 yd			61
Lateral shuffle with arm swing	2 × 10 yd per side			62
Backpedal	2 × 10 yd			63
Workout				
Exercise	**Sets × reps at RPE**	**Notes**		**Page #**
Objective: Steady-state aerobic conditioning Pick one: erg rower, air bike, ski erg, or treadmill	Total duration: 30-40 minutes Target heart rate: 130-150 bpm Target RPE: 6-7 (60-70% of max HR)			232
Recovery				
Exercise	**Reps/time**	**Notes**		**Page #**
Hamstring floss	12 per side			N/A
Book opener isometric	20 sec per side			N/A
Rear foot elevated half-kneeling hip flexor stretch	20 sec per side			N/A

(continued)

Table 12.1 Strength Training Program: Phase 1 (Weeks 1-4) *(continued)*

DAY 5: FRIDAY				
Warm-up				
Exercise	Reps/time/distance	Notes		Page #
Band cat-cow	8			42
Heels-up single-leg bridge isometric with knee drive isometric	15 sec per side			43
Catcher rockback isometric with reach and rotate	5 per side			44
Floor bent-knee Copenhagen plank	15 sec per side			45
Alternating Spiderman	3 per side			46
Split squat isometric	15 sec per side			47
Squat rack Kang squat	5			48
Extensive pogo hop	15			49
Drop squat to stick	8			50
Linear skip	20 yd			51
Workout				
Exercise	Sets × reps at RPE	Notes		Page #
Power block • A1: 90-degree rotational single-leg hop with stick • A2: MB half-kneeling around-the-world slam	3 × 5 per side at RPE 6-7 3 × 5 per side at RPE 6-7	Complete A block (A1 and A2) with no rest between exercises, then rest for 45-60 sec. That equals 1 set. Complete all sets in this way, then move on to B block.		202 203
Strength block • B1: Trap bar deadlift • B2: PB push–pull	3 × 6 at RPE 8 3 × 12 at RPE 7-8	Complete B block (B1 and B2) with no rest between exercises, then rest for 45-60 sec. That equals 1 set. Complete all sets in this way, then move on to C block.		122 123
Hypertrophy block • C1: Two DB foam roller hack squat against a wall • C2: Cable half-kneeling high row with 1-second isometric	3 × 10 at RPE 8 3 × 8 per side at RPE 8	Complete C block (C1 and C2) with no rest between exercises, then rest for 45-60 sec. That equals 1 set. Complete all sets in this way, then move on to D block.		124 125
Accessory block • D1: Cable double-arm single-leg RDL with knee drive and row • D2: Band standing triceps extension	3 × 6 per side at RPE 7-8 3 × 15 at RPE 7-8	Complete D block (D1 and D2) with no rest between exercises, then rest for 45-60 sec. That equals 1 set. Complete all sets in this way, then move on to recovery.		190 127
Recovery				
Exercise	Reps/time	Notes		Page #
Hamstring floss	12 per side			N/A
Book opener isometric	20 sec per side			N/A
Rear foot elevated half-kneeling hip flexor stretch	20 sec per side			N/A

Table 12.2 Strength Training Program: Phase 2 (Weeks 5-8)

DAY 1: MONDAY			
Warm-up			
Exercise	Reps/time/distance	Notes	Page #
Cat-cow	8		64
Single-leg bridge isometric with bent-knee leg whip	5 per side		65
Catcher rockback	5 per side		66
Elevated bent-knee Copenhagen plank	15 sec per side		67
Alternating Spiderman to yoga pike	3		68
Heels-up split squat isometric	15 sec per side		69
MB hug Kang squat	5		70
Extensive single-leg pogo hop	10 per side		71
Drop reverse lunge to stick	3 per side		72
Lateral skip	20 yd per side		73
Workout			
Exercise	Sets × reps at RPE	Notes	Page #
Strength and power block • A1: DB step-up • A2: Band-resisted acceleration power step	3 × 6 per side at RPE 7-8 3 × 3 per side at RPE 6-7	Complete A block (A1 and A2) with no rest between exercises, then rest for 45-60 sec. That equals 1 set. Complete all sets in this way, then move on to B block.	128 204
Strength and power block • B1: DB heels-up three-point row with 3-second eccentric • B2: Barbell explosive inverted row with hip thrust isometric	3 × 8 per side at RPE 7-8 3 × 5 at RPE 6-7	Complete B block (B1 and B2) with no rest between exercises, then rest for 45-60 sec. That equals 1 set. Complete all sets in this way, then move on to C block.	129 205
Hypertrophy block • C1: DB cyclist squat (2 DB) • C2: Cable seated lat pull-down with 3-second eccentric	3 × 10 at RPE 8 3 × 12 at RPE 7	Complete C block (C1 and C2) with no rest between exercises, then rest for 45-60 sec. That equals 1 set. Complete all sets in this way, then move on to D block.	130 131
Accessory block • D1: KB front rack carry • D2: Cable tall-kneeling rope triceps extension	3 × 40 yd at RPE 7-8 3 × 12 at RPE 7-8	Complete D block (D1 and D2) with no rest between exercises, then rest for 45-60 sec. That equals 1 set. Complete all sets in this way, then move on to recovery.	132 133
Recovery			
Exercise	Reps/time	Notes	Page #
Band single-leg lower	8 per side		N/A
Band Brettzel stretch	20 sec per side		N/A
Rear foot elevated half-kneeling hip flexor stretch with single-arm overhead reach	20 sec per side		N/A

(continued)

Table 12.2 Strength Training Program: Phase 2 (Weeks 5-8) *(continued)*

DAY 2: TUESDAY			
Warm-up			
Exercise	Reps/time/distance	Notes	Page #
Single-leg long bridge isometric with knee drive isometric	15 sec per side		74
Cross-connect dead bug (opposite side)	8 sec per side		75
Mini-band stork	15 sec per side		76
Wall bent-knee single-leg heel raise isometric	15 sec per side		77
Alternating yoga plex to yoga pike	3 per side		78
Walking inchworm	3		79
Hinge to squat with alternating rotation	3		80
Wall linear double exchange	5 per side		81
Walking alternating hamstring scoop	2 × 10 yd		82
Walking alternating Spiderman to reach and rotate	2 × 10 yd		83
Double lateral shuffle with alternating lateral squat	2 × 10 yd per side		84
Backward reach run	2 × 10 yd		85
Workout			
Exercise	Reps at RPE	Notes	Page #
A. 10-yard sprint and rehearsed Y-turn	3 per side at RPE 8-9	Complete 1 rep, then rest for 30-45 sec. That equals 1 set. Complete all sets in this way, then move on to the next exercise.	223
B. 10-yard sprint from lateral half-kneeling start	3 per side at RPE 8-9	Complete 1 rep per side, then rest for 30-45 sec. That equals 1 set. Complete all sets in this way, then move on to the next exercise.	224
C. 20-yard dash	4 @ 100% effort	Rest 60-75 sec between reps.	225
Recovery			
Exercise	Reps/time	Notes	Page #
Band single-leg lower	8 per side		N/A
Band Brettzel stretch	20 sec per side		N/A
Rear foot elevated half-kneeling hip flexor stretch with single-arm overhead reach	20 sec per side		N/A

DAY 3: WEDNESDAY				
Warm-up				
Exercise	**Reps/time/distance**	**Notes**		**Page #**
Cat-cow	8			64
Single-leg bridge isometric with bent-knee leg whip	5 per side			65
Catcher rockback	5 per side			66
Elevated bent-knee Copenhagen plank	15 sec per side			67
Alternating Spiderman to yoga pike	3			68
Heels-up split squat isometric	15 sec per side			69
MB hug Kang squat	5			70
Extensive single-leg pogo hop	10 per side			71
Drop reverse lunge to stick	3 per side			72
Lateral skip	20 yd per side			73
Workout				
Exercise	**Sets × reps at RPE**	**Notes**		**Page #**
Strength and power block • A1: Weighted neutral-grip pull-up • A2: MB standing double clutch slam	3 × 6-10 (AMGRAP) 3 × 5 at RPE 6-7	Complete A block (A1 and A2) with no rest between exercises, then rest for 45-60 sec. That equals 1 set. Complete all sets in this way, then move on to B block.		191 206
Strength and power block • B1: Landmine goblet lateral squat • B2: Band-resisted skater hop with stick (lateral orientation)	3 × 6 per side at RPE 7-8 3 × 5 per side at RPE 6-7	Complete B block (B1 and B2) with no rest between exercises, then rest for 45-60 sec. That equals 1 set. Complete all sets in this way, then move on to C block.		135 208
Hypertrophy block • C1: DB captain stance single-arm shoulder press • C2: Cable plank single-arm row to triceps extension	3 × 8 per side at RPE 8 3 × 8 per side at RPE 8	Complete C block (C1 and C2) with no rest between exercises, then rest for 45-60 sec. That equals 1 set. Complete all sets in this way, then move on to D block.		136 137
Accessory block • D1: KB suitcase carry • D2: DB incline bench trap raise (Y) with 3-second eccentric	3 × 40 yd per side at RPE 7-8 3 × 12 at RPE 7-8	Complete D block (D1 and D2) with no rest between exercises, then rest for 45-60 sec. That equals 1 set. Complete all sets in this way, then move on to recovery.		138 139
Recovery				
Exercise	**Reps/time**	**Notes**		**Page #**
Band single-leg lower	8 per side			N/A
Band Brettzel stretch	20 sec per side			N/A
Rear foot elevated half-kneeling hip flexor stretch with single-arm overhead reach	20 sec per side			N/A

(continued)

Table 12.2 Strength Training Program: Phase 2 (Weeks 5-8) *(continued)*

DAY 4: THURSDAY			
Warm-up			
Exercise	Reps/time/distance	Notes	Page #
Single-leg long bridge isometric with knee drive isometric	15 sec per side		74
Cross-connect dead bug (opposite side)	8 sec per side		75
Mini-band stork	15 sec per side		76
Wall bent-knee single-leg heel raise isometric	15 sec per side		77
Alternating yoga plex to yoga pike	3 per side		78
Walking inchworm	3		79
Hinge to squat with alternating rotation	3		80
Wall linear double exchange	5 per side		81
Walking alternating hamstring scoop	2 × 10 yd		82
Walking alternating Spiderman to reach and rotate	2 × 10 yd		83
Double lateral shuffle with alternating lateral squat	2 × 10 yd per side		84
Backward reach run	2 × 10 yd		85
Workout			
Exercise	Sets × reps at RPE	Notes	Page #
Objective: Aerobic conditioning intervals Pick one: erg rower, air bike, ski erg, or treadmill	Total duration: 15-20 minutes Interval protocol: 15 sec of hard work (RPE 8-9; 80-90% of max HR) followed by 45 sec of easy work (RPE 5; 50% of max HR)		233
Recovery			
Exercise	Reps/time	Notes	Page #
Band single-leg lower	8 per side		N/A
Band Brettzel stretch	20 sec per side		N/A
Rear foot elevated half-kneeling hip flexor stretch with single-arm overhead reach	20 sec per side		N/A

DAY 5: FRIDAY			
Warm-up			
Exercise	Reps/time/distance	Notes	Page #
Cat-cow	8		64
Single-leg bridge isometric with bent-knee leg whip	5 per side		65
Catcher rockback	5 per side		66
Elevated bent-knee Copenhagen plank	15 sec per side		67
Alternating Spiderman to yoga pike	3		68
Heels-up split squat isometric	15 sec per side		69
MB hug Kang squat	5		70
Extensive single-leg pogo hop	10 per side		71
Drop reverse lunge to stick	3 per side		72
Lateral skip	20 yd per side		73
Workout			
Exercise	Sets × reps at RPE	Notes	Page #
Strength and power block • A1: DB hand-supported ipsilateral single-leg RDL • A2: Single-leg broad jump to double-leg stick	3 × 6 per side at RPE 7-8 3 × 3 per side at RPE 6-7	Complete A block (A1 and A2) with no rest between exercises, then rest for 45-60 sec. That equals 1 set. Complete all sets in this way, then move on to B block.	192 209
Strength and power block • B1: DB single-arm bench press with single-leg hip thrust isometric • B2: MB step-through wall chest pass (staggered-stance start)	3 × 8 per side at RPE 7-8 3 × 3 per side at RPE 6-7	Complete B block (B1 and B2) with no rest between exercises, then rest for 45-60 sec. That equals 1 set. Complete all sets in this way, then move on to C block.	141 211
Hypertrophy block • C1: Cable pull-through • C2: DB seal row	3 × 12 at RPE 8 3 × 10 at RPE 8	Complete C block (C1 and C2) with no rest between exercises, then rest for 45-60 sec. That equals 1 set. Complete all sets in this way, then move on to D block.	142 143
Accessory block • D1: Band wide-stance vertical Pallof press • D2: Cable tall-kneeling straight bar biceps curl	3 × 8 per side at RPE 7-8 3 × 12 at RPE 7-8	Complete D block (D1 and D2) with no rest between exercises, then rest for 45-60 sec. That equals 1 set. Complete all sets in this way, then move on to recovery.	144 145
Recovery			
Exercise	Reps/time	Notes	Page #
Band single-leg lower	8 per side		N/A
Band Brettzel stretch	20 sec per side		N/A
Rear foot elevated half-kneeling hip flexor stretch with single-arm overhead reach	20 sec per side		N/A

Table 12.3 The Strength Training Program: Phase 3 (Weeks 9-12)

DAY 1: MONDAY				
Warm-up				
Exercise	Reps/time/distance	Notes		Page #
Segmental cat-cow	5			86
Bridge isometric with alternating reach	5 per side			87
Catcher rockback with toe turn	6 per side			88
Floor bent-knee Copenhagen plank with liftoff	5 per side			89
Alternating Spiderman to stationary inchworm	3 per side			90
Rear foot elevated split squat isometric	15 sec per side			91
KB goblet Kang squat	5			92
Intensive pogo hop	10			93
Drop skater squat to stick	5 per side			94
Lateral crossover skip	20 yd per side			95
Workout				
Exercise	Sets × reps at RPE	Notes		Page #
Strength and power block • A1: Landmine single-leg RDL (lateral orientation) • A2: Continuous broad jump	3 × 6 per side at RPE 8 3 × 4 at RPE 7	Complete A block (A1 and A2) with no rest between exercises, then rest for 45-60 sec. That equals 1 set. Complete all sets in this way, then move on to B block.		146 212
Strength and power block • B1: DB alternating bench press (bottom) • B2: MB step-back rotational single-arm wall chest pass	3 × 8 per side at RPE 8 3 × 4 per side at RPE 7	Complete B block (B1 and B2) with no rest between exercises, then rest for 45-60 sec. That equals 1 set. Complete all sets in this way, then move on to C block.		193 214
Strength block • C1: DB neutral grip kickstand RDL • C2: Cable split-stance single-arm mid row with opposite hand reach	3 × 8 per side at RPE 7-8 3 × 8 per side at RPE 7-8	Complete C block (C1 and C2) with no rest between exercises, then rest for 45-60 sec. That equals 1 set. Complete all sets in this way, then move on to D block.		148 149
Accessory block • D1: DB bent-over lateral raise • D2: Band-resisted tall-kneeling ab wheel rollout	3 × 12 at RPE 7-8 3 × 10 at RPE 7-8	Complete D block (D1 and D2) with no rest between exercises, then rest for 45-60 sec. That equals 1 set. Complete all sets in this way, then move on to recovery.		150 194
Recovery				
Exercise	Reps/time	Notes		Page #
Three-way hamstring floss	5 each direction per side			N/A
Brettzel stretch with breathing	8 breaths per side			N/A
Rear foot elevated half-kneeling hip flexor stretch with single-arm overhead reach and rotation	20 sec per side			N/A

DAY 2: TUESDAY			
Warm-up			
Exercise	**Reps/time/distance**	**Notes**	**Page #**
Single-leg long bridge isometric with power switch	3 per side		96
Wall press with single-leg lower	8 per side		97
Mini-band stork with clam lift	8 per side		98
Tempo wall heel raise (3 seconds up/3 seconds iso/3 seconds down)	6		99
Hand-supported alternating reverse lunge with single-arm overhead reach	3 per side		100
Walking inchworm to push-up	3		101
Hinge to squat isometric with alternating rotation	3 per side		102
Wall press single-leg RDL with power drive	3 per side		103
Reverse walking single-leg RDL	2 × 10 yd		104
Walking alternating Spiderman to yoga push-up	2 × 10 yd		105
5-yard lateral shuffle to turn and 10-yard sprint	2 × 15 yd per side		106
5-yard backpedal to turn and 10-yard sprint	2 × 15 yd per side		107
Workout			
Exercise	**Sets × reps at RPE**	**Notes**	**Page #**
A. 10-yard sprint and rehearsed T-turn	3 per side at RPE 8-9	Complete 1 rep, then rest for 30-45 sec. That equals 1 set. Complete all sets in this way, then move on to the next exercise.	226
B: 5-10-5 pro agility shuttle	3 per side at RPE 8-9	Complete 1 rep per side, then rest for 30-45 sec. That equals 1 set. Complete all sets in this way, then move on to the next exercise.	227
C: 20-yard curvilinear sprint	3 per side at 100% effort (60-75 sec rest between reps)	Rest 60-75 sec between reps.	228
Recovery			
Exercise	**Reps/time**	**Notes**	**Page #**
Three-way hamstring floss	5 each direction per side		N/A
Brettzel stretch with breathing	8 breaths per side		N/A
Rear foot elevated half-kneeling hip flexor stretch with single-arm overhead reach and rotation	20 sec per side		N/A

(continued)

Table 12.3 The Strength Training Program: Phase 3 (Weeks 9-12) *(continued)*

DAY 3: WEDNESDAY				
Warm-up				
Exercise	**Reps/time/distance**	**Notes**		**Page #**
Segmental cat-cow	5			86
Bridge isometric with alternating reach	5 per side			87
Catcher rockback with toe turn	6 per side			88
Floor bent-knee Copenhagen plank with liftoff	5 per side			89
Alternating Spiderman to stationary inchworm	3 per side			90
Rear foot elevated split squat isometric	15 sec per side			91
KB goblet Kang squat	5			92
Intensive pogo hop	10			93
Drop skater squat to stick	5 per side			94
Lateral crossover skip	20 yd per side			95
Workout				
Exercise	**Sets × reps at RPE**	**Notes**		**Page #**
Strength and power block • A1: Barbell bench press • A2: Band standing continuous power punch	3 × 6 at RPE 8 3 × 5 at RPE 7	Complete A block (A1 and A2) with no rest between exercises, then rest for 45-60 sec. That equals 1 set. Complete all sets in this way, then move on to B block.		152 215
Strength and power block • B1: DB single-arm offset band slider lateral lunge • B2: Plate skater hop with quick, stick, and punch	3 × 8 per side at RPE 8 3 × 3 per side at RPE 7	Complete B block (B1 and B2) with no rest between exercises, then rest for 45-60 sec. That equals 1 set. Complete all sets in this way, then move on to C block.		153 216
Strength block • C1: Landmine standing Viking shoulder press • C2: Band wide-stance crossbody long chop	3 × 8 at RPE 7-8 3 × 8 per side at RPE 7-8	Complete C block (C1 and C2) with no rest between exercises, then rest for 45-60 sec. That equals 1 set. Complete all sets in this way, then move on to D block.		154 155
Accessory block • D1: KB towel standing hammer curl • D2: Bent-knee star plank with clamshell	3 × 12 at RPE 7-3 3 × 10 per side at RPE 7-8	Complete D block (D1 and D2) with no rest between exercises, then rest for 45-60 sec. That equals 1 set. Complete all sets in this way, then move on to recovery.		156 157
Recovery				
Exercise	**Reps/time**	**Notes**		**Page #**
Three-way hamstring floss	5 each direction per side			N/A
Brettzel strength with breathing	8 breaths per side			N/A
Rear foot elevated half-kneeling hip flexor stretch with single-arm overhead reach and rotation	20 sec per side			N/A

DAY 4: THURSDAY

Warm-up

Exercise	Reps/time/distance	Notes	Page #
Single-leg long bridge isometric with power switch	3 per side		96
Wall press with single-leg lower	8 per side		97
Mini-band stork with clam lift	8 per side		98
Tempo wall heel raise (3 seconds up/3 seconds iso/3 seconds down)	6		99
Hand-supported alternating reverse lunge with single-arm overhead reach	3 per side		100
Walking inchworm to push-up	3		101
Hinge to squat isometric with alternating rotation	3 per side		102
Wall press single-leg RDL with power drive	3 per side		103
Reverse walking single-leg RDL	2 × 10 yd		104
Walking alternating Spiderman to yoga push-up	2 × 10 yd		105
5-yard lateral shuffle to turn and 10-yard sprint	2 × 15 yd per side		106
5-yard backpedal to turn and 10-yard sprint	2 × 15 yd per side		107

Workout

Exercise	Sets × reps at RPE	Notes	Page #
Objective: High-intensity sprint intervals Pick one: Incline treadmill (20%-30% incline), outdoor hill (20%-30% incline), or empty sled (no weight added)	Total duration: 8-12 sets Interval protocol: 6-8 sec of all-out sprint (RPE 10; 100% of max HR) followed by 45-60 sec of complete rest (goal is to bring HR back down during this time)		234

Recovery

Exercise	Reps/time	Notes	Page #
Three-way hamstring floss	5 each direction per side		N/A
Brettzel stretch with breathing	8 breaths per side		N/A
Rear foot elevated half-kneeling hip flexor stretch with single-arm overhead reach and rotation	20 sec per side		N/A

(continued)

Table 12.3 The Strength Training Program: Phase 3 (Weeks 9-12) *(continued)*

DAY 5: FRIDAY				
Warm-up				
Exercise	Reps/time/distance	Notes		Page #
Segmental cat-cow	5			86
Bridge isometric with alternating reach	5 per side			87
Catcher rockback with toe turn	6 per side			88
Floor bent-knee Copenhagen plank with liftoff	5 per side			89
Alternating Spiderman to stationary inchworm	3 per side			90
Rear foot elevated split squat isometric	15 sec per side			91
KB goblet Kang squat	5			92
Intensive pogo hop	10			93
Drop skater squat to stick	5 per side			94
Lateral crossover skip	20 yd per side			95
Workout				
Exercise	Sets × reps at RPE	Notes		Page #
Strength and power block • A1: DB rear foot elevated split squat • A2: DB reactive split squat jump	3 × 6 per side at RPE 8 3 × 5 per side at RPE 7	Complete A block (A1 and A2) with no rest between exercises, then rest for 45-60 sec. That equals 1 set. Complete all sets in this way, then move on to B block.		158 217
Strength and power block • B1: DB single-arm row • B2: Cable split-stance single-arm low row with box stomp	3 × 8 per side at RPE 8 3 × 4 per side at RPE 7	Complete B block (B1 and B2) with no rest between exercises, then rest for 45-60 sec. That equals 1 set. Complete all sets in this way, then move on to C block.		159 218
Strength block • C1: KB goblet kickstand squat (2 DB) • C2: Cable half-kneeling single-arm high row	3 × 6 per side at RPE 8 3 × 8 per side at RPE 7-8	Complete C block (C1 and C2) with no rest between exercises, then rest for 45-60 sec. That equals 1 set. Complete all sets in this way, then move on to D block.		186 161
Accessory block • D1: DB floor skull crusher • D2: DB floor prone Superman isometric	3 × 12 at RPE 7-8 3 × 15 sec at RPE 7-8	Complete D block (D1 and D2) with no rest between exercises, then rest for 45-60 sec. That equals 1 set. Complete all sets in this way, then move on to recovery.		162 163
Recovery				
Exercise	Reps/time	Notes		Page #
Three-way hamstring floss	5 each direction per side			N/A
Brettzel stretch with breathing	8 breaths per side			N/A
Rear foot elevated half-kneeling hip flexor stretch with single-arm overhead reach and rotation	20 sec per side			N/A

CHAPTER 13

The Power Training Program

This 12-week training program has three consecutive phases (four-week training blocks) that build off each other. In all three phases, the primary emphasis is on power development. The goal is to help you increase your overall power and explosive capabilities in order to show those qualities off in competition!

The power training program complements the initial flagship program, Train Like a Pro. If your goal is to tap into your inner athlete while becoming the most powerful and explosive version of yourself, this is the program for you. This training program is the perfect fit for directly before the season begins—it will help you peak right in time!

Table 13.1 Power Training Program: Phase 1 (Weeks 1-4)

DAY 1: MONDAY			
Warm-up			
Exercise	Reps/time/distance	Notes	Page #
Band cat-cow	8		42
Heels-up single-leg bridge isometric with knee drive isometric	15 sec per side		43
Catcher rockback isometric with reach and rotate	5 per side		44
Floor bent-knee Copenhagen plank	15 sec per side		45
Alternating Spiderman	3 per side		46
Split squat isometric	15 sec per side		47
Squat rack Kang squat	5		48
Extensive pogo hop	15		49
Drop squat to stick	8		50
Linear skip	20 yd		51
Workout			
Exercise	Sets × reps at RPE	Notes	Page #
Power block • A1: Band-assisted continuous squat jump • A2: MB tall-kneeling slam with hip hinge	3 × 6 at RPE 6-7 3 × 4 at RPE 7-8	Complete A block (A1 and A2) with no rest between exercises, then rest for 45-60 sec. That equals 1 set. Complete all sets in this way, then move on to B block.	198 199
Strength block • B1: KB goblet squat with 3-second isometric • B2: Band tall-kneeling Pallof press isometric	3 × 8 at RPE 8 3 × 20 sec per side at RPE 7-8	Complete B block (B1 and B2) with no rest between exercises, then rest for 45-60 sec. That equals 1 set. Complete all sets in this way, then move on to C block.	110 111
Hypertrophy block • C1: DB RDL • C2: KB half-kneeling shoulder press with 3-second isometric	3 × 10, 12, 15 at RPE 8, 7, 7 3 × 8 per side at RPE 8	Complete C block (C1 and C2) with no rest between exercises, then rest for 45-60 sec. That equals 1 set. Complete all sets in this way, then move on to D block.	112 113
Accessory block • D1: Suspension skater squat with 3-second isometric • D2: DB standing hammer curl	3 × 8 per side at RPE 7-8 3 × 15 at RPE 7-8	Complete D block (D1 and D2) with no rest between exercises, then rest for 45-60 sec. That equals 1 set. Complete all sets in this way, then move on to recovery.	114 115
Recovery			
Exercise	Reps/time	Notes	Page #
Hamstring floss	12 per side		N/A
Book opener isometric	20 sec per side		N/A
Rear foot elevated half-kneeling hip flexor stretch	20 sec per side		N/A

DAY 2: TUESDAY

Warm-up

Exercise	Reps/time/distance	Notes	Page #
Long bridge isometric	15 sec		52
Wall press with alternating dead bug	8 per side		53
Wall stork	15 sec per side		54
Wall single-leg heel raise isometric	15 sec per side		55
Alternating yoga plex	3 per side		56
Stationary inchworm	3		57
Hinge to squat	5		58
Wall linear single exchange	5 per side		59
Stationary hamstring scoop	5 per side		60
Walking alternating Spiderman	2 × 10 yd		61
Lateral shuffle with arm swing	2 × 10 yd per side		62
Backpedal	2 × 10 yd		63

Workout

Exercise	Sets × reps at RPE	Notes	Page #
A. 10-yard sprint and rehearsed stop	3 per side at RPE 8-9	Complete 1 rep, then rest for 30-45 sec. That equals 1 set. Complete all sets in this way, then move on to the next exercise.	220
B. Multidirectional plyo step from half-kneeling start to 5-yard sprint	2 each direction (4 directions total) at RPE 8-9	Complete 1 rep per side, then rest for 30-45 sec. That equals 1 set. Complete all sets in this way, then move on to the next exercise.	221
C. 100-yard tempo run	6 @ 80% effort	Rest 60-75 sec between reps.	222

Recovery

Exercise	Reps/time	Notes	Page #
Hamstring floss	12 per side		N/A
Book opener isometric	20 sec per side		N/A
Rear foot elevated half-kneeling hip flexor stretch	20 sec per side		N/A

(continued)

Table 13.1 Power Training Program: Phase 1 (Weeks 1-4) *(continued)*

DAY 3: WEDNESDAY			
Warm-up			
Exercise	Reps/time/distance	Notes	Page #
Band cat-cow	8		42
Heels-up single-leg bridge isometric with knee drive isometric	15 sec per side		43
Catcher rockback isometric with reach and rotate	5 per side		44
Floor bent-knee Copenhagen plank	15 sec per side		45
Alternating Spiderman	3 per side		46
Split squat isometric	15 sec per side		47
Squat rack Kang squat	5		48
Extensive pogo hop	15		49
Drop squat to stick	8		50
Linear skip	20 yd		51
Workout			
Exercise	Sets × reps at RPE	Notes	Page #
Power block • A1: MB skater hop with chop and stick • A2: MB half-kneeling lateral wall toss	3 × 6 per side at RPE 6-7 3 × 6 per side at RPE 6-7	Complete A block (A1 and A2) with no rest between exercises, then rest for 45-60 sec. That equals 1 set. Complete all sets in this way, then move on to B block.	200 201
Strength block • B1: DB bench press with 3-second isometric (top) • B2: Bent-knee star plank with top leg long	3 × 8 at RPE 8 3 × 15 sec per side at RPE 7-8	Complete B block (B1 and B2) with no rest between exercises, then rest for 45-60 sec. That equals 1 set. Complete all sets in this way, then move on to C block.	116 117
Hypertrophy block • C1: DB chest-supported row • C2: KB single-arm offset lateral squat with 1-second isometric	3 × 10, 12, 15 at RPE 8, 7, 7 3 × 8 per side at RPE 8	Complete C block (C1 and C2) with no rest between exercises, then rest for 45-60 sec. That equals 1 set. Complete all sets in this way, then move on to D block.	118 119
Accessory block • D1: KB goblet carry • D2: Band tall-kneeling pull-apart	3 × 40 yd at RPE 7-8 3 × 15 at RPE 7-8	Complete D block (D1 and D2) with no rest between exercises, then rest for 45-60 sec. That equals 1 set. Complete all sets in this way, then move on to recovery.	120 121
Recovery			
Exercise	Reps/time	Notes	Page #
Hamstring floss	12 per side		N/A
Book opener isometric	20 sec per side		N/A
Rear foot elevated half-kneeling hip flexor stretch	20 sec per side		N/A

DAY 4: THURSDAY

Warm-up

Exercise	Reps/time/distance	Notes	Page #
Long bridge isometric	15 sec		52
Wall press with alternating dead bug	8 per side		53
Wall stork	15 sec per side		54
Wall single-leg heel raise isometric	15 sec per side		55
Alternating yoga plex	3 per side		56
Stationary inchworm	3		57
Hinge to squat	5		58
Wall linear single exchange	5 per side		59
Stationary hamstring scoop	5 per side		60
Walking alternating Spiderman	2 × 10 yd		61
Lateral shuffle with arm swing	2 × 10 yd per side		62
Backpedal	2 × 10 yd		63

Workout

Exercise	Sets × reps at RPE	Notes	Page #
Objective: Steady-state aerobic conditioning Pick one: erg rower, air bike, ski erg, or treadmill	Total duration: 30-40 minutes Target heart rate: 130-150 bpm Target RPE: 6-7 (60-70% of max HR)		232

Recovery

Exercise	Reps/time	Notes	Page #
Hamstring floss	12 per side		N/A
Book opener isometric	20 sec per side		N/A
Rear foot elevated half-kneeling hip flexor stretch	20 sec per side		N/A

(continued)

Table 13.1 Power Training Program: Phase 1 (Weeks 1-4) *(continued)*

DAY 5: FRIDAY			
Warm-up			
Exercise	Reps/time/distance	Notes	Page #
Band cat-cow	8		42
Heels-up single-leg bridge isometric with knee drive isometric	15 sec per side		43
Catcher rockback isometric with reach and rotate	5 per side		44
Floor bent-knee Copenhagen plank	15 sec per side		45
Alternating Spiderman	3 per side		46
Split squat isometric	15 sec per side		47
Squat rack Kang squat	5		48
Extensive pogo hop	15		49
Drop squat to stick	8		50
Linear skip	20 yd		51
Workout			
Exercise	Sets × reps at RPE	Notes	Page #
Power block • A1: 90-degree rotational single-leg hop with stick • A2: MB half-kneeling around-the-world slam	3 × 5 per side at RPE 6-7 3 × 6 per side at RPE 6-7	Complete A block (A1 and A2) with no rest between exercises, then rest for 45-60 sec. That equals 1 set. Complete all sets in this way, then move on to B block.	202 203
Strength block • B1: Trap bar deadlift • B2: PB push–pull	3 × 6 at RPE 8 3 × 12 at RPE 7-8	Complete B block (B1 and B2) with no rest between exercises, then rest for 45-60 sec. That equals 1 set. Complete all sets in this way, then move on to C block.	122 123
Hypertrophy block • C1: Two DB foam roller hack squat against a wall • C2: Cable half-kneeling high row with 1-second isometric	3 × 10, 12, 15 at RPE 8, 7, 7 3 × 8 per side at RPE 8	Complete C block (C1 and C2) with no rest between exercises, then rest for 45-60 sec. That equals 1 set. Complete all sets in this way, then move on to D block.	124 125
Accessory block • D1: Cable double-arm single-leg RDL with knee drive and row • D2: Band standing triceps extension	3 × 8 per side at RPE 7-8 3 × 15 at RPE 7-8	Complete D block (D1 and D2) with no rest between exercises, then rest for 45-60 sec. That equals 1 set. Complete all sets in this way, then move on to recovery.	190 127
Recovery			
Exercise	Reps/time	Notes	Page #
Hamstring floss	12 per side		N/A
Book opener isometric	20 sec per side		N/A
Rear foot elevated half-kneeling hip flexor stretch	20 sec per side		N/A

Table 13.2 Power Training Program: Phase 2 (Weeks 5-8)

DAY 1: MONDAY			
Warm-up			
Exercise	**Reps/time/distance**	**Notes**	**Page #**
Cat-cow	8		64
Single-leg bridge isometric with bent-knee leg whip	5 per side		65
Catcher rockback	5 per side		66
Elevated bent-knee Copenhagen plank	15 sec per side		67
Alternating Spiderman to yoga pike	3		68
Heels-up split squat isometric	15 sec per side		69
MB hug Kang squat	5		70
Extensive single-leg pogo hop	10 per side		71
Drop reverse lunge to stick	3 per side		72
Lateral skip	20 yd per side		73
Workout			
Exercise	**Sets × reps at RPE**	**Notes**	**Page #**
Strength and power block • A1: Barbell power step-up • A2: Band-resisted acceleration power step	3 × 5 per side at RPE 8 3 × 3 per side at RPE 6-7	Complete A block (A1 and A2) with no rest between exercises, then rest for 45-60 sec. That equals 1 set. Complete all sets in this way, then move on to B block.	195 204
Strength and power block • B1: DB heels-up three-point row with 3-second eccentric • B2: Barbell explosive inverted row with hip thrust isometric	3 × 8 per side at RPE 7-8 3 × 5 at RPE 6-7	Complete B block (B1 and B2) with no rest between exercises, then rest for 45-60 sec. That equals 1 set. Complete all sets in this way, then move on to C block.	129 205
Hypertrophy block • C1: DB cyclist squat (2 DB) • C2: Cable seated lat pull-down with 3-second eccentric	3 × 8, 10, 12 at RPE 8, 7, 7 3 × 8, 10, 12 at RPE 8, 7, 7	Complete C block (C1 and C2) with no rest between exercises, then rest for 45-60 sec. That equals 1 set. Complete all sets in this way, then move on to D block.	130 131
Accessory block • D1: KB front rack carry • D2: Cable tall-kneeling rope triceps extension	3 × 40 yd at RPE 7-8 3 × 12 at RPE 7-8	Complete D block (D1 and D2) with no rest between exercises, then rest for 45-60 sec. That equals 1 set. Complete all sets in this way, then move on to recovery.	132 133
Recovery			
Exercise	**Reps/time**	**Notes**	**Page #**
Band single-leg lower	8 per side		N/A
Band Brettzel stretch	20 sec per side		N/A
Rear foot elevated half-kneeling hip flexor stretch with single-arm overhead reach	20 sec per side		N/A

(continued)

Table 13.2 Power Training Program: Phase 2 (Weeks 5-8) *(continued)*

DAY 2: TUESDAY			
Warm-up			
Exercise	Reps/time/distance	Notes	Page #
Single-leg long bridge isometric with knee drive isometric	15 sec per side		74
Cross-connect dead bug (opposite side)	8 sec per side		75
Mini-band stork	15 sec per side		76
Wall bent-knee single-leg heel raise isometric	15 sec per side		77
Alternating yoga plex to yoga pike	3 per side		78
Walking inchworm	3		79
Hinge to squat with alternating rotation	3		80
Wall linear double exchange	5 per side		81
Walking alternating hamstring scoop	2 × 10 yd		82
Walking alternating Spiderman to reach and rotate	2 × 10 yd		83
Double lateral shuffle with alternating lateral squat	2 × 10 yd per side		84
Backward reach run	2 × 10 yd		85
Workout			
Exercise	Sets × reps at RPE	Notes	Page #
A: 10-yard sprint and rehearsed Y-turn	3 per side at RPE 8-9	Complete 1 rep, then rest for 30-45 sec. That equals 1 set. Complete all sets in this way, then move on to the next exercise.	223
B: 10-yard sprint from lateral half-kneeling start	3 per side at RPE 8-9	Complete 1 rep per side, then rest for 30-45 sec. That equals 1 set. Complete all sets in this way, then move on to the next exercise.	224
C: 20-yard dash	4 @ 100% effort	Rest 60-75 sec between reps.	225
Recovery			
Exercise	Reps/time	Notes	Page #
Band single-leg lower	8 per side		N/A
Band Brettzel stretch	20 sec per side		N/A
Rear foot elevated half-kneeling hip flexor stretch with single-arm overhead reach	20 sec per side		N/A

DAY 3: WEDNESDAY

Warm-up

Exercise	Reps/time/distance	Notes	Page #
Cat-cow	8		64
Single-leg bridge isometric with bent-knee leg whip	5 per side		65
Catcher rockback	5 per side		66
Elevated bent-knee Copenhagen plank	15 sec per side		67
Alternating Spiderman to yoga pike	3		68
Heels-up split squat isometric	15 sec per side		69
MB hug Kang squat	5		70
Extensive single-leg pogo hop	10 per side		71
Drop reverse lunge to stick	3 per side		72
Lateral skip	20 yd per side		73

Workout

Exercise	Sets × reps at RPE	Notes	Page #
Strength and power block • A1: Weighted eccentric-only neutral grip pull-up with 5-second eccentric • A2: MB standing double clutch slam	3 × 5 at RPE 7-8 3 × 4 at RPE 7-8	Complete A block (A1 and A2) with no rest between exercises, then rest for 45-60 sec. That equals 1 set. Complete all sets in this way, then move on to B block.	134 206
Strength and power block • B1: Landmine goblet lateral squat • B2: Band-resisted skater hop with stick (lateral orientation)	3 × 6 per side at RPE 7-8 3 × 4 per side at RPE 7-8	Complete B block (B1 and B2) with no rest between exercises, then rest for 45-60 sec. That equals 1 set. Complete all sets in this way, then move on to C block.	135 208
Hypertrophy block • C1: DB captain stance single-arm shoulder press • C2: Cable plank single-arm row to triceps extension	3 × 8, 10, 12 per side at RPE 8, 7, 7 3 × 8 per side at RPE 8	Complete C block (C1 and C2) with no rest between exercises, then rest for 45-60 sec. That equals 1 set. Complete all sets in this way, then move on to D block.	136 137
Accessory block • D1: KB suitcase carry • D2: DB incline bench trap raise (Y) with 3-second eccentric	3 × 40 yd per side at RPE 7-8 3 × 12 at RPE 7-8	Complete D block (D1 and D2) with no rest between exercises, then rest for 45-60 sec. That equals 1 set. Complete all sets in this way, then move on to recovery.	138 139

Recovery

Exercise	Reps/time	Notes	Page #
Band single-leg lower	8 per side		N/A
Band Brettzel stretch	20 sec per side		N/A
Rear foot elevated half-kneeling hip flexor stretch with single-arm overhead reach	20 sec per side		N/A

(continued)

Table 13.2 Power Training Program: Phase 2 (Weeks 5-8) *(continued)*

DAY 4: THURSDAY			
Warm-up			
Exercise	Reps/time/distance	Notes	Page #
Single-leg long bridge isometric with knee drive isometric	15 sec per side		74
Cross-connect dead bug (opposite side)	8 sec per side		75
Mini-band stork	15 sec per side		76
Wall bent-knee single-leg heel raise isometric	15 sec per side		77
Alternating yoga plex to yoga pike	3 per side		78
Walking inchworm	3		79
Hinge to squat with alternating rotation	3		80
Wall linear double exchange	5 per side		81
Walking alternating hamstring scoop	2 × 10 yd		82
Walking alternating Spiderman to reach and rotate	2 × 10 yd		83
Double lateral shuffle with alternating lateral squat	2 × 10 yd per side		84
Backward reach run	2 × 10 yd		85
Workout			
Exercise	Sets × reps at RPE	Notes	Page #
Objective: Aerobic conditioning intervals. Pick one: erg rower, air bike, ski erg, or treadmill	Total duration: 15-20 minutes. Interval protocol: 15 sec of hard work (RPE 8-9; 80-90% of max HR) followed by 45 sec of easy work (RPE 5; 50% of max HR)		233
Recovery			
Exercise	Reps/time	Notes	Page #
Band single-leg lower	8 per side		N/A
Band Brettzel stretch	20 sec per side		N/A
Rear foot elevated half-kneeling hip flexor stretch with single-arm overhead reach	20 sec per side		N/A

DAY 5: FRIDAY			
Warm-up			
Exercise	Reps/time/distance	Notes	Page #
Cat-cow	8		64
Single-leg bridge isometric with bent-knee leg whip	5 per side		65
Catcher rockback	5 per side		66
Elevated bent-knee Copenhagen plank	15 sec per side		67
Alternating Spiderman to yoga pike	3		68
Heels-up split squat isometric	15 sec per side		69
MB hug Kang squat	5		70
Extensive single-leg pogo hop	10 per side		71
Drop reverse lunge to stick	3 per side		72
Lateral skip	20 yd per side		73
Workout			
Exercise	Sets × reps at RPE	Notes	Page #
Strength and power block • A1: DB single-leg RDL • A2: DB release squat jump to broad jump with stick	3 × 6 per side at RPE 7-8 3 × 3 at RPE 6-7	Complete A block (A1 and A2) with no rest between exercises, then rest for 45-60 sec. That equals 1 set. Complete all sets in this way, then move on to B block.	140 210
Strength and power block • B1: DB single-arm bench press with single-leg hip thrust isometric • B2: MB step-through wall chest pass (staggered-stance start)	3 × 8 per side at RPE 7-8 3 × 4 per side at RPE 6-7	Complete B block (B1 and B2) with no rest between exercises, then rest for 45-60 sec. That equals 1 set. Complete all sets in this way, then move on to C block.	141 211
Hypertrophy block • C1: Cable pull-through • C2: DB seal row	3 × 12, 15, 20 at RPE 8, 7, 6 3 × 8, 10, 12 at RPE 8, 7, 7	Complete C block (C1 and C2) with no rest between exercises, then rest for 45-60 sec. That equals 1 set. Complete all sets in this way, then move on to D block.	142 143
Accessory block • D1: Band wide-stance vertical Pallof press • D2: Cable tall-kneeling straight bar biceps curl	3 × 8 per side at RPE 7-8 3 × 12 at RPE 7-8	Complete D block (D1 and D2) with no rest between exercises, then rest for 45-60 sec. That equals 1 set. Complete all sets in this way, then move on to recovery.	144 145
Recovery			
Exercise	Reps/time	Notes	Page #
Band single-leg lower	8 per side		N/A
Band Brettzel stretch	20 sec per side		N/A
Rear foot elevated half-kneeling hip flexor stretch with single-arm overhead reach	20 sec per side		N/A

Table 13.3 Power Training Program: Phase 3 (Weeks 9-12)

DAY 1: MONDAY				
Warm-up				
Exercise	Reps/time/distance	Notes		Page #
Segmental cat-cow	5			86
Bridge isometric with alternating reach	5 per side			87
Catcher rockback with toe turn	6 per side			88
Floor bent-knee Copenhagen plank with liftoff	5 per side			89
Alternating Spiderman to stationary inchworm	3 per side			90
Rear foot elevated split squat isometric	15 sec per side			91
KB goblet Kang squat	5			92
Intensive pogo hop	10			93
Drop skater squat to stick	5 per side			94
Lateral crossover skip	20 yd per side			95
Workout				
Exercise	Sets × reps at RPE	Notes		Page #
Strength and power block • A1: Landmine single-leg RDL (lateral orientation) • A2: Continuous broad jump	3 × 6 per side at RPE 8 3 × 3 at RPE 7	Complete A block (A1 and A2) with no rest between exercises, then rest for 45-60 sec. That equals 1 set. Complete all sets in this way, then move on to B block.		146 212
Strength and power block • B1: DB single-arm bench press with single-arm fixed (top) • B2: MB step-back rotational single-arm wall chest pass	3 × 8 per side at RPE 8 3 × 5 per side at RPE 7	Complete B block (B1 and B2) with no rest between exercises, then rest for 45-60 sec. That equals 1 set. Complete all sets in this way, then move on to C block.		147 214
Strength block • C1: DB neutral grip kickstand RDL • C2: Cable split-stance single-arm mid row with opposite hand reach	3 × 8 per side at RPE 7-8 3 × 8 per side at RPE 7-8	Complete C block (C1 and C2) with no rest between exercises, then rest for 45-60 sec. That equals 1 set. Complete all sets in this way, then move on to D block.		148 149
Accessory block • D1: DB bent-over lateral raise • D2: Ab wheel tall-kneeling rollout	3 × 12 at RPE 7-8 3 × 10 at RPE 7-8	Complete D block (D1 and D2) with no rest between exercises, then rest for 45-60 sec. That equals 1 set. Complete all sets in this way, then move on to recovery.		150 151
Recovery				
Exercise	Reps/time	Notes		Page #
Three-way hamstring floss	5 each direction per side			N/A
Brettzel stretch with breathing	8 breaths per side			N/A
Rear foot elevated half-kneeling hip flexor stretch with single-arm overhead reach and rotation	20 sec per side			N/A

DAY 2: TUESDAY			
Warm-up			
Exercise	**Reps/time/distance**	**Notes**	**Page #**
Single-leg long bridge isometric with power switch	3 per side		96
Wall press with single-leg lower	8 per side		97
Mini-band stork with clam lift	8 per side		98
Tempo wall heel raise (3 seconds up/3 seconds iso/3 seconds down)	6		99
Hand-supported alternating reverse lunge with single-arm overhead reach	3 per side		100
Walking inchworm to push-up	3		101
Hinge to squat isometric with alternating rotation	3 per side		102
Wall press single-leg RDL with power drive	3 per side		103
Reverse walking single-leg RDL	2 × 10 yd		104
Walking alternating Spiderman to yoga push-up	2 × 10 yd		105
5-yard lateral shuffle to turn and 10-yard sprint	2 × 15 yd per side		106
5-yard backpedal to turn and 10-yard sprint	2 × 15 yd per side		107
Workout			
Exercise	**Sets × reps at RPE**	**Notes**	**Page #**
A: 10-yard sprint and rehearsed T-turn	3 per side at RPE 8-9	Complete 1 rep, then rest for 30-45 sec. That equals 1 set. Complete all sets in this way, then move on to the next exercise.	226
B: 5-10-5 pro agility shuttle	3 per side at RPE 8-9	Complete 1 rep per side, then rest for 30-45 sec. That equals 1 set. Complete all sets in this way, then move on to the next exercise.	227
C: 20-yard curvilinear sprint	3 per side @ 100% effort	Rest 60-75 sec between reps.	228
Recovery			
Exercise	**Reps/time**	**Notes**	**Page #**
Three-way hamstring floss	5 each direction per side		N/A
Brettzel stretch with breathing	8 breaths per side		N/A
Rear foot elevated half-kneeling hip flexor stretch with single-arm overhead reach and rotation	20 sec per side		N/A

(continued)

Table 13.3 Power Training Program: Phase 3 (Weeks 9-12) *(continued)*

DAY 3: WEDNESDAY				
Warm-up				
Exercise	Reps/time/distance	Notes		Page #
Segmental cat-cow	5			86
Bridge isometric with alternating reach	5 per side			87
Catcher rockback with toe turn	6 per side			88
Floor bent-knee Copenhagen plank with liftoff	5 per side			89
Alternating Spiderman to stationary inchworm	3 per side			90
Rear foot elevated split squat isometric	15 sec per side			91
KB goblet Kang squat	5			92
Intensive pogo hop	10			93
Drop skater squat to stick	5 per side			94
Lateral crossover skip	20 yd per side			95
Workout				
Exercise	Sets × reps at RPE	Notes		Page #
Strength and power block • A1: Barbell speed bench press • A2: Band standing continuous power punch	3 × 5 at RPE 8 3 × 5 at RPE 7	Complete A block (A1 and A2) with no rest between exercises, then rest for 45-60 sec. That equals 1 set. Complete all sets in this way, then move on to B block.		196 215
Strength and power block • B1: DB single-arm offset band slider lateral lunge • B2: Plate skater hop with quick, stick, and punch	3 × 8 per side at RPE 8 3 × 3 per side at RPE 7	Complete B block (B1 and B2) with no rest between exercises, then rest for 45-60 sec. That equals 1 set. Complete all sets in this way, then move on to C block.		153 216
Strength block • C1: Landmine standing Viking shoulder press • C2: Band wide-stance crossbody long chop	3 × 8 at RPE 7-8 3 × 10 per side at RPE 7-8	Complete C block (C1 and C2) with no rest between exercises, then rest for 45-60 sec. That equals 1 set. Complete all sets in this way, then move on to D block.		154 155
Accessory block • D1: KB towel standing hammer curl • D2: Bent-knee star plank with clamshell	3 × 12 at RPE 7-8 3 × 8 per side at RPE 7-8	Complete D block (D1 and D2) with no rest between exercises, then rest for 45-60 sec. That equals 1 set. Complete all sets in this way, then move on to recovery.		156 157
Recovery				
Exercise	Reps/time	Notes		Page #
Three-way hamstring floss	5 each direction per side			N/A
Brettzel stretch with breathing	8 breaths per side			N/A
Rear foot elevated half-kneeling hip flexor stretch with single-arm overhead reach and rotation	20 sec per side			N/A

DAY 4: THURSDAY

Warm-up

Exercise	Reps/time/distance	Notes	Page #
Single-leg long bridge isometric with power switch	3 per side		96
Wall press with single-leg lower	8 per side		97
Mini-band stork with clam lift	8 per side		98
Tempo wall heel raise (3 seconds up/3 seconds iso/3 seconds down)	6		99
Hand-supported alternating reverse lunge with single-arm overhead reach	3 per side		100
Walking inchworm to push-up	3		101
Hinge to squat isometric with alternating rotation	3 per side		102
Wall press single-leg RDL with power drive	3 per side		103
Reverse walking single-leg RDL	2 × 10 yd		104
Walking alternating Spiderman to yoga push-up	2 × 10 yd		105
5-yard lateral shuffle to turn and 10-yard sprint	2 × 15 yd per side		106
5-yard backpedal to turn and 10-yard sprint	2 × 15 yd per side		107

Workout

Exercise	Sets × reps at RPE	Notes	Page #
Objective: High-intensity sprint intervals Pick one: Incline treadmill (20%-30% incline), outdoor hill (20%-30% incline), or empty sled (no weight added)	Total duration: 8-12 sets Interval protocol: 6-8 sec of all-out sprint (RPE 10; 100% of max HR) followed by 45-60 sec of complete rest (goal is to bring HR back down during this time)		234

Recovery

Exercise	Reps/time	Notes	Page #
Three-way hamstring floss	5 each direction per side		N/A
Brettzel stretch with breathing	8 breaths per side		N/A
Rear foot elevated half-kneeling hip flexor stretch with single-arm overhead reach and rotation	20 sec per side		N/A

(continued)

Table 13.3 Power Training Program: Phase 3 (Weeks 9-12) *(continued)*

DAY 5: FRIDAY			
Warm-up			
Exercise	Reps/time/distance	Notes	Page #
Segmental cat-cow	5		86
Bridge isometric with alternating reach	5 per side		87
Catcher rockback with toe turn	6 per side		88
Floor bent-knee Copenhagen plank with liftoff	5 per side		89
Alternating Spiderman to stationary inchworm	3 per side		90
Rear foot elevated split squat isometric	15 sec per side		91
KB goblet Kang squat	5		92
Intensive pogo hop	10		93
Drop skater squat to stick	5 per side		94
Lateral crossover skip	20 yd per side		95
Workout			
Exercise	Sets × reps at RPE	Notes	Page #
Strength and power block • A1: DB rear foot elevated split squat • A2: DB reactive split squat jump	3 × 6 per side at RPE 8 3 × 5 per side at RPE 7	Complete A block (A1 and A2) with no rest between exercises, then rest for 45-60 sec. That equals 1 set. Complete all sets in this way, then move on to B block.	158 217
Strength and power block • B1: DB single-arm row • B2: Cable split-stance single-arm low row with box stomp	3 × 8 per side at RPE 8 3 × 4 per side at RPE 7	Complete B block (B1 and B2) with no rest between exercises, then rest for 45-60 sec. That equals 1 set. Complete all sets in this way, then move on to C block.	159 218
Strength • C1: KB goblet kickstand squat (2 DB) • C2: Cable half-kneeling single-arm high row	3 × 8 per side at RPE 7-8 3 × 8 per side at RPE 7-8	Complete C block (C1 and C2) with no rest between exercises, then rest for 45-60 sec. That equals 1 set. Complete all sets in this way, then move on to D block.	186 161
Accessory block • D1: DB floor skull crusher • D2: DB floor prone Superman isometric	3 × 12 at RPE 7-8 3 × 15 sec at RPE 7-8	Complete D block (D1 and D2) with no rest between exercises, then rest for 45-60 sec. That equals 1 set. Complete all sets in this way, then move on to recovery.	162 163
Recovery			
Exercise	Reps/time	Notes	Page #
Three-way hamstring floss	5 each direction per side		N/A
Brettzel stretch with breathing	8 breaths per side		N/A
Rear foot elevated half-kneeling hip flexor stretch with single-arm overhead reach and rotation	20 sec per side		N/A

EXERCISE FINDER

Exercise	Page #
CHANGE OF DIRECTION AND AGILITY SKILLS	
Novice Series: Change of Direction and Agility	
5-Yard Sprint and Rehearsed Stop	21
5-Yard Sprint, Rehearsed Stop and Go	21
5-Yard Sprint and Rehearsed Y-Turn	21
5-Yard Sprint and Rehearsed T-Turn	22
Sprint and Reactionary Stop	23
Sprint and Reactionary Y-Turn	23
Sprint and Reactionary T-Turn	24
Advanced Series: Change of Direction and Agility	
5-Yard Sprint to Rehearsed Curved Run	25
5-Yard Backpedal to Rehearsed Turn and Sprint	25
5-Yard Lateral Shuffle to Rehearsed Turn and Sprint	26
5-Yard Partner Chase and Hip Tap Reactionary T-Turn (Sprinter Reacts to Chaser)	27
5-Yard Partner Chase and Verbal Reactionary T-Turn (Sprinter Reacts to Chaser)	27
5-Yard Partner Chase and Non-Verbal Reactionary T-Turn (Chaser Reacts to Sprinter)	28
5-Yard Partner Chase and Verbal Reactionary T-Turn (Chaser Reacts to Sprinter)	29
WARM-UP EXERCISES	
Band Cat-Cow	42
Heels-Up Single-Leg Bridge Isometric With Knee Drive Isometric	43
Catcher Rockback Isometric With Reach and Rotate	44
Floor Bent-Knee Copenhagen Plank	45
Alternating Spiderman	46
Split Squat Iso	47
Squat Rack Kang Squat	48
Extensive Pogo Hop	49
Drop Squat to Stick	50
Linear Skip	51
Long Bridge Iso	52
Wall Press With Alternating Dead Bug	53
Wall Stork	54
Wall Single-Leg Heel Raise Iso	55
Alternating Yoga Plex	56
Stationary Inchworm	57
Hinge to Squat	58
Wall Linear Single Exchange	59
Stationary Hamstring Scoop	60

Exercise	Page #
WARM-UP EXERCISES (continued)	
Walking Alternating Spiderman	61
Lateral Shuffle With Arm Swing	62
Backpedal	63
Cat-Cow	64
Single-Leg Bridge Isometric With Bent-Knee Leg Whip	65
Catcher Rockback	66
Elevated Bent-Knee Copenhagen Plank	67
Alternating Spiderman to Yoga Pike	68
Heels-Up Split Squat Isometric	69
MB Hug Kang Squat	70
Extensive Single-Leg Pogo Hop	71
Drop Reverse Lunge to Stick	72
Lateral Skip	73
Single-Leg Long Bridge Isometric With Knee Drive Isometric	74
Cross-Connect Dead Bug (Opposite Side)	75
Mini-Band Stork	76
Wall Bent-Knee Single-Leg Heel Raise Isometric	77
Alternating Yoga Plex to Yoga Pike	78
Walking Inchworm	79
Hinge to Squat With Alternating Rotation	80
Wall Linear Double Exchange	81
Walking Alternating Hamstring Scoop	82
Walking Alternating Spiderman to Reach and Rotate	83
Double Lateral Shuffle With Alternating Lateral Squat	84
Backward Reach Run	85
Segmental Cat-Cow	86
Bridge Isometric With Alternating Reach	87
Catcher Rockback With Toe Turn	88
Floor Bent-Knee Copenhagen Plank With Liftoff	89
Alternating Spiderman to Stationary Inchworm	90
Rear Foot Elevated Split Squat Isometric	91
KB Goblet Kang Squat	92
Intensive Pogo Hop	93
Drop Skater Squat to Stick	94
Lateral Crossover Skip	95
Single-Leg Long Bridge Isometric With Power Switch	96
Wall Press With Single-Leg Lower	97
Mini-Band Stork With Clam Lift	98
Tempo Wall Heel Raise (3 Seconds Up/3 Seconds Iso/3 Seconds Down)	99
Hand-Supported Alternating Reverse Lunge With Single-Arm Overhead Reach	100
Walking Inchworm to Push-Up	101

Exercise	Page #
Hinge to Squat Isometric With Alternating Rotation	102
Wall Press Single-Leg RDL With Power Drive	103
Reverse Walking Single-Leg RDL	104
Walking Alternating Spiderman to Yoga Push-Up	105
5-Yard Lateral Shuffle to Turn and 10-Yard Sprint	106
5-Yard Backpedal to Turn and 10-Yard Sprint	107
STRENGTH EXERCISES	
KB Goblet Squat With 3-Second Isometric	110
Band Tall-Kneeling Pallof Press Isometric	111
DB Romanian Deadlift (RDL)	112
KB Half-Kneeling Shoulder Press With 3-Second Isometric	113
Suspension Skater Squat With 3-Second Isometric	114
DB Standing Hammer Curl	115
DB Bench Press With 3-Second Isometric (Top)	116
Bent-Knee Star Plank With Top Leg Long	117
DB Chest-Supported Row	118
KB Single-Arm Offset Lateral Squat With 1-Second Isometric	119
KB Goblet Carry	120
Band Tall-Kneeling Pull-Apart	121
Trap Bar Deadlift	122
Physioball Push–Pull	123
Two DB Foam Roller Hack Squat Against a Wall	124
Cable Half-Kneeling High Row With 1-Second Isometric	125
Cable Double-Arm Single-Leg Romanian Deadlift (RDL)	126
Band Standing Triceps Extension	127
DB Step-Up	128
DB Heels-Up Three-Point Row With 3-Second Eccentric	129
Two DB Cyclist Squat	130
Cable Seated Lat Pull-Down With 3-Second Eccentric	131
KB Front Rack Carry	132
Cable Tall-Kneeling Rope Triceps Extension	133
Weighted Eccentric-Only Neutral Grip Pull-Up With 5-Second Eccentric	134
Landmine Goblet Lateral Squat	135
DB Captain Stance Single-Arm Shoulder Press	136
Cable Plank Single-Arm Row to Triceps Extension	137
KB Suitcase Carry	138
DB Incline Bench Trap Raise (Y) With 3-Second Eccentric	139
DB Single-Leg RDL	140
DB Single-Arm Bench Press With Single-Leg Hip Thrust Isometric	141
Cable Pull-Through	142
DB Seal Row	143
Band Wide-Stance Vertical Pallof Press	144
Cable Tall-Kneeling Straight Bar Biceps Curl	145

Exercise	Page #
STRENGTH EXERCISES (continued)	
Landmine Single-Leg RDL (Lateral Orientation)	146
DB Single-Arm Bench Press With Single-Arm Fixed (Top)	147
DB Neutral Grip Kickstand RDL	148
Cable Split-Stance Single-Arm Mid Row With Opposite Hand Reach	149
DB Bent-Over Lateral Raise	150
Ab Wheel Tall-Kneeling Rollout	151
Barbell Bench Press	152
DB Single-Arm Offset Band Slider Lateral Lunge	153
Landmine Standing Viking Shoulder Press	154
Band Wide-Stance Crossbody Long Chop	155
KB Towel Standing Hammer Curl	156
Bent-Knee Star Plank With Clamshell	157
DB Rear Foot–Elevated Split Squat	158
DB Single-Arm Row	159
Two DB Kickstand Squat	160
Cable Half-Kneeling Single-Arm High Row	161
DB Floor Skull Crusher	162
DB Floor Prone Superman Isometric	163
DB Goblet Squat	164
Band Standing Pallof Press	165
Barbell RDL	166
KB Seated Shoulder Press (Back Supported)	167
Walking Lunge	168
DB Standing Biceps Curl	169
DB Bench Press	170
Side Plank	171
KB Goblet Lateral Squat	172
Standing Band Pull-Apart	173
KB Deadlift	174
Band-Assisted Pull-Up	175
DB Captain Stance Shoulder Press	176
DB Single-Leg RDL (2 DB)	177
DB Single-Arm Bench Press	178
DB Frankenstein Floor Press	179
Cable Seated Mid Row	180
Band Resisted Bent-Over DB Lateral Raise	181
Band Wide-Stance Crossbody Short Chop	182
KB Horns-Grip Tall-Kneeling Biceps Curl	183
Mini-Band Bent-Knee Star Plank	184
DB Split Squat	185
KB Goblet Kickstand Squat	186

Exercise	Page #
Barbell Front Squat	187
Band Tall-Kneeling Pallof Press	188
DB Skater Squat	189
Cable Double-Arm Single-Leg RDL With Knee Drive and Row	190
Weighted Neutral-Grip Pull-Up	191
DB Hand-Supported Ipsilateral Single-Leg RDL	192
DB Alternating Bench Press (Bottom)	193
Band-Resisted Tall-Kneeling Ab Wheel Rollout	194
Barbell Power Step-Up	195
Barbell Speed Bench Press	196
PLYOMETRICS AND POWER EXERCISES	
Band-Assisted Continuous Squat Jump	198
MB Tall-Kneeling Slam With Hip Hinge	199
MB Skater Hop With Chop and Stick	200
MB Half-Kneeling Lateral Wall Toss	201
90-Degree Rotational Single-Leg Hop With Stick	202
MB Half-Kneeling Around-the-World Slam	203
Band-Resisted Acceleration Power Step	204
Barbell Explosive Inverted Row With Hip Thrust Isometric	205
MB Standing Double Clutch Slam	206
Band-Resisted Skater Hop With Stick (Lateral Orientation)	208
Single-Leg Broad Jump to Double-Leg Stick	209
DB Release Squat Jump to Broad Jump With Stick	210
MB Step-Through Wall Chest Pass (Staggered-Stance Start)	211
Continuous Broad Jump	212
MB Step-Back Rotational Single-Arm Wall Chest Pass	214
Band Standing Continuous Power Punch	215
Plate Skater Hop With Quick, Stick, and Punch	216
DB Reactive Split Squat Jump	217
Cable Split-Stance Single-Arm Low Row With Box Stomp	218
CHANGE OF DIRECTION, AGILITY, AND SPEED EXERCISES	
10-Yard Sprint and Rehearsed Stop	220
Multidirectional Plyo Step From Half-Kneeling Start to 5-Yard Sprint	221
100-Yard Tempo Run	222
10-Yard Sprint and Rehearsed Y-Turn	223
10-Yard Sprint From Lateral Half-Kneeling Start	224
20-Yard Dash	225
10-Yard Sprint and Rehearsed T-Turn	226
5-10-5 Pro Agility Shuttle	227
20-Yard Curvilinear Sprint	228
CONDITIONING EXERCISES AND PROTOCOLS	
Steady-State Aerobic Conditioning	232
Aerobic Conditioning Intervals	233
High-Intensity Sprint Intervals	234

ABOUT THE AUTHOR

Matthew S. Ibrahim is a strength and conditioning coach, college professor, public speaker, and author. His professional journey is marked by a series of pivotal roles, including gym co-owner, director of strength and conditioning, and internship coordinator. Currently, he serves as clinical coordinator and as an instructor of exercise science at Endicott College, and he volunteers as a strength and conditioning coach for their NCAA Division III student-athletes. He also serves as co-advisor of the Exercise Science Club and co-advisor of The Hidden Opponent at Endicott College. In addition, he is an adjunct instructor of exercise science and an advisory board member at Maryville University.

As the founder of Athletic Performance University (APU), Matthew has created an impactful online mentorship program designed to elevate the career cornerstone skills of coaching, creating, and communicating for strength and conditioning coaches as well as exercise science students. APU is a leading education company approved by the National Strength & Conditioning Association (NSCA) for 1.4 continuing education units (CEUs).

Matthew's influence extends nationally and internationally as a sought-after public speaker who has presented in over 25 U.S. states for the NSCA, Perform Better, EXOS at Google, Sports Academy (formerly Mamba), UFC Performance Institute, Duke University, Stanford University, and Equinox, along with several engagements in Europe. His professional work and expertise have been featured in leading platforms and publications, including *Muscle & Fitness*, *Men's Journal*, *Personal Training Quarterly*, *Science for Sport*, and *T Nation*.

Matthew is deeply committed to education and professional development. He holds a bachelor's degree in exercise and health sciences from University of Massachusetts Boston and a master's degree in sport performance from Rocky Mountain University of Health Professions (RMU). He is currently a PhD candidate in human and sport performance at RMU and a master's student in sport leadership at Endicott College. Matthew is a member of the NSCA, holds their Certified Strength and Conditioning Specialist (CSCS) credential, and serves as a Massachusetts state advisory board member. He also holds the Licensed Massage Therapist (LMT) credential through Cortiva Institute, and he is beginning studies in organizational leadership from Harvard Business School in 2025.

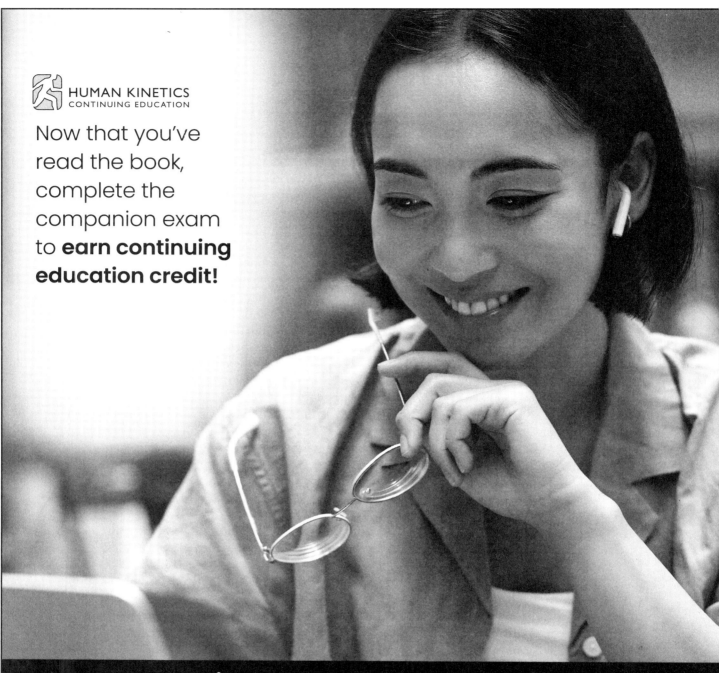

HUMAN KINETICS
CONTINUING EDUCATION

Now that you've read the book, complete the companion exam to **earn continuing education credit!**

Find your CE exam here:
US & International: US.HumanKinetics.com/collections/Continuing-Education
Canada: Canada.HumanKinetics.com/collections/Continuing-Education

Subscribe to our newsletters today!

Get exclusive offers and stay apprised of CE opportunities.

US   Canada